DNA AND RNA: PROPERTIES AND MODIFICATIONS, FUNCTIONS
AND INTERACTIONS, RECOMMENDATIONS AND APPLICATIONS

# MICRORNAS IN SOLID CANCER

## FROM BIOMARKERS TO THERAPEUTIC TARGETS

# DNA AND RNA: PROPERTIES AND MODIFICATIONS, FUNCTIONS AND INTERACTIONS, RECOMMENDATIONS AND APPLICATIONS

Additional books in this series can be found on Nova's website under the Series tab.

Additional E-books in this series can be found on Nova's website under the E-books tab.

# CANCER ETIOLOGY, DIAGNOSIS AND TREATMENTS

Additional books in this series can be found on Nova's website under the Series tab.

Additional E-books in this series can be found on Nova's website under the E-books tab.

DNA AND RNA: PROPERTIES AND MODIFICATIONS, FUNCTIONS
AND INTERACTIONS, RECOMMENDATIONS AND APPLICATIONS

# MicroRNAs in Solid Cancer

## From Biomarkers to Therapeutic Targets

**Ondrej Slaby**
Editor

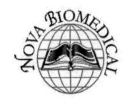

Nova Science Publishers, Inc.
*New York*

Copyright © 2012 by Nova Science Publishers, Inc.

**All rights reserved.** No part of this book may be reproduced, stored in a retrieval system or transmitted in any form or by any means: electronic, electrostatic, magnetic, tape, mechanical photocopying, recording or otherwise without the written permission of the Publisher.

For permission to use material from this book please contact us:
Telephone 631-231-7269; Fax 631-231-8175
Web Site: http://www.novapublishers.com

## NOTICE TO THE READER

The Publisher has taken reasonable care in the preparation of this book, but makes no expressed or implied warranty of any kind and assumes no responsibility for any errors or omissions. No liability is assumed for incidental or consequential damages in connection with or arising out of information contained in this book. The Publisher shall not be liable for any special, consequential, or exemplary damages resulting, in whole or in part, from the readers' use of, or reliance upon, this material. Any parts of this book based on government reports are so indicated and copyright is claimed for those parts to the extent applicable to compilations of such works.

Independent verification should be sought for any data, advice or recommendations contained in this book. In addition, no responsibility is assumed by the publisher for any injury and/or damage to persons or property arising from any methods, products, instructions, ideas or otherwise contained in this publication.

This publication is designed to provide accurate and authoritative information with regard to the subject matter covered herein. It is sold with the clear understanding that the Publisher is not engaged in rendering legal or any other professional services. If legal or any other expert assistance is required, the services of a competent person should be sought. FROM A DECLARATION OF PARTICIPANTS JOINTLY ADOPTED BY A COMMITTEE OF THE AMERICAN BAR ASSOCIATION AND A COMMITTEE OF PUBLISHERS.

Additional color graphics may be available in the e-book version of this book.

**Library of Congress Cataloging-in-Publication Data**

MicroRNAs in solid cancer : from biomarkers to therapeutic targets / editor, Ondrej Slaby.
 p. ; cm.
Includes bibliographical references and index.
ISBN 978-1-61324-514-9 (hardcover : alk. paper) 1. Small interfering RNA. 2. Cancer--Gene therapy. I. Slab}, Ondrej, 1981-
 [DNLM: 1. MicroRNAs--physiology. 2. Molecular Targeted Therapy. 3. Neoplasms--physiopathology. 4. Neoplasms--therapy. 5. Tumor Markers, Biological. QU 58.7]
QP623.5.S63M535 2011
572.8'8--dc23
 2011013685

*Published by Nova Science Publishers, Inc. † New York*

# Contents

| | | |
|---|---|---|
| **Preface** | | vii |
| **Chapter I** | MicroRNAs Biogenesis, Function and Decay | 1 |
| | *Ondrej Slaby and Jiri Sana* | |
| **Chapter II** | MicroRNAs and Genetic Polymorphisms in Cancer | 21 |
| | *Ondrej Slaby* | |
| **Chapter III** | Methods for MicroRNAs Discovery and Detection | 29 |
| | *Ondrej Slaby and Jiri Sana* | |
| **Chapter IV** | MicroRNAs and the Hallmarks of Cancer | 47 |
| | *Ondrej Slaby* | |
| **Chapter V** | MicroRNAs and Colorectal Cancer | 65 |
| | *Ondrej Slaby, Marek Svoboda and Rostislav Vyzula* | |
| **Chapter VI** | MicroRNAs and Breast Cancer | 81 |
| | *Martina Redova, Marek Svoboda and Rostislav Vyzula* | |
| **Chapter VII** | MicroRNAs and Lung Cancer | 95 |
| | *Jiri Sana and Ondrej Slaby* | |
| **Chapter VIII** | MicroRNAs and Prostate Cancer | 111 |
| | *Jiri Sana* | |
| **Chapter IX** | MicroRNAs and Renal Cell Carcinoma | 121 |
| | *Martina Redova, Jaroslav Michalek, Ondrej Slaby* | |
| **Chapter X** | MicroRNAs and Hepatocellular Carcinoma | 129 |
| | *Martina Redova* | |
| **Chapter XI** | MicroRNAs and Pancreatic Cancer | 141 |
| | *Martina Redova* | |
| **Chapter XII** | MicroRNAs and Gastric Cancer | 149 |
| | *Ondrej Slaby* | |
| **Chapter XIII** | MicroRNAs and Thyroid Cancer | 161 |
| | *Martina Redova* | |
| **Chapter XIV** | MicroRNAs and Glioblastoma | 169 |
| | *Jiri Sana, Radek Lakomy, Marian Hajduch and Ondrej Slaby* | |
| **Abbreviations** | | 177 |
| Index | | 185 |

# Preface

MicroRNAs (miRNAs) were discovered in the early 1990s by Victor Ambros and colleagues. They found that *lin-4*, a known gene involved in development of the nematode *C. elegans*, does not code a protein but, instead, gives origin to a small RNA that is 22 nucleotides in length and which was subsequently shown to interact with the 3' untranslated region (UTR) of the *lin-14* mRNA and to repress its expression. This fascinating form of gene regulation – where a small RNA binds to another RNA – had been largely overlooked for more than 30 years. miRNAs had perhaps escaped detection because of their size as avid gene hunters were mainly interested in long mRNAs and disregarded very short RNAs. Because miRNAs' function had not been clarified, this small molecule RNA was initially considered to be "junk" RNA. Understanding of miRNAs has grown since that early report, and in 2006 Andrew Z. Fire and Craig C. Mello won the Nobel Prize in Physiology or Medicine for their work in understanding how miRNAs regulate gene expression.

MiRNA is extremely fast growing field, and miRNA knowledge is now believed to be a pivotal element of cancer biology. An individual miRNA interferes with a broad range of mRNAs; conversely, a single mRNA could be targeted by a variety of miRNAs. The complexity of miRNA:mRNA interaction is far-reaching and a bit beyond our understanding to date. It is already evident that the discovery of miRNA has created a paradigm shift in post-genomics biology, not only for scientists accustomed to traditional central dogma of molecular biology but also for researchers studying human diseases and accustomed to traditional genetics approach of studying one gene at the time. The ability of miRNAs to control large groups of genes and impose global post-transcriptional regulation of many (if not all) important cellular processes in development, cell proliferation and differentiation has opened up a new dimension and uncovered complexity of intracellular regulatory processes. This book is expected to provide introduction to the basic principles of miRNA biology, overview of miRNA significance in the hallmarks of cancer, experimental techniques used in miRNA research, and in special part - miRNAs importance in wide range of solid cancers with a special focus on its potential usage in molecular pathology, predictive oncology or as a novel therapeutic targets.

I would like to express my sincerest gratitude to the co-authors, especially Martina Redova and Jiri Sana, who made this book possible — for their enthusiastic support of this project, and to many authors whose works are cited in the reference lists. They have contributed importantly, and without them this review volume would not have been realized. Finally, I dedicate this book to my wife Katerina and son Jakub for their patience and unwavering support.

*Ondrej Slaby*
*Brno, February 2011*

In: MicroRNAs in Solid Cancer
Editor: Ondrej Slaby

ISBN: 978-61324-514-9
©2012 Nova Science Publishers, Inc.

*Chapter I*

# MicroRNAs Biogenesis, Function and Decay

### *Ondrej Slaby and Jiri Sana*
Masaryk Memorial Cancer Institute, Brno, Czech Republic
Central European Institute of Technology, Masaryk University, Brno, Czech Republic

## Abstract

MicroRNAs (miRNAs) are important regulators of gene expression that control both physiological and pathological processes such as development and cancer. Research during the past decade has identified major factors participating in miRNA biogenesis and has established basic principles of miRNA function. Recent studies, however, have introduced a paradigm shift in our understanding of the miRNA biogenesis pathway, which was previously believed to be universal to all miRNAs. It has become apparent that miRNA regulators themselves are subject to sophisticated control, which takes place at the levels of both miRNA metabolism and function. In this chapter we focus on the recent advances in knowledge of the miRNA biogenesis pathways and regulatory mechanisms involved in miRNA gene transcription, processing, maturation and functionality. Potential impact of the alterations in miRNA biogenesis pathways on cancer pathogenesis is discussed.

## 1.1. Introduction

MiRNAs comprise an abundant class of endogenous, small non-coding RNAs, 18–25 nucleotides in length, that repress protein translation through binding to target mRNAs, and have revolutionized our comprehension of the post-transcriptional regulation of gene expression [1]. The number of verified human miRNAs is still expanding. The latest version of miRBase (release 16.0, September 2010) has annotated over 800 miRNA sequences in the human genome [2]. This number is predicted to double as more miRNAs are awaiting experimental validation. Bioinformatics and cloning studies have estimated that miRNAs may regulate 50% of all human genes and each miRNA can control hundreds of gene targets. MiRNAs are highly conserved in sequence between distantly related organisms, indicating their participation in essential biological processes. It is well known today that miRNAs have very important regulatory functions in such basic biological processes as development, cellular differentiation, proliferation and apoptosis that affect such major biological systems as stemness, immunity and cancer [3-8]. A large fraction of miRNAs exhibit strict developmental stage-specific and tissue-specific expression patterns and the levels of many of these miRNAs are altered during disease. Although the final synthesis rate of a miRNA can, in principle, be controlled at any step of miRNA biogenesis, from transcription to mature miRNA turn over, recent findings have uncovered a significant role for posttranscriptional mechanisms in the regulation of miRNA biogenesis and activity [9-15].

## 1.2. Overview of Canonical miRNA Biogenesis and Function

Many previous seminal studies have revealed abundant knowledge about miRNAs biogenesis and mechanism of action [4,9,10]. Compared with the regulators of gene expression found previously, miRNAs are different in their production and biogenesis. Early annotation for the genomic position of miRNAs indicated that most miRNAs are located in intergenic regions (>1 kb away from annotated or predicted genes), although a sizeable minority was found in the intronic regions of known genes (mirtrons) in the sense or antisense orientation. This led to the postulation that most miRNA genes are transcribed as autonomous transcription units [4]. A detailed analysis of miRNA gene expression showed that miRNA genes can be transcribed from their own promoters and that miRNAs are generated by RNA polymerase II as primary transcripts (pri-miRNAs). These are processed to short 70-nucleotide stem-loop structures known as pre-miRNAs by the ribonuclease called Drosha and the double-stranded-RNA-binding protein known as Pasha (or DGCR8 – DiGeorge critical region 8), which together compose a multiprotein complex termed a microprocessor. The pre-miRNAs are transported to cytoplasm by the RAN GTP-dependent transporter exportin 5 (XPO5). In the cytoplasm, the pre-miRNAs are processed to mature miRNA duplexes by their interaction with the endonuclease enzyme Dicer in complex with dsRNA binding protein TRBP [13]. One strand ("guide strand") of the resulting 18–25-nucleotide mature miRNA duplex ultimately gets integrated into the miRNA-induced silencing complex (miRISC) with the central part formed by proteins of the Argonaute family (Ago), whereas the other strand ("passenger" or miRNA*) is released and degraded. The retained ("guide") strand is the one that has the less stably base-paired 5' end in the miRNA/miRNA* duplex. The position of Drosha and Dicer cleavage sites determines the identity of 5'-terminal and/or 3'-terminal miRNA nucleotides [10]. Notably, processing of some precursors by these enzymes is not uniform and generates miRNA isoforms with different termini. Heterogeneity at the 5' end in particular can have important functional consequences, because the thermodynamic stability of the miRNA duplex ends determines which strand, miRNA or miRNA*, is preferentially loaded into miRISC, moreover, it affects the seed register of miRNAs and, consequently, changes the identity of targeted mRNAs [16]. Generally, most miRNA genes produce one dominant miRNA species. However, the ratio of miRNA to miRNA* can vary in different tissues or developmental stages, which probably depends on specific properties of the pre-miRNA or miRNA duplex, or on the activity of different accessory processing factors [9,16]. Moreover, the ratio might be modulated by the availability of mRNA targets as a result of enhanced destabilization of either miRNA or miRNA* occurring in the absence of respective complementary mRNAs [17]. Mature miRNAs in miRISC exert their regulatory effects by binding to imperfect complementary sites within the 3' untranslated region (3-UTR) of their mRNA targets. The 3' UTR controls many aspects of mRNA metabolism, such as transport, localization, efficiency of translation and stability. 3' UTRs can extend over several kilobases and generally contain binding sites for various regulatory proteins and miRNAs allowing dynamic and combinatorial regulation [10]. MiRNAs repress target-gene expression post-transcriptionally, apparently at the level of translation, through a miRISC complex that is similar to, or possibly identical with, that used for the RNAi pathway (comparison in Table 1.1) [18].

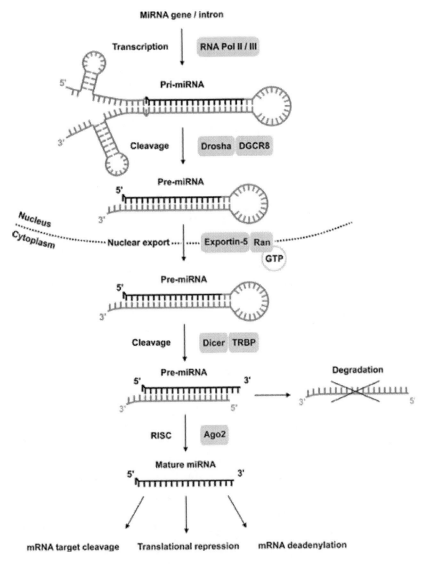

Figure 1.1. Linear "canonical" pathway of miRNA processing.

**Table 1.1. Comparison of siRNA and miRNA characteristics**

| miRNA | siRNA |
|---|---|
| Always endogenous | Can be endogenous or exogenous |
| Usually derived from genomic loci distinct from recognised genes | Usually derived from mRNAs, transposons, viruses or heterochromatic DNA |
| Formed from local RNA hairpin structures | Produced from long exogenous or endogenous dsRNA molecules (very long hairpins or biomolecular duplexes) |
| A single miRNA:miRNA* duplex is generated from each hairpin precursor | Multiple duplexes are generated |
| Highly conserved among species | Rarely conserved |
| Hetero-silencing; ie, target remote loci | Auto-silencing; ie, target the same locus |
| Processed in the nucleus by Drosha and in the cytoplasm by Dicer | Processed in the cytoplasm by Dicer |
| Perform function by either suppressing protein synthesis or mRNA cleavage | Perform function by mRNA cleavage |

Perfect complementarity of mRNA-miRNA allows Ago-catalyzed cleavage of the mRNA strand, whereas central mismatches exclude cleavage and promote repression of mRNA translation. Consistent with translational control, miRNAs that use this mechanism reduce the protein levels of their target genes, but the mRNA levels of these genes are barely affected (see Figure 1.1).

## 1.3. MiRNA Gene Transcription

The promoter regions of autonomously expressed miRNA genes are highly similar to those of protein-coding genes. The presence of CpG islands, TATA box sequences, initiation elements and certain histone modifications indicate that the promoters of miRNA genes are controlled by transcription factors (TFs), enhancers, silencing elements, methylation and chromatin modifications, which is similar to protein-coding genes [19]. MiRNA genes are transcribed by either RNA polymerase II or RNA polymerase III into primary miRNA transcripts (pri-miRNA). Many pri-miRNAs are polyadenylated and capped - hallmarks of polymerase II transcription [20]. Their transcription is sensitive to treatment with the polymerase II inhibitor α-amanitin, and polymerase II binds to promoter sequences upstream of the miR-23a/miR-27a/miR-24-2 cluster [21]. In contrast, miRNAs encoded by the largest human miRNA cluster, C19MC, are transcribed by polymerase III [22]. Both RNA polymerases are regulated differently and recognize specific promoter and terminator elements, facilitating a wide variety of regulatory options [9]. A significant number of TFs have been mechanistically characterized and showed to activate or repress the synthesis of pri-miRNAs in mammalian cells (Table 1.2) [23]. Some examples of such regulation are briefly discussed below (see Figure 1.2).

MYC and MYCN both stimulate expression of the miR-17-92 oncogenic cluster in lymphoma cells and miR-9 in neuroblastoma cells, but inhibit expression of several tumor suppressor miRNAs (for example, miR-15a), which promote MYC-mediated tumorigenesis

[24]. p53 stimulates the expression of numerous miRNAs: miR-34 family, miR-17-92, miR-145 and miR-107 family, which enhances cell cycle arrest and apoptosis [25]. MiR-21 is regulated by transcription factors including the androgen receptor, AP1, Gfi1, REST, and STAT3.

These factors contribute to miR-21 expression patterns in different contexts. For example, REST suppresses miR-21 to maintain self-renewal and pluripotency in mouse embryonic stem cells, while STAT3 induces miR-21 in multiple myeloma cells. Transcription of miR-148a, miR-34b/c, miR-9 and let-7 is dependent on their gene promoter methylation status, which is regulated by the DNMT1 and DNMT3b DNA methyltransferases [26].

**Table 1.2. Examples of transcription factors regulating miRNA levels in mammalian cell (extended from [23])**

| miRNAs | Transcription factors | Comments | Refs. |
|---|---|---|---|
| miR-1, 133a | SRF, MyoD, Mef2, myogenin | Muscle-specific | [27] |
| miR-7 | HoxD10 | Role in invasivness of breast cancer | [28] |
| miR-10b | Twist | Suggested role in breast cancer | [29] |
| miR-15a | c-myb | Regulatory feedback loop in hematopoietic cells | [30] |
| miR-17-92 | E2F, c-Myc, p53, STAT3 | Oncogene and role in development | [31, 32] |
| miR-21 | AR, AP-1, STAT3, REST | Up-regulated in wide range of solid cancers | [33] |
| miR-23a/b | c-Myc, NFATc3 | Regulation of cardiac hypertrophy | [34] |
| miR-34 | p53, ELK1 | Tumor suppressor function | [35] |
| miR-106b-25 | E2F1 | Homologous to the miR-17-92 cluster | [36] |
| miR-124a, 9 | REST | Neuronal specific | [37] |
| miR-132 | CREB | Molecular representation of memory | [38] |
| miR-133b | Pitx3 | Dopaminergic transmission in midbrain | [39] |
| miR-143 | NF-kappaB | Tumor suppressor function | [40] |
| miR-143, 145 | SRF, myocardin, Nkx2-5 | Smooth muscle cell plasticity | [41] |
| miR-145 | p53 | Tumor suppressor function | [42] |
| miR-146a | NF-kappaB | Signaling of innate immunity | [43] |
| miR-155 | Foxp3, NF-kappaB, AP-1 | Critical regulator of the immune system | [44] |
| miR-192, 215 | p53 | Cell cycle regulation | [45] |
| miR-194-2 | HNF-1alfa | Epithelial cell differentiation | [46] |
| miR-196b | Gfi1 | Control of the myelopoiesis | [47] |
| miR-199a/214 | Twist-1 | Development of specific neural cell populations | [48] |
| miR-200 | ZEB1-SIP1, ZEB1, ZEB2 | Roles in development and cancer | [49] |
| miR-223 | C/EBPs, PU.1, NFI-A | Granulocyte differentiation | [50] |
| miR-302 | Oct4/Sox2 | Embryonic stem cell specific | [51] |
| miR-342 | PU.1, IRFs | Granulocyte differentiation | [52] |
| miR-424 | PU.1 | Monocyte/macrophage differentiation | [53] |

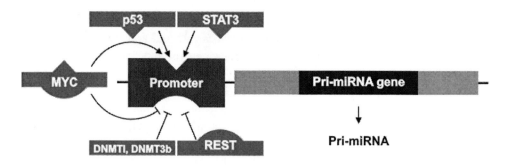

Figure 1.2. Regulation of pri-miRNA gene transcription.

The involvement of TFs in pri-miRNA production largely accounts for the temporally and spatially specific expression patterns of miRNAs, and it is indeed becoming increasingly clear that a critical aspect of the biological functions of TFs is to regulate the expression of particular miRNAs. Furthermore, many TFs are themselves subject to extensive regulation, which couples the expression of the target miRNAs to the physiological status of the cells. Consequently, these miRNAs execute the functions of the TFs and relay the upstream signals by regulating the expression of their downstream target genes [23].

## 1.4. MiRNA Editing

RNA editing of primary transcripts by ADARs (adenosine deaminases acting on RNA) modifies adenosine (A) into inosine (I). Because the base-pairing properties of inosine are similar to those of guanosine (G), A-to-I editing of miRNA precursors may change their sequence, base-pairing and structural properties and can influence their further Drosha-mediated and Dicer-mediated cleavage, pre-miRNAs export as well as their target recognition abilities [9]. Selective editing by ADAR1 and ADAR2 inhibits cleavage of human pri-miR-142 by Drosha and contributes to its degradation by the nuclease Tudor-SN, which has affinity for dsRNA containing inosine-uracil pairs [54]. Editing of pre-miR-151 prevents Dicer processing, resulting in accumulation of pre-miR-151 (Figure 1.3) [55]. However, editing can also enhance Drosha processing. Interestingly, pri-miR-376a-2 processing in *Drosophila melanogaster* is inhibited even by catalytically inactive ADAR2, which binds pri-miRNA and inhibits Drosha activity [56]. In addition to altering miRNA processing, miRNA editing can have an impact on miRNA target specificity. For example, a single A-to-I change in the miR-376 precursor redirects the mature miRNA to a new target, resulting in altered protein expression in mice [57].

## 1.5. Regulation of miRNA Processing in Nucleus

Number of mechanisms exists to regulate miRNA processing in nucleus consisting highly complex regulatory system of miRNA biogenesis.

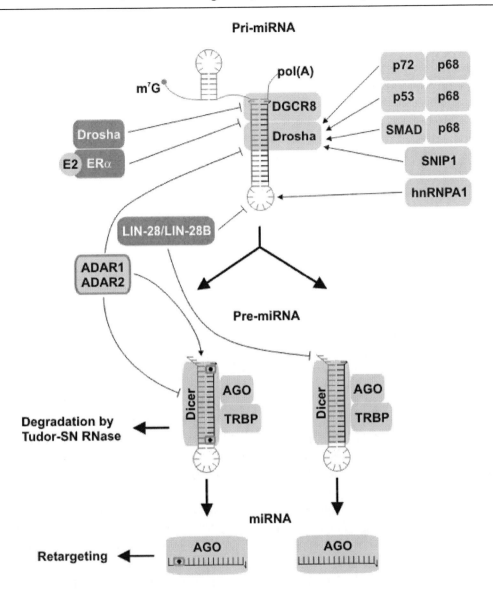

Figure 1.3. Regulation of miRNA processing.

## Reciprocal Regulation of Drosha and DGCR8

Two components of microprocessor complex, Drosha and DGCR8, operate in cooperation and regulate each other. Both the levels and activity of these proteins are subject to regulation that affects the accumulation of miRNAs. DGCR8 has a stabilizing effect on Drosha through the interaction with its middle domain, whereas Drosha controls DGCR8 levels by cleaving hairpins present in the *DGCR8* mRNA, thereby inducing its degradation [58,59], resulting in negative feedback loop reducing DGCR8 expression when sufficient microprocessor activity is available. Keeping the Drosha to DGCR8 ratio in check may be important, as a threefold excess of DGCR8 dramatically inhibits Drosha processing activity *in vitro* [60].

## p68 and p72

The p68 and p72 helicases, identified as components of the Drosha microprocessor complex, are thought to stimulate processing of one third of murine pri-miRNAs [61]. These helicases are conserved across eukaryotes and are implicated in diverse RNA processing pathways (for review [62]). In p68 or p72 knock-out cells, levels of pre-miRNAs, but not pri-miRNAs, are significantly reduced as a consequence of attenuated Drosha binding and pri-miRNA processing. It seems that they are required to properly recruit the microprocessor to some pri-miRNAs. Now, it is clear that multiple critical cellular signaling pathways use the p68 and p72 association with microprocessor to effect regulation of pri-miRNA processing. The p68-mediated interaction of the Drosha complex with the tumor suppressor p53 has a stimulatory effect on pri-miR-16-1, pri-miR-143 and pri-miR-145 processing in response to DNA damage in cancer cells [63].

## Transforming Growth Factor-β/Bone Morphogenetic Protein (TGFβ/BMP)

The signal transducers of the transforming growth factor-β (TGFβ) and bone morphogenetic protein (BMP) signaling cascade, SMADs, regulate gene expression at the level of transcription, but also control Drosha-mediated miRNA processing (see Figure 1.3). SMADs are present, together with Drosha and p68, in a complex interacting with pri-miR-21. Up-regulation of miR-21, induced by TGFβ and BMP4, facilitates differentiation of vascular smooth muscle cells into contractile cells [64]. It is unclear how SMADs control miRNA biogenesis. Davis and co-workers reasoned that SMAD proteins might be the intermediaries responsible for connecting these signaling pathways with miR-21 processing, as they are translocated into the nucleus upon TGFβ or BMP signaling and are known to bind DNA [64]. Furthermore, a previous study reported that SMAD1, or a SMAD nuclear interacting protein 1 (SNIP1), interact directly with the RNA helicase p68 and enhances processing of pri-miRNAs, as well as the accumulation of mature miRNAs. Accordingly, depletion of receptor-specific SMADs (SMAD1 and SMAD5) or p68 abrogated the BMP and TGFβ-driven increase in pri-miR-21 processing [65].

The full complement of miRNAs that are regulated by this pathway is presently unknown. Since the TGFβ and BMP signaling pathways regulate many biological phenomena, it is possible that these pathways stimulate processing of other pri-miRNAs; indeed, pri-miR-199a was observed to be processed in this manner [64]. This is not surprising, since these signaling pathways converge on miRNA processing via p68, and this helicase has been shown to modulate a number of miRNAs [11].

## ERα/Estrogen

Estrogen hormones are well known regulators for transcription and post-transcriptional events of a number of genes through binding to their specific nuclear estrogen receptors (ERs), ERα or ERβ. Although both receptors exhibit a similar affinity toward estrogen, a distinction in tissue distribution between ERα and ERβ has long been recognized. ERα is mainly found in endometrium, breast cancer cells, ovarian stroma cells, and in the hypothalamus, whereas ERβ appears to be ubiquitously expressed [11]. Interesting report revealed how ERα signaling cascade can negatively regulate pri-miRNA processing. Kato and colleagues [66] noticed that ERα was shown previously to interact with p68 and p72. Augmentation of the ERα signaling pathway produced a striking pattern of changes in certain miRNAs; many miRNAs were increased in ERα-/- mice: including miR-16, miR-26a, miR-29a, miR-125a, miR-143, miR-145, miR-195, etc. [67]. The physiological importance of ERα-regulated miRNA biogenesis was evident from the observation that the 3′ UTR of VEGF, an ERα target gene, is targeted by ERα-repressed miRNAs. Further, it was demonstrated *in vitro* that estrogen (E2)-bound ERα could directly inhibit Drosha processing of ERα target pri-miRNAs and determined that p68 and/or p72 bridge the interaction between Drosha and E2-bound ERα [67]. Thus, when ERα is recruited to the large Drosha complex in an E2-dependent manner, Drosha is dissociated from ERα-targeted pri-miRNA loci. It remains to determine whether ERα/E2 weakens the overall integrity of the large Drosha complex, or simply its affinity for certain pri-miRNAs [15]. Taken together, these data suggest that E2-ERα signaling is antagonistic for miRNA processing, possibly through direct interaction between ERα and p68/p72, leading to dissociation of the Drosha microprocessor from a subset of pri-miRNAs.

The evidence showing inhibitory roles of ERα on the biogenesis of a select subset of miRNAs provides a new explanation for the molecular mechanisms of the ERα positive breast cancers. Due to its negative regulation on some of these tumor suppressor-like miRNAs, including miR-16 and miR-26a, ERα can amplify the tumorigenic signals from VEGF [67], EZH2 [68] and some oncogenes that are targeted by miR-16 or miR-26a in breast epithelial cells. Thus, there is strong indication for pursuing an ERα-based therapeutic approach. First, suppression of the ERα signaling by selective ERα modulators, such as tamoxifen, can inactivate transcriptional regulation of ERα on some growth factors important for the transformation of the cells. Second, blocking ERα signaling will enhance the tumor suppressive potential of the cells by promoting the biogenesis of those tumor suppressor-like miRNAs, which limit the growth and vascularization of the tumors [15].

## hnRNP Proteins

Drosha-mediated cleavage can also be regulated for individual miRNAs: the heterogeneous nuclear ribonucleoprotein A1 (hnRNP A1) binds specifically to loop region of pri-miR-18a and facilitates its processing. This protein has been well established as a component of many hnRNPs and performs essential functions in many RNA processing and transport pathways [69]. MiR-18a is one of six miRNA stem-loops on the oncogenic polycistron miR-17-92. Loss of hnRNP A1 diminishes the abundance of mature miR-18a (Figure 1.3), but hnRNP A1 does not have any impact on other miRNAs that are located in the same miR-17 genomic cluster, demonstrating the extraordinary specificity of miR-18a biogenesis [70]. hnRNP A1 binds to the conserved loop of the pri-miR-18a and changes the hairpin conformation to create a more favourable cleavage site for Drosha. About 14% of the human pri-miRNA loops are conserved between different species and could provide anchor points for similar regulatory mechanisms [71]. The general physiological functions of hnRNP-miRNA loop interactions remain to be elucidated; ultimately, it will be important to understand the global distribution of hnRNP proteins between miRNAs and non-miRNA-containing substrates.

### LIN-28–Let-7 Regulatory System

LIN-28 is the best-studied master regulator of let-7 production. Let-7 is one of the most abundant miRNA families in mammals, with high expression in essentially all adult tissues. In embryonic cells, in contrast, mature let-7 is present at 1000-fold lower levels. Unexpectedly, pri-let-7 expression is constant throughout development, thus providing a dramatic illustration of post-transcriptional regulation of a miRNA [72]. Research published over the past two years has demonstrated that the RNA-binding protein LIN28 blocks let-7 miRNA maturation in early embryonic cells, and contributes to let-7 reduction in cancer (for review [73]). The processing failure is due to LIN-28 binding to the terminal loop of pri-let-7, which interferes with cleavage by Drosha. Binding of LIN-28 to pre-let-7 can also block its processing by Dicer. In the latter case, LIN-28 induces the 3′-terminal polyuridylation of pre-let-7 by attracting the poly(U) polymerase, terminal (U) transferase (TUT4) [73]. Uridylation prevents Dicer processing and targets pre-let-7 for degradation by an as yet unknown RNAse. Repression of LIN-28 is highly specific and affects only members of the let-7 family [74]. The LIN-28–let-7 regulatory system is highly conserved in evolution and plays an important role in maintaining the pluripotency of embryonic stem cells (eSCs), and also in development and oncogenesis. Inhibition of let-7 maturation by LIN-28 is essential for maintaining self-renewal of eSCs and for blocking their differentiation; during differentiation LIN-28 levels decrease and let-7 miRNAs accumulate. Let-7 functions as a tumor suppressor by targeting several oncogenes, including *MYC*, *KRAS* and cyclin D1 (*CCND1*) [75]. By repressing maturation of let-7 miRNAs, LIN-28 acts as an oncogene; indeed, activation of LIN-28 is found in many human tumors [76]. Interestingly, LIN-28 itself is targeted by let-7, indicating that LIN-28 and let-7 control the levels of each other following differentiation. The miRNA binding site of the Drosha competitor LIN-28 maps to conserved bases in the terminal loop of pri-let-7 (see Figure 1.4). Intriguingly, although the loop region is considered dispensable for microprocessor action, many miRNAs have evolutionarily conserved loops potentially containing regulatory information [71].

## 1.6. Regulation of miRNA Maturation and Function in Cytoplasm

MiRISC is the cytoplasmic effector machine of the miRNA pathway and contains a single-stranded miRNA guiding it to its target mRNAs. Cytoplasmic miRNA processing and miRISC assembly are mediated by the miRISC loading complex (mRLC). mRLC is a multi-protein complex composed of the RNase Dicer, the double-stranded RNA-binding domain proteins TRBP (Tar RNA binding protein) and PACT (protein activator of PKR), and the core component Ago2, which also mediates miRISC effects on mRNA targets [77-80]. TRBP and PACT are not essential for Dicer-mediated cleavage of the pre-miRNA but they facilitate it, and TRBP stabilizes [81]. Depletion of TRBP or PACT reduces the efficiency of post-transcriptional gene silencing.

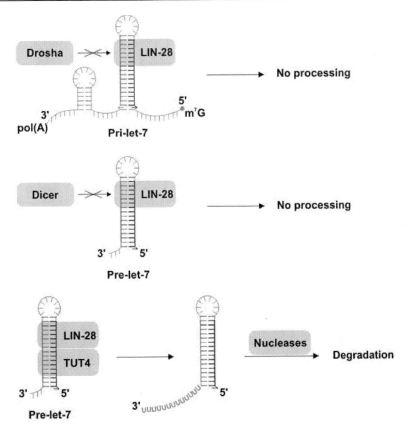

Figure 1.4. Schematic overview of LIN-28–let-7 regulatory system.

In mammals, Ago2 has robust RNase H-like endonuclease activity, and in case of miRNAs which display a high degree of complementarity along the hairpin stem, an additional endonucleolytic cleavage step occurs before Dicer-mediated cleavage. The slicer activity of Ago2 cleaves the 3' arm of the hairpin - the prospective passenger strand - in the middle to generate a nicked hairpin, producing the Ago2-cleaved precursor miRNA (ac-pre-miRNA) [82]. Dicer can process this precursor as efficiently as the pre-miRNAs, but the Ago2-mediated step most probably facilitates subsequent strand dissociation and miRISC activation, in a similar manner to its function in the siRNA pathway [83]. Processing of pre-miR-451 also requires cleavage by Ago2, but is independent of Dicer and the 3' end is generated by exonucleolytic trimming [84].

Ago proteins in general exerts multiple functions in the miRNA pathway. They participate in miRNA processing by generating the ac-pre-miRNA, and they are the miRISC effector proteins mediating the mRNA degradation, destabilization or translational inhibition [4,15,60]. In addition, Ago proteins regulate miRNA abundance post-transcriptionally, and loss of endogenous Ago2 diminishes the expression and activity of mature miRNA [82]. This particular function of Ago2 is independent of its slicer function and endonuclease activity. Most probably, the capacity of Ago proteins to bind to mature miRNAs stabilizes these short molecules [9]. Several mechanisms have been described that regulate Ago2 levels in mammalian cells, including stabilization of Ago2 by the chaperone heat shock protein 90 (HSP90) [85], and modulating effects of protein modifications [86-88]. The TRIM-NHL protein TRIM71 promotes Ago2 polyubiquitylation and subsequent proteasomal degradation, resulting in impaired miRNA mediated silencing [87]. Hydroxylation of the Ago2 Pro700 by type I collagen prolyl-4-hydroxylase C-P4H(I) stabilizes Ago2 and increases its localization to processing bodies (P-bodies) [86]. P-bodies function in both storage and decay of repressed mRNAs. Consequently, they are enriched in proteins involved in translational repression, and in mRNA deadenylation, decapping and degradation [89,90]. P-bodies are dynamic structures, with proteins and mRNAs continuously moving in and out of them, and the number and size of P-bodies varies depending on the translational activity of the cell. Argonaute proteins, mature miRNAs and repressed mRNAs are all enriched in P-bodies, and the inhibition of miRNA biogenesis causes the disappearance of P-bodies [90]. Moreover, a positive correlation exists between miRNA-mediated repression and the accumulation of target mRNAs in P-bodies. For example, miR-29a interacts with the 3' UTR of the HIV-1 mRNA and targets it to P-bodies in human T-lymphocytes, and the artificial disruption of P-bodies enhances HIV-1 infection [91]. Increased recruitment of Ago2 to P-bodies was also observed on Ser387 phosphorylation, which occurs in response to stress and mediated by the MAPK/p38 kinase signaling pathway [88].

The RNase III Dicer cleaves off the loop of the pre-miRNA or the nicked ac-pre-miRNA and generates a roughly 22-nucleotide miRNA duplex with two nucleotides protruding as overhangs at each 3' end. This cleavage is essential for miRNA processing. Deletion of Dicer decreases or abrogates the production of mature miRNAs [92,93]. Several modes of Dicer cleavage activity regulation have been described. The amino-terminal DExD/H-box helicase domain of human Dicer inhibits its cleavage activity; TRBP binds to Dicer in this region and activates Dicer through a conformational rearrangement [94]. Dicer is also regulated by its product let-7, which targets *Dicer* mRNA, creating a negative feedback loop [95]. Additional mechanisms to regulate Dicer activity may exist: pre-miR-138 is expressed ubiquitously but its mature form is restricted to certain cell types, indicating tissue-specific processing of this miRNA [9].

The miRNA acts as an adaptor for miRISC to specifically recognize and regulate particular mRNAs. With few exceptions, miRNA binding sites in animal mRNAs lie in the 3' UTR and are usually present in multiple copies. Most animal miRNAs bind with mismatches and bulges, although a key feature of recognition involves Watson-Crick base pairing of miRNA nucleotides 2–8, representing the seed region. In contrast, most plant miRNAs bind with near-perfect complementarity to sites within the coding sequence of their targets [4]. The degree of miRNA-mRNA complementarity has been considered a key determinant of the regulatory mechanism. Perfect complementarity allows Ago-catalyzed cleavage of the mRNA strand, whereas central mismatches exclude cleavage and promote repression of mRNA translation. The mechanisms by which miRISC regulates translation have been subject to ongoing debate. The fundamental issue of whether repression occurs at translation initiation or post-initiation has not yet been resolved. Non-repressed mRNAs recruit eIF4 initiation factors and ribosomal subunits and form circularized mRNA structures that enhance translation. When miRISCs bind to mRNAs, they can repress initiation at the cap recognition stage (by competing with eIF4E [96]) or the 60S recruitment stage [97]. Alternatively, they can induce deadenylation of the mRNA and thereby inhibit circularization of the mRNA [98]. They can repress a post-initiation stage of translation by inducing ribosomes to drop off prematurely. Finally, they can promote degradation by inducing mRNA deadenylation followed by decapping [98] (see Figure 1.5).

Interestingly, several reports indicate that miRNAs not only act as repressors but can also act as activators of translation under conditions of serum starvation (or general growth arrest, or at the G0 stage) the Ago2-miRISC complex has been shown to switch from a translational repressor to an activator. The switch required fragile X-related protein 1 (FXR1), a paralogue of FMRP [99,100].

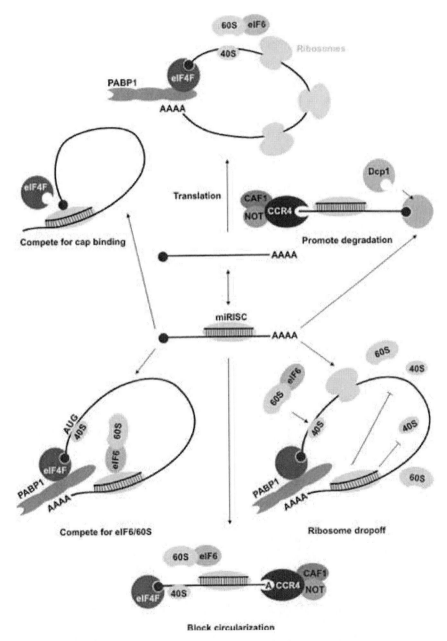

Figure 1.5. Mechanisms of miRISC mediated repression. (adapted from [4]).

## 1.7. Half-Life and Decay of miRNA

In comparison to our increasing knowledge about miRNA processing, surprisingly little is known about the half-life and degradation of individual miRNAs. It is generally thought that miRNAs represent highly stable molecules and, indeed, experimentation using RNA polymerase II inhibitors or depletion of miRNA processing enzymes, have indicated that the half-lives of miRNAs in cell lines or in organs such as liver or heart correspond to many hours or even days [101,102]. However, such slow turnover is unlikely to be a universal feature of miRNAs as they often play a role in developmental transitions or act as on and off switches, conditions that require more active metabolism [10].

Several examples of accelerated or regulated miRNA turnover are now known. MiR-29b decays faster in cycling mammalian cells than in cells arrested in mitosis. MiR-27a stability can be modulated by viral infection [103]. The marked decrease in miR-122 within 1 h after treatment of liver cells with interferon supports this notion [104]. In addition, miRNA activity could also be regulated after processing by blocking the miRNA binding sites on their target mRNA by RNA-binding proteins [105]. Nevertheless, general mechanisms that may control miRNA turnover remain unidentified for now.

## Acknowledgment

This work was supported by grants NS 10361-3/2009, NR/9814-4/2008, NS 10352-3/2009, NT/11214-4/2010 of Czech Ministry of Health, Project No. MZ0MOU2005 of the Czech Ministry of Health and by the project "CEITEC – Central European Institute of Technology" (CZ.1.05/1.1.00/02.0068).

## References

[1] Bartel DP: MicroRNAs: genomics, biogenesis, mechanism, and function. *Cell* 2004 116:281-97.

[2] Griffiths-Jones S, Saini HK, van Dongen S, Enright AJ: miRBase: tools for microRNA genomics. *Nucleic Acids Res* 2008 36:D154-8.

[3] Hatfield S, Ruohola-Baker H: microRNA and stem cell function. *Cell Tissue Res.* 2008 331:57-66.

[4] Carthew RW, Sontheimer EJ: Origins and Mechanisms of miRNAs and siRNAs. *Cell* 2009 136:642-55.

[5] Winter J, Diederichs S: MicroRNA biogenesis and cancer. *Methods Mol. Biol. 2011* 676:3-22.

[6] Croce CM: Causes and consequences of microRNA dysregulation in cancer. *Nat. Rev. Genet* 2009 10:704-14.

[7] Alvarez-Garcia I, Miska EA: MicroRNA functions in animal development and human disease. *Development* 2005 132:4653-62.

[8] Xiao C, Rajewsky K: MicroRNA control in the immune system: basic principles. *Cell* 2009 136:26-36.

[9] Winter J, Jung S, Keller S, Gregory RI, Diederichs S: Many roads to maturity: microRNA biogenesis pathways and their regulation. *Nat. Cell Biol.* 2009 11:228-34.

[10] Krol J, Loedige I, Filipowicz W: The widespread regulation of microRNA biogenesis, function and decay. *Nat. Rev Genet.* 11:597-610.

[11] Newman MA, Hammond SM: Emerging paradigms of regulated microRNA processing. *Genes Dev.* 24:1086-92.

[12] Davis BN, Hata A: Regulation of MicroRNA Biogenesis: A miRiad of mechanisms. *Cell Commun. Signal* 2009 7:18.

[13] Siomi H, Siomi MC: Posttranscriptional regulation of microRNA biogenesis in animals. *Mol. Cell* 38:323-32.

[14] Miyoshi K, Miyoshi T, Siomi H: Many ways to generate microRNA-like small RNAs: non-canonical pathways for microRNA production. *Mol. Genet Genomics* 284:95-103.

[15] Beezhold KJ, Castranova V, Chen F: Microprocessor of microRNAs: regulation and potential for therapeutic intervention. *Mol. Cancer* 2010 9:134.

[16] Chiang HR, Schoenfeld LW, Ruby JG, Auyeung VC, Spies N, Baek D, Johnston WK, Russ C, Luo S, Babiarz JE, Blelloch R, Schroth GP, Nusbaum C, Bartel DP: Mammalian microRNAs: experimental evaluation of novel and previously annotated genes. *Genes Dev.* 2010 24:992-1009.

[17] Chatterjee S, Grosshans H: Active turnover modulates mature microRNA activity in Caenorhabditis elegans. *Nature* 2009 461:546-9.

[18] Lederman L: siRNA and microRNA. *Biotechniques* 2009 46:257-9.

[19] Ozsolak F, Poling LL, Wang Z, Liu H, Liu XS, Roeder RG, Zhang X, Song JS, Fisher DE: Chromatin structure analyses identify miRNA promoters. *Genes Dev.* 2008 22:3172-83.

[20] Lee Y, Kim M, Han J, Yeom KH, Lee S, Baek SH, Kim VN: MicroRNA genes are transcribed by RNA polymerase II. *EMBO J.* 2004 23:4051-60.

[21] Cai X, Hagedorn CH, Cullen BR: Human microRNAs are processed from capped, polyadenylated transcripts that can also function as mRNAs. *RNA* 2004 10:1957-66.

[22] Borchert GM, Lanier W, Davidson BL: RNA polymerase III transcribes human microRNAs. *Nat. Struct. Mol. Biol.* 2006 13:1097-101.

[23] Zhang X, Zeng Y: Regulation of mammalian microRNA expression. *J. Cardiovasc. Transl Res.* 2010 3:197-203.

[24] Chang TC, Yu D, Lee YS, Wentzel EA, Arking DE, West KM, Dang CV, Thomas-Tikhonenko A, Mendell JT: Widespread microRNA repression by Myc contributes to tumorigenesis. *Nat. Genet.* 2008 40:43-50.

[25] He L, He X, Lim LP, de Stanchina E, Xuan Z, Liang Y, Xue W, Zender L, Magnus J, Ridzon D, Jackson AL, Linsley PS, Chen C, Lowe SW, Cleary MA, Hannon GJ: A microRNA component of the p53 tumour suppressor network. *Nature* 2007 447:1130-4.

[26] Han L, Witmer PD, Casey E, Valle D, Sukumar S: DNA methylation regulates MicroRNA expression. *Cancer Biol. Ther.* 2007 6:1284-8.

[27] Rao PK, Kumar RM, Farkhondeh M, Baskerville S, Lodish HF: Myogenic factors that regulate expression of muscle-specific microRNAs. *Proc. Natl. Acad. Sci. USA* 2006 103:8721-6.

[28] Slaby O, Svoboda M, Michalek J, Vyzula R: MicroRNAs in colorectal cancer: translation of molecular biology into clinical application. *Mol. Cancer* 2009 8:102.

[29] Ma L, Teruya-Feldstein J, Weinberg RA: Tumour invasion and metastasis initiated by microRNA-10b in breast cancer. *Nature* 2007 449:682-8.
[30] Zhao H, Kalota A, Jin S, Gewirtz AM: The c-myb proto-oncogene and microRNA-15a comprise an active autoregulatory feedback loop in human hematopoietic cells. *Blood* 2009 113:505-16.
[31] O'Donnell KA, Wentzel EA, Zeller KI, Dang CV, Mendell JT: c-Myc-regulated microRNAs modulate E2F1 expression. *Nature* 2005 435:839-43.
[32] Yan HL, Xue G, Mei Q, Wang YZ, Ding FX, Liu MF, Lu MH, Tang Y, Yu HY, Sun SH: Repression of the miR-17-92 cluster by p53 has an important function in hypoxia-induced apoptosis. *EMBO J.* 2009 28:2719-32.
[33] Ribas J, Lupold SE: The transcriptional regulation of miR-21, its multiple transcripts, and their implication in prostate cancer. *Cell Cycle* 2010 9:923-9.
[34] Lin Z, Murtaza I, Wang K, Jiao J, Gao J, Li PF: miR-23a functions downstream of NFATc3 to regulate cardiac hypertrophy. *Proc. Natl. Acad. Sci. USA* 2009 106:12103-8.
[35] Hermeking H: The miR-34 family in cancer and apoptosis. *Cell Death Differ.* 2010 17:193-9.
[36] Petrocca F, Visone R, Onelli MR, Shah MH, Nicoloso MS, de Martino I, Iliopoulos D, Pilozzi E, Liu CG, Negrini M, Cavazzini L, Volinia S, Alder H, Ruco LP, Baldassarre G, Croce CM, Vecchione A: E2F1-regulated microRNAs impair TGFbeta-dependent cell-cycle arrest and apoptosis in gastric cancer. *Cancer Cell* 2008 13:272-86.
[37] Conaco C, Otto S, Han JJ, Mandel G: Reciprocal actions of REST and a microRNA promote neuronal identity. *Proc. Natl. Acad. Sci. USA* 2006 103:2422-7.
[38] Nudelman AS, DiRocco DP, Lambert TJ, Garelick MG, Le J, Nathanson NM, Storm DR: Neuronal activity rapidly induces transcription of the CREB-regulated microRNA-132, in vivo. *Hippocampus* 2010 20:492-8.
[39] Kim J, Inoue K, Ishii J, Vanti WB, Voronov SV, Murchison E, Hannon G, Abeliovich A: A MicroRNA feedback circuit in midbrain dopamine neurons. *Science* 2007 317:1220-4.
[40] Zhang X, Liu S, Hu T, He Y, Sun S: Up-regulated microRNA-143 transcribed by nuclear factor kappa B enhances hepatocarcinoma metastasis by repressing fibronectin expression. *Hepatology* 2009 50:490-9.
[41] 41. Cordes KR, Sheehy NT, White MP, Berry EC, Morton SU, Muth AN, Lee TH, Miano JM, Ivey KN, Srivastava D: miR-145 and miR-143 regulate smooth muscle cell fate and plasticity. *Nature* 2009 460:705-10.
[42] Sachdeva M, Zhu S, Wu F, Wu H, Walia V, Kumar S, Elble R, Watabe K, Mo YY: p53 represses c-Myc through induction of the tumor suppressor miR-145. *Proc. Natl. Acad. Sci. USA* 2009 106:3207-12.
[43] Taganov KD, Boldin MP, Chang KJ, Baltimore D: NF-kappaB-dependent induction of microRNA miR-146, an inhibitor targeted to signaling proteins of innate immune responses. *Proc. Natl. Acad. Sci. USA* 2006 103:12481-6.
[44] Faraoni I, Antonetti FR, Cardone J, Bonmassar E: miR-155 gene: a typical multifunctional microRNA. *Biochim. Biophys. Acta* 2009 1792:497-505.
[45] Georges SA, Biery MC, Kim SY, Schelter JM, Guo J, Chang AN, Jackson AL, Carleton MO, Linsley PS, Cleary MA, Chau BN: Coordinated regulation of cell cycle

transcripts by p53-Inducible microRNAs, miR-192 and miR-215. *Cancer Res.* 2008 68:10105-12.

[46] Hino K, Tsuchiya K, Fukao T, Kiga K, Okamoto R, Kanai T, Watanabe M: Inducible expression of microRNA-194 is regulated by HNF-1alpha during intestinal epithelial cell differentiation. *RNA* 2008 14:1433-42.

[47] Velu CS, Baktula AM, Grimes HL: Gfi1 regulates miR-21 and miR-196b to control myelopoiesis. *Blood* 2009 113:4720-8.

[48] Lee YB, Bantounas I, Lee DY, Phylactou L, Caldwell MA, Uney JB: Twist-1 regulates the miR-199a/214 cluster during development. *Nucleic. Acids Res.* 2009 37:123-8.

[49] Bracken CP, Gregory PA, Kolesnikoff N, Bert AG, Wang J, Shannon MF, Goodall GJ: A double-negative feedback loop between ZEB1-SIP1 and the microRNA-200 family regulates epithelial-mesenchymal transition. *Cancer Res.* 2008 68:7846-54.

[50] Fazi F, Rosa A, Fatica A, Gelmetti V, De Marchis ML, Nervi C, Bozzoni I: A minicircuitry comprised of microRNA-223 and transcription factors NFI-A and C/EBPalpha regulates human granulopoiesis. *Cell* 2005 123:819-31.

[51] Card DA, Hebbar PB, Li L, Trotter KW, Komatsu Y, Mishina Y, Archer TK: Oct4/Sox2-regulated miR-302 targets cyclin D1 in human embryonic stem cells. *Mol. Cell Biol.* 2008 28:6426-38.

[52] De Marchis ML, Ballarino M, Salvatori B, Puzzolo MC, Bozzoni I, Fatica A: A new molecular network comprising PU.1, interferon regulatory factor proteins and miR-342 stimulates ATRA-mediated granulocytic differentiation of acute promyelocytic leukemia cells. *Leukemia* 2009 23:856-62.

[53] Rosa A, Ballarino M, Sorrentino A, Sthandier O, De Angelis FG, Marchioni M, Masella B, Guarini A, Fatica A, Peschle C, Bozzoni I: The interplay between the master transcription factor PU.1 and miR-424 regulates human monocyte/macrophage differentiation. *Proc. Natl. Acad. Sci. USA* 2007 104:19849-54.

[54] Scadden AD: The RISC subunit Tudor-SN binds to hyper-edited double-stranded RNA and promotes its cleavage. *Nat Struct Mol Biol* 2005 12:489-96.

[55] Kawahara Y, Zinshteyn B, Chendrimada TP, Shiekhattar R, Nishikura K: RNA editing of the microRNA-151 precursor blocks cleavage by the Dicer-TRBP complex. *EMBO Rep.* 2007 8:763-9.

[56] Heale BS, Keegan LP, McGurk L, Michlewski G, Brindle J, Stanton CM, Caceres JF, O'Connell MA: Editing independent effects of ADARs on the miRNA/siRNA pathways. *EMBO J.* 2009 28:3145-56.

[57] Kawahara Y, Zinshteyn B, Sethupathy P, Iizasa H, Hatzigeorgiou AG, Nishikura K: Redirection of silencing targets by adenosine-to-inosine editing of miRNAs. *Science* 2007 315:1137-40.

[58] Han J, Pedersen JS, Kwon SC, Belair CD, Kim YK, Yeom KH, Yang WY, Haussler D, Blelloch R, Kim VN: Posttranscriptional crossregulation between Drosha and DGCR8. *Cell* 2009 136:75-84.

[59] Triboulet R, Chang HM, Lapierre RJ, Gregory RI: Post-transcriptional control of DGCR8 expression by the Microprocessor. *RNA* 2009 15:1005-11.

[60] Gregory RI, Yan KP, Amuthan G, Chendrimada T, Doratotaj B, Cooch N, Shiekhattar R: The Microprocessor complex mediates the genesis of microRNAs. *Nature* 2004 432:235-40.

[61] Fukuda T, Yamagata K, Fujiyama S, Matsumoto T, Koshida I, Yoshimura K, Mihara M, Naitou M, Endoh H, Nakamura T, Akimoto C, Yamamoto Y, Katagiri T, Foulds C, Takezawa S, Kitagawa H, Takeyama K, O'Malley BW, Kato S: DEAD-box RNA helicase subunits of the Drosha complex are required for processing of rRNA and a subset of microRNAs. *Nat. Cell Biol.* 2007 9:604-11.

[62] Fuller-Pace FV: DExD/H box RNA helicases: multifunctional proteins with important roles in transcriptional regulation. *Nucleic. Acids Res.* 2006 34:4206-15.

[63] Suzuki HI, Yamagata K, Sugimoto K, Iwamoto T, Kato S, Miyazono K: Modulation of microRNA processing by p53. *Nature* 2009 460:529-33.

[64] Davis BN, Hilyard AC, Lagna G, Hata A: SMAD proteins control DROSHA-mediated microRNA maturation. *Nature* 2008 454:56-61.

[65] Warner DR, Bhattacherjee V, Yin X, Singh S, Mukhopadhyay P, Pisano MM, Greene RM: Functional interaction between Smad, CREB binding protein, and p68 RNA helicase. *Biochem Biophys Res Commun* 2004 324:70-6.

[66] Endoh H, Maruyama K, Masuhiro Y, Kobayashi Y, Goto M, Tai H, Yanagisawa J, Metzger D, Hashimoto S, Kato S: Purification and identification of p68 RNA helicase acting as a transcriptional coactivator specific for the activation function 1 of human estrogen receptor alpha. *Mol. Cell Biol.* 1999 19:5363-72.

[67] Yamagata K, Fujiyama S, Ito S, Ueda T, Murata T, Naitou M, Takeyama K, Minami Y, O'Malley BW, Kato S: Maturation of microRNA is hormonally regulated by a nuclear receptor. *Mol. Cell* 2009 36:340-7.

[68] Wong CF, Tellam RL: MicroRNA-26a targets the histone methyltransferase Enhancer of Zeste homolog 2 during myogenesis. *J. Biol. Chem.* 2008 283:9836-43.

[69] He Y, Smith R: Nuclear functions of heterogeneous nuclear ribonucleoproteins A/B. *Cell Mol. Life Sci.* 2009 66:1239-56.

[70] Guil S, Caceres JF: The multifunctional RNA-binding protein hnRNP A1 is required for processing of miR-18a. *Nat. Struct. Mol. Biol.* 2007 14:591-6.

[71] Michlewski G, Guil S, Semple CA, Caceres JF: Posttranscriptional regulation of miRNAs harboring conserved terminal loops. *Mol. Cell* 2008 32:383-93.

[72] Thomson JM, Newman M, Parker JS, Morin-Kensicki EM, Wright T, Hammond SM: Extensive post-transcriptional regulation of microRNAs and its implications for cancer. *Genes Dev* 2006 20:2202-7.

[73] Viswanathan SR, Daley GQ: Lin28: A microRNA regulator with a macro role. *Cell* 140:445-9.

[74] Heo I, Joo C, Cho J, Ha M, Han J, Kim VN: Lin28 mediates the terminal uridylation of let-7 precursor MicroRNA. *Mol. Cell* 2008 32:276-84.

[75] Roush S, Slack FJ: The let-7 family of microRNAs. *Trends Cell Biol.* 2008 18:505-16.

[76] Viswanathan SR, Powers JT, Einhorn W, Hoshida Y, Ng TL, Toffanin S, O'Sullivan M, Lu J, Phillips LA, Lockhart VL, Shah SP, Tanwar PS, Mermel CH, Beroukhim R, Azam M, Teixeira J, Meyerson M, Hughes TP, Llovet JM, Radich J, Mullighan CG, Golub TR, Sorensen PH, Daley GQ: Lin28 promotes transformation and is associated with advanced human malignancies. *Nat. Genet.* 2009 41:843-8.

[77] Gregory RI, Chendrimada TP, Cooch N, Shiekhattar R: Human RISC couples microRNA biogenesis and posttranscriptional gene silencing. *Cell* 2005 123:631-40.

[78] Haase AD, Jaskiewicz L, Zhang H, Laine S, Sack R, Gatignol A, Filipowicz W: TRBP, a regulator of cellular PKR and HIV-1 virus expression, interacts with Dicer and functions in RNA silencing. *EMBO Rep.* 2005 6:961-7.

[79] Lee Y, Hur I, Park SY, Kim YK, Suh MR, Kim VN: The role of PACT in the RNA silencing pathway. *EMBO J.* 2006 25:522-32.

[80] MacRae IJ, Ma E, Zhou M, Robinson CV, Doudna JA: In vitro reconstitution of the human RISC-loading complex. *Proc. Natl. Acad. Sci. USA* 2008 105:512-7.

[81] Chendrimada TP, Gregory RI, Kumaraswamy E, Norman J, Cooch N, Nishikura K, Shiekhattar R: TRBP recruits the Dicer complex to Ago2 for microRNA processing and gene silencing. *Nature* 2005 436:740-4.

[82] Diederichs S, Haber DA: Dual role for argonautes in microRNA processing and posttranscriptional regulation of microRNA expression. *Cell* 2007 131:1097-108.

[83] Rand TA, Petersen S, Du F, Wang X: Argonaute2 cleaves the anti-guide strand of siRNA during RISC activation. *Cell* 2005 123:621-9.

[84] Cifuentes D, Xue H, Taylor DW, Patnode H, Mishima Y, Cheloufi S, Ma E, Mane S, Hannon GJ, Lawson ND, Wolfe SA, Giraldez AJ: A novel miRNA processing pathway independent of Dicer requires Argonaute2 catalytic activity. *Science* 2010 328:1694-8.

[85] Johnston M, Geoffroy MC, Sobala A, Hay R, Hutvagner G: HSP90 protein stabilizes unloaded argonaute complexes and microscopic P-bodies in human cells. *Mol. Biol. Cell* 2010 21:1462-9.

[86] Qi HH, Ongusaha PP, Myllyharju J, Cheng D, Pakkanen O, Shi Y, Lee SW, Peng J: Prolyl 4-hydroxylation regulates Argonaute 2 stability. *Nature* 2008 455:421-4.

[87] Rybak A, Fuchs H, Hadian K, Smirnova L, Wulczyn EA, Michel G, Nitsch R, Krappmann D, Wulczyn FG: The let-7 target gene mouse lin-41 is a stem cell specific E3 ubiquitin ligase for the miRNA pathway protein Ago2. *Nat. Cell Biol.* 2009 11:1411-20.

[88] Zeng Y, Sankala H, Zhang X, Graves PR: Phosphorylation of Argonaute 2 at serine-387 facilitates its localization to processing bodies. *Biochem. J.* 2008 413:429-36.

[89] Eulalio A, Behm-Ansmant I, Schweizer D, Izaurralde E: P-body formation is a consequence, not the cause, of RNA-mediated gene silencing. *Mol. Cell Biol.* 2007 27:3970-81.

[90] Parker R, Sheth U: P bodies and the control of mRNA translation and degradation. *Mol. Cell* 2007 25:635-46.

[91] Nathans R, Chu CY, Serquina AK, Lu CC, Cao H, Rana TM: Cellular microRNA and P bodies modulate host-HIV-1 interactions. *Mol. Cell* 2009 34:696-709.

[92] Grishok A, Pasquinelli AE, Conte D, Li N, Parrish S, Ha I, Baillie DL, Fire A, Ruvkun G, Mello CC: Genes and mechanisms related to RNA interference regulate expression of the small temporal RNAs that control C. elegans developmental timing. *Cell* 2001 106:23-34.

[93] Hutvagner G, McLachlan J, Pasquinelli AE, Balint E, Tuschl T, Zamore PD: A cellular function for the RNA-interference enzyme Dicer in the maturation of the let-7 small temporal RNA. *Science* 2001 293:834-8.

[94] Ma E, MacRae IJ, Kirsch JF, Doudna JA: Autoinhibition of human dicer by its internal helicase domain. *J. Mol. Biol.* 2008 380:237-43.

[95] Forman JJ, Legesse-Miller A, Coller HA: A search for conserved sequences in coding regions reveals that the let-7 microRNA targets Dicer within its coding sequence. *Proc. Natl. Acad. Sci. USA* 2008 105:14879-84.

[96] 96. Mathonnet G, Fabian MR, Svitkin YV, Parsyan A, Huck L, Murata T, Biffo S, Merrick WC, Darzynkiewicz E, Pillai RS, Filipowicz W, Duchaine TF, Sonenberg N: MicroRNA inhibition of translation initiation in vitro by targeting the cap-binding complex eIF4F. *Science* 2007 317:1764-7.

[97] Chendrimada TP, Finn KJ, Ji X, Baillat D, Gregory RI, Liebhaber SA, Pasquinelli AE, Shiekhattar R: MicroRNA silencing through RISC recruitment of eIF6. *Nature* 2007 447:823-8.

[98] Behm-Ansmant I, Rehwinkel J, Doerks T, Stark A, Bork P, Izaurralde E: mRNA degradation by miRNAs and GW182 requires both CCR4:NOT deadenylase and DCP1:DCP2 decapping complexes. *Genes Dev.* 2006 20:1885-98.

[99] Vasudevan S, Steitz JA: AU-rich-element-mediated upregulation of translation by FXR1 and Argonaute 2. *Cell* 2007 128:1105-18.

[100] Vasudevan S, Tong Y, Steitz JA: Switching from repression to activation: microRNAs can up-regulate translation. *Science* 2007 318:1931-4.

[101] van Rooij E, Sutherland LB, Qi X, Richardson JA, Hill J, Olson EN: Control of stress-dependent cardiac growth and gene expression by a microRNA. *Science* 2007 316:575-9.

[102] Gatfield D, Le Martelot G, Vejnar CE, Gerlach D, Schaad O, Fleury-Olela F, Ruskeepaa AL, Oresic M, Esau CC, Zdobnov EM, Schibler U: Integration of microRNA miR-122 in hepatic circadian gene expression. *Genes Dev.* 2009 23:1313-26.

[103] Buck AH, Perot J, Chisholm MA, Kumar DS, Tuddenham L, Cognat V, Marcinowski L, Dolken L, Pfeffer S: Post-transcriptional regulation of miR-27 in murine cytomegalovirus infection. *RNA* 16:307-15.

[104] Pedersen IM, Cheng G, Wieland S, Volinia S, Croce CM, Chisari FV, David M: Interferon modulation of cellular microRNAs as an antiviral mechanism. *Nature* 2007 449:919-22.

[105] Kedde M, Strasser MJ, Boldajipour B, Oude Vrielink JA, Slanchev K, le Sage C, Nagel R, Voorhoeve PM, van Duijse J, Orom UA, Lund AH, Perrakis A, Raz E, Agami R: RNA-binding protein Dnd1 inhibits microRNA access to target mRNA. *Cell* 2007 131:1273-86.

In: MicroRNAs in Solid Cancer
Editor: Ondrej Slaby

ISBN: 978-61324-514-9
©2012 Nova Science Publishers, Inc.

*Chapter II*

# MicroRNAs and Genetic Polymorphisms in Cancer

### *Ondrej Slaby*
Masaryk Memorial Cancer Institute, Brno, Czech Republic
Central European Institute of Technology, Masaryk University, Brno, Czech Republic

## Abstract

Single nucleotide polymorphisms (SNPs) may occur at the level of miRNA biogenesis pathway genes, pri-miRNA, pre-miRNA or the mature miRNA sequence. Such SNPs may be functional in the biogenesis and action of the mature miRNA. SNPs located to predicted miRNA target sites within 3' UTR of mRNAs have the potential to affect the efficiency of miRNA binding on its target site, create or destroy binding sites. Resulting gene deregulation can involve changes in phenotype and be eventually critical not only for the susceptibility and the onset of cancer, but also for its prognosis and therapy response prediction.

## 2.1. Introduction

From the mechanistic point of view, miRNAs represent ideal candidates for cancer predisposition loci because small variation in quantity may have an effect on thousands of target mRNAs and result in diverse functional consequences [1]. The initial demonstration that miRNA-related SNPs can affect phenotype was elegantly depicted by Abelson and co-workers who found that a mutation in the miR-189 binding site of SLITRK1 was associated with Tourette's syndrome [2]. The first evidence that point mutations in miRNA genes can have a functional effect and confer cancer susceptibility comes from a pioneering study of Carlo Croce's group in which a germline mutation in pri-mir-16-1 resulted in low levels of miR-16-1 expression and was found in familial chronic lymphocytic leukemia [3]. Since then, several studies have used systematic sequencing or *in silico* approaches to identify SNPs in miRNA-related genes, catalogues of which have been created and made public [4-6]. Taken together these facts provide sufficient theoretical basis for follow-up case-control studies to determine the association between these genetic markers and cancer risk. This chapter provides brief outlook on functional effects of miRNA-related SNPs, and to our knowledge, complete summary of case-control studies performed in the field of solid cancer and miRNA-associated SNPs.

## 2.2. Classification of miRNA-Related SNPs

SNPs have been widely implicated in cancer development [7,8]. However, polymorphisms in the miRNA regulatory pathway are a novel class of functional polymorphisms present in the human genome. In principal, SNPs in miRNA genes are thought to affect function in one of three ways: first, through the transcription of the primary transcript (pri-miRNA SNPs and SNPs in miRNA biogenesis genes); second, through pri-miRNA and pre-miRNA processing (pri-, pre-miRNA SNPs and SNPs in miRNA biogenesis genes); and third, through effects on miRNA-mRNA interactions (SNPs in mature miRNA sequences and miRNA binding sites) [9,10].

### SNPs in miRNA Processing Machinery

MiRNA genes are first transcribed by RNA polymerase II/III into primary miRNAs (pri-miRNAs) with several hundred nucleotides. Processing of pri-miRNA by the nuclear RNase Drosha within the microprocessor complex also including DGCR8/Pasha produces the 70- to 100-nt pre-miRNAs. The pre-miRNAs are then exported into the cytoplasm by the Exportin-5 (XPO5)/Ran-GTP complex [11]. The pre-miRNA is further cleaved in the cytoplasm by an RNase III endonuclease, Dicer, to release two complementary short RNA molecules. The Argonaute proteins (Ago1-4) form complex together with GEMIN3 and GEMIN4 and selectively binds to the guide strand and facilitates the formation of a miRNA-RNA-induced silencing complex (miRISC) [11]. Upon miRNA binding, the miRISC complex is activated, and by a mechanism that is still unclear, locates its binding site in the 3' UTR of the target mRNA and contributes to regulation of the gene expression.

Polymorphisms that affect expression of miRNA biogenesis proteins may affect miRNA-mediated regulation within the cell. SNPs in core components of the silencing machinery might affect the overall efficacy of silencing. Mutations that drastically perturb RNA silencing will obviously be rare, according to their predictable highly deleterious consequences. Nevertheless, SNPs with subtle effects on gene function might occur. Because distinct targets might be more or less sensitive to variations in miRNA concentration or silencing efficiency, such SNPs might affect some pathways more than others. Thus, SNPs affecting the silencing machinery may contribute to the genetic variation observed for specific phenotypes [9]. Recently a few reports focused on the SNPs in silencing machinery and their association with cancer. Some of these SNPs in these genes, including GEMIN4, GEMIN3, XPO5, AGO1, AGO2, TRBP, and RAN had a role in cancer risk [12,13].

The first study to evaluate significance of SNPs in miRNA processing pathway genes in cancer predisposition realized Yang and co-workers in 2008 [12]. In this case-control study, they tested the hypothesis that common sequence variants in genes of miRNA and of the miRNA biogenesis pathway affect bladder cancer susceptibility. To better understand this effect, they genotyped 41 SNPs from 24 miRNA genes in a study conducted in 746 Caucasian patients with bladder cancer and 746 matched controls. The homozygous variant genotype of a non-synonymous SNP in the GEMIN3 gene (rs197414) was associated with significantly increased bladder cancer risk (2.40 odds ratio (OR); 95% confidential interval (CI) 1.04-5.56).

## SNPs in Pri-, Pre-, Mat-miRNAs

In general, sequence variations in miRNA genes, including pri-miRNAs, pre-miRNAs and mature miRNAs, could potentially influence the processing and/or target selection of miRNAs. As a consequence, SNPs present in pri-, pre- and mature-miRNA can potentially result in aberrant expression of hundreds of genes and pathways, broadly affecting miRNA function [14]. There are three options how to interfere with miRNA function on the basis of SNPs in miRNA sequences: 1) mutations in the pri- or pre-miRNA might affect their stability or processing efficiency; 2) mutations acting in *cis* or *trans* on the pri-miRNA promoter might influence its transcription rate; 3) sequence of the mat-miRNA might be altered, thereby stabilizing or destabilizing its interaction with mRNA targets; SNPs in mat-miRNA sequences can be further subclassified in following two categories: (i) SNPs within miRNA 5'-seed region, from positions 2-7, which is responsible for the target recognition specificity; (ii) SNPs within miRNA 3'-mismatch tolerant region, which is able to tolerate mismatches to a certain extent.

In the study focusing occurrence of SNPs within pre-miRNAs sequences, Saunders and co-workers identified 65 SNPs in 474 pre-miRNAs using publicly available SNP database (dbSNP).

Pre-miRNAs were found with the SNP density of 1.3 SNPs per kb. As the regions flanking miRNAs are most often intergenic regions, likely with weak or no functional constraint, these regions show a higher SNP density of 3 SNPs per kb. Consequently, a relatively low level of variation in functional regions of miRNAs was found [5]. Examples of the most frequently studied SNPs within miRNA sequences associated with solid cancer are summarized in Table 2.1.

## SNPs in miRNA Binding Sites

In contrast to the SNPs in pri-, pre-, and mat-miRNA, sequence variations within the 3' UTR of a target (coding) gene are more abundant in the human genome and have a more defined and limited range of effects. SNPs within miRNA target sites impact only its encoded target mRNA and its downstream effectors, hence, are more specific. A recent genome-wide association study (GWAS) suggests that a gene with more than two miRNA target sites will have increased expression variability as compared with a gene that is not regulated by a miRNA. The variability is further induced by SNPs in the miRNA target sites [30].

**Table 2.1. The most frequently studied SNPs within miRNA sequences associated with susceptibility and the onset of cancer**

| SNP Id | miRNA | Allele | Association with susceptibility of cancer |
|---|---|---|---|
| rs11614913 | miR-196-a2 | T/C | breast [15], lung [16], gastric [17], esophageal [18], head and neck [19] and liver cancer [20], glioma [21] |
| rs2910164 | miR-146a | G/C | breast [22], ovarian [22], esophageal [23], liver [24] and thyroideal cancer [25] |
| rs6505162 | miR-423 | A/C | breast [26], ovarian [26], bladder [17] and esophageal cancer [18] |
| rs7372209 | miR-26a-1 | C/T | bladder [17] and esophageal cancer [18] |
| rs895819 | miR-27a | A/G | breast [27] and gastric cancer [28] |
| rs2289030 | miR-492 | C/G | colorectal [29] and esophageal cancer [18] |

There are two possible mechanistic consequences of SNPs within miRNA binding region [10]: 1) SNPs might affect functional target sites, thereby destabilizing or stabilizing the interaction with the miRNA; 2) mutations might create illegitimate miRNA target sites (in the 3′ UTR or even in other segments of the transcript) that will be particularly relevant if occurring in anti-targets (see Figure 2.1).

Pioneering design in the field of miRNA associated SNPs indicated study of Landi and co-workers [31] who selected the 3' UTRs of 104 genes candidate for colorectal carcinoma (CRC) and identified putative miRNA-binding sites by specialized algorithms (PicTar, DianaMicroT, miRBase, miRanda, TargetScan). Fifty-seven SNPs were identified in miRNA-binding sites and evaluated for their ability to affect the binding of the miRNA with its target, by assessing the variation of Gibbs free energy between the two alleles of each SNP.

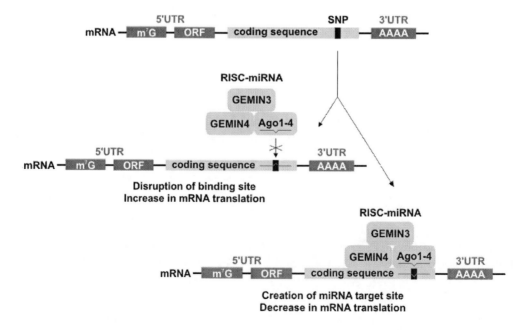

Figure 2.1. SNPs in miRNA binding sites.

Eight common SNPs were found that were further investigated in a case-control association study. The study was carried out on a series of 968 cases and 697 controls from Czech Republic, a population with the highest worldwide incidence of CRC. Statistically significant associations were found between risk of CRC and variant alleles of CD86 (OR 2.74; 95% CI, 1.24-6.04, for the variant homozygotes) and INSR genes (OR 1.94; 95% CI, 1.03-3.66, for the variant homozygotes). These observations are the first to report positive association between SNPs in miRNA-binding regions and cancer risk [31]. Several reports came after indicating SNPs in miRNA binding sites as a new risk factors of breast cancer (ITGB4 [32], ESR1 [33], SET8 [34] and BMPR1B [35]), colorectal (KRAS [36]) and lung cancer (KRAS [37]).

## Acknowledgment

This work was supported by grants NS 10361-3/2009, NR/9814-4/2008, NS 10352-3/2009, NT/11214-4/2010 of Czech Ministry of Health, Project No. MZ0MOU2005 of the Czech Ministry of Health and by the project "CEITEC – Central European Institute of Technology" (CZ.1.05/1.1.00/02.0068).

## References

[1] Xu W, Zhao W, Qi C, Qi X: MicroRNA Polymorphisms, MicroRNA Pharmacogenomics and Cancer Susceptibility. *Current Pharmacogenomics and Personalized Medicine* 2010 8:289-305.

[2] Abelson JF, Kwan KY, O'Roak BJ, Baek DY, Stillman AA, Morgan TM, Mathews CA, Pauls DL, Rasin MR, Gunel M, Davis NR, Ercan-Sencicek AG, Guez DH, Spertus JA, Leckman JF, Dure LS 4th, Kurlan R, Singer HS, Gilbert DL, Farhi A, Louvi A, Lifton RP, Sestan N, State MW: Sequence variants in SLITRK1 are associated with Tourette's syndrome. *Science* 2005 310:317-20.

[3] Sevignani C, Calin GA, Nnadi SC, Shimizu M, Davuluri RV, Hyslop T, Demant P, Croce CM, Siracusa LD: MicroRNA genes are frequently located near mouse cancer susceptibility loci. *Proc. Natl. Acad. Sci. USA* 2007 104:8017-22.

[4] Bao L, Zhou M, Wu L, Lu L, Goldowitz D, Williams RW, Cui Y: PolymiRTS Database: linking polymorphisms in microRNA target sites with complex traits. *Nucleic Acids Res* 2007 35:D51-4.

[5] Saunders MA, Liang H, Li WH: Human polymorphism at microRNAs and microRNA target sites. *Proc. Natl. Acad. Sci. USA* 2007 104:3300-5.

[6] Glinsky GV: An SNP-guided microRNA map of fifteen common human disorders identifies a consensus disease phenocode aiming at principal components of the nuclear import pathway. *Cell Cycle* 2008 7:2570-83.

[7] McLeod HL, Yu J: Cancer pharmacogenomics: SNPs, chips, and the individual patient. *Cancer Invest* 2003 21:630-40.

[8] Erichsen HC, Chanock SJ: SNPs in cancer research and treatment. *Br. J. Cancer* 2004 90:747-51.

[9]  Ryan BM, Robles AI, Harris CC: Genetic variation in microRNA networks: the implications for cancer research. *Nat. Rev. Cancer* 10:389-402.
[10] Mishra PJ, Bertino JR: MicroRNA polymorphisms: the future of pharmacogenomics, molecular epidemiology and individualized medicine. *Pharmacogenomics* 2009 10:399-416.
[11] Bartel DP: MicroRNAs: genomics, biogenesis, mechanism, and function. *Cell* 2004 116:281-97.
[12] Yang H, Dinney CP, Ye Y, Zhu Y, Grossman HB, Wu X: Evaluation of genetic variants in microRNA-related genes and risk of bladder cancer. *Cancer Res.* 2008 68:2530-7.
[13] Horikawa Y, Wood CG, Yang H, Zhao H, Ye Y, Gu J, Lin J, Habuchi T, Wu X: Single nucleotide polymorphisms of microRNA machinery genes modify the risk of renal cell carcinoma. *Clin. Cancer Res.* 2008 14:7956-62.
[14] Georges M, Coppieters W, Charlier C: Polymorphic miRNA-mediated gene regulation: contribution to phenotypic variation and disease. *Curr. Opin. Genet. Dev.* 2007 17:166-76.
[15] Hu Z, Liang J, Wang Z, Tian T, Zhou X, Chen J, Miao R, Wang Y, Wang X, Shen H: Common genetic variants in pre-microRNAs were associated with increased risk of breast cancer in Chinese women. *Hum. Mutat.* 2009 30:79-84.
[16] Tian T, Shu Y, Chen J, Hu Z, Xu L, Jin G, Liang J, Liu P, Zhou X, Miao R, Ma H, Chen Y, Shen H: A functional genetic variant in microRNA-196a2 is associated with increased susceptibility of lung cancer in Chinese. *Cancer Epidemiol. Biomarkers Prev.* 2009 18:1183-7.
[17] Peng S, Kuang Z, Sheng C, Zhang Y, Xu H, Cheng Q: Association of microRNA-196a-2 gene polymorphism with gastric cancer risk in a Chinese population. *Dig. Dis. Sci.* 2010 55:2288-93.
[18] Ye Y, Wang KK, Gu J, Yang H, Lin J, Ajani JA, Wu X: Genetic variations in microRNA-related genes are novel susceptibility loci for esophageal cancer risk. *Cancer Prev. Res. (Phila Pa)* 2008 1:460-9.
[19] Christensen BC, Avissar-Whiting M, Ouellet LG, Butler RA, Nelson HH, McClean MD, Marsit CJ, Kelsey KT: Mature microRNA sequence polymorphism in MIR196A2 is associated with risk and prognosis of head and neck cancer. *Clin. Cancer Res.* 16:3713-20.
[20] Qi P, Dou TH, Geng L, Zhou FG, Gu X, Wang H, Gao CF: Association of a variant in MIR 196A2 with susceptibility to hepatocellular carcinoma in male Chinese patients with chronic hepatitis B virus infection. *Hum. Immunol.* 71:621-6.
[21] Dou T, Wu Q, Chen X, Ribas J, Ni X, Tang C, Huang F, Zhou L, Lu D: A polymorphism of microRNA196a genome region was associated with decreased risk of glioma in Chinese population. *J. Cancer Res. Clin. Oncol.* 2010 136:1853-9.
[22] Shen J, Ambrosone CB, DiCioccio RA, Odunsi K, Lele SB, Zhao H: A functional polymorphism in the miR-146a gene and age of familial breast/ovarian cancer diagnosis. *Carcinogenesis* 2008 29:1963-6.
[23] Guo H, Wang K, Xiong G, Hu H, Wang D, Xu X, Guan X, Yang K, Bai Y: A functional varient in microRNA-146a is associated with risk of esophageal squamous cell carcinoma in Chinese Han. *Fam. Cancer* 2010 9:599-603.

[24] Xu T, Zhu Y, Wei QK, Yuan Y, Zhou F, Ge YY, Yang JR, Su H, Zhuang SM: A functional polymorphism in the miR-146a gene is associated with the risk for hepatocellular carcinoma. *Carcinogenesis* 2008 29:2126-31.

[25] Jazdzewski K, Murray EL, Franssila K, Jarzab B, Schoenberg DR, de la Chapelle A: Common SNP in pre-miR-146a decreases mature miR expression and predisposes to papillary thyroid carcinoma. *Proc. Natl. Acad. Sci. USA* 2008 105:7269-74.

[26] Kontorovich T, Levy A, Korostishevsky M, Nir U, Friedman E: Single nucleotide polymorphisms in miRNA binding sites and miRNA genes as breast/ovarian cancer risk modifiers in Jewish high-risk women. *Int. J. Cancer* 2010 127:589-97.

[27] Yang R, Schlehe B, Hemminki K, Sutter C, Bugert P, Wappenschmidt B, Volkmann J, Varon R, Weber BH, Niederacher D, Arnold N, Meindl A, Bartram CR, Schmutzler RK, Burwinkel B: A genetic variant in the pre-miR-27a oncogene is associated with a reduced familial breast cancer risk. *Breast Cancer Res. Treat.* 2010 121:693-702.

[28] Sun Q, Gu H, Zeng Y, Xia Y, Wang Y, Jing Y, Yang L, Wang B: Hsa-mir-27a genetic variant contributes to gastric cancer susceptibility through affecting miR-27a and target gene expression. *Cancer Sci.* 2010 101:2241-7.

[29] Lee HC, Kim JG, Chae YS, Sohn SK, Kang BW, Moon JH, Jeon SW, Lee MH, Lim KH, Park JY, Choi GS, Jun SH: Prognostic impact of microRNA-related gene polymorphisms on survival of patients with colorectal cancer. *J. Cancer Res. Clin. Oncol.* 2010 136:1073-8.

[30] Liu J, Rivas FV, Wohlschlegel J, Yates JR, Parker R, Hannon GJ: A role for the P-body component GW182 in microRNA function. *Nat. Cell Biol.* 2006 7:1261-6.

[31] Landi D, Gemignani F, Naccarati A, Pardini B, Vodicka P, Vodickova L, Novotny J, Forsti A, Hemminki K, Canzian F, Landi S: Polymorphisms within micro-RNA-binding sites and risk of sporadic colorectal cancer. *Carcinogenesis* 2008 29:579-84.

[32] Brendle A, Lei H, Brandt A, Johansson R, Enquist K, Henriksson R, Hemminki K, Lenner P, Forsti A: Polymorphisms in predicted microRNA-binding sites in integrin genes and breast cancer: ITGB4 as prognostic marker. *Carcinogenesis* 2008 29:1394-9.

[33] Tchatchou S, Jung A, Hemminki K, Sutter C, Wappenschmidt B, Bugert P, Weber BH, Niederacher D, Arnold N, Varon-Mateeva R, Ditsch N, Meindl A, Schmutzler RK, Bartram CR, Burwinkel B: A variant affecting a putative miRNA target site in estrogen receptor (ESR) 1 is associated with breast cancer risk in premenopausal women. *Carcinogenesis* 2009 30:59-64.

[34] Song F, Zheng H, Liu B, Wei S, Dai H, Zhang L, Calin GA, Hao X, Wei Q, Zhang W, Chen K: An miR-502-binding site single-nucleotide polymorphism in the 3'-untranslated region of the SET8 gene is associated with early age of breast cancer onset. *Clin. Cancer Res.* 2009 15:6292-300.

[35] Saetrom P, Biesinger J, Li SM, Smith D, Thomas LF, Majzoub K, Rivas GE, Alluin J, Rossi JJ, Krontiris TG, Weitzel J, Daly MB, Benson AB, Kirkwood JM, O'Dwyer PJ, Sutphen R, Stewart JA, Johnson D, Larson GP: A risk variant in an miR-125b binding site in BMPR1B is associated with breast cancer pathogenesis. *Cancer Res.* 2009 69:7459-65.

[36] Zhang W, Winder T, Ning Y, Pohl A, Yang D, Kahn M, Lurje G, Labonte MJ, Wilson PM, Gordon MA, Hu-Lieskovan S, Mauro DJ, Langer C, Rowinsky EK, Lenz HJ: A let-7 microRNA-binding site polymorphism in 3'-untranslated region of KRAS gene

predicts response in wild-type KRAS patients with metastatic colorectal cancer treated with cetuximab monotherapy. *Ann. Oncol.* 2011 22:104-9.

[37] Chin LJ, Ratner E, Leng S, Zhai R, Nallur S, Babar I, Muller RU, Straka E, Su L, Burki EA, Crowell RE, Patel R, Kulkarni T, Homer R, Zelterman D, Kidd KK, Zhu Y, Christiani DC, Belinsky SA, Slack FJ, Weidhaas JB: A SNP in a let-7 microRNA complementary site in the KRAS 3' untranslated region increases non-small cell lung cancer risk. *Cancer Res.* 2008 68:8535-40.

In: MicroRNAs in Solid Cancer
Editor: Ondrej Slaby

ISBN: 978-61324-514-9
©2012 Nova Science Publishers, Inc.

*Chapter III*

# Methods for MicroRNAs Discovery and Detection

### *Ondrej Slaby and Jiri Sana*
Masaryk Memorial Cancer Institute, Brno, Czech Republic
Central European Institute of Technology, Masaryk University, Brno, Czech Republic

## Abstract

The identification of new microRNAs (miRNAs), which is the foundation of miRNA research, led to the development of increasingly sophisticated computational prediction approaches of miRNA genes (and their targets) and experimental techniques enabling accurate and precise miRNA quantification. However, significant progress in the miRNA field, mainly in translational cancer research, requires the development of new, more quantitative methods for the rapid, and high-troughput multiplexed detection of all miRNAs that are present in a particular cell or tissue sample. In this chapter, we present an overview of the current state of the art for miRNA discovery and detection techniques.

## 3.1. MiRNA Discovery and Target Identification

Molecular biological approaches to miRNAs discovery [1] are summarized and sorted in chronogical sequence, from classical forward genetics to next generation sequencing. The discovery that miRNAs are synthesized as hairpin-containing precursors and share many features has stimulated the development of several computational approaches for identifying new miRNA genes in various animal species [2]. Many of these approaches rely heavily on conservation of sequence within and between species, whereas others emphasize machine-learning methods to screen hairpin candidates for structural features shared with known miRNA precursors. The identification of animal miRNA targets is a particularly difficult problem because an exact match to the target sequence is not required. The most recently devised algorithms for miRNA and their targets discovery are discussed [2].

## 1) Molecular Biological Approaches

### Classical Forward Genetics

In forward genetic experiments mutant genes are isolated from an organism showing abnormal phenotypic characteristics. The first known miRNA, lin-4, was discovered in 1993 by Victor Ambros and his colleagues through the study of heterochronic gene lin-14 in worms by classic forward genetics. They discovered that lin-4 in *C. elegans* did not code for a protein but instead produced a pair of short RNA transcripts that each regulate the timing of larval development by translational repression of lin-14 which encodes for a nuclear protein [3]. In 2000, almost 7 years later, the second miRNA, let-7, was discovered, also using forward genetics in worms [4]. However, this method is also tedious, time-consuming and costly for miRNA discovery, primarily owing to the enormous effort required to identify each gene responsible for a particular phenotype [1,5].

### MiRNAs Cloning

Subsequently, a breakthrough in miRNA identification was made when directional cloning was used to construct a cDNA library for endogenous small RNAs [6]. Direct cloning and sequencing of short RNA molecules has enabled the identification of many miRNAs. Several research groups identified more than a hundred miRNAs by cDNA cloning and subsequent sequence analysis [6]. This approach has the advantage that it can be applied to any organism, even if little or no genomic information is available. In addition, miRNAs can be identified independently of their function, thus also allowing the identification of redundant miRNAs. By cDNA cloning, miRNAs have now been identified in diverse animals, plants and viruses [7-9]. Several different methods have been applied for miRNA cloning [9,10], but their basic principles and procedures are similar. First, small RNA molecules are isolated by denaturing polyacrylamide gel electrophoresis, the 3' and 5' ends of the small RNA molecules are ligated with adaptor sequences that contain restriction sites and PCR primers are then designed based on the adaptor sequences. Then, the PCR products obtained from RT-PCR amplification are transferred into the vectors for further cloning and sequencing analysis (see Figure 3.1). A limitation of this approach, however, is that miRNA expressed at a low level or only in a specific condition or specific cell types would be difficult to find [11].

### Next Generation Sequencing

With the advent of next generation sequencing (NGS, also called deep sequencing), new opportunities have arisen to identify and quantify miRNAs and elucidate their function [12]. The millions of short sequence reads generated by NGS, like the SOLiD (AppliedBiosystems) and Illumina Genome Analyzer, are particularly useful for small RNA transcription profiling. NGS provides miRNA expression profiling at an unprecedented sensitivity and resolution. Compared to available miRNA microarray platforms, the NGS systems are not limited by a predefined number of features, probe design, probe cross hybridization or array background issues. Moreover, the NGS systems directly count the number of transcripts found as a measure for expression abundance, have high multiplexing potential, are species independent, show high sensitivity towards low abundant transcripts and display excellent reproducibility [13,14].

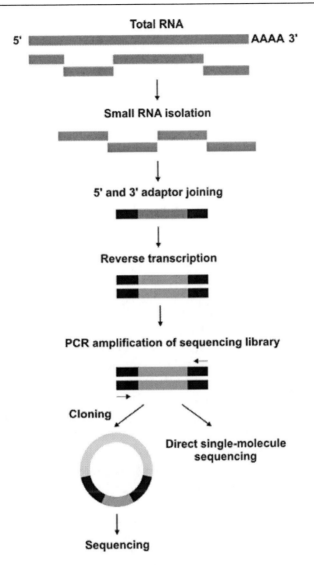

Figure 3.1. Overview of miRNA cloning.

In this overview, it is not aim to describe sophisticated NGS technogies in detail. Just for example, the Illumina/Solexa technology is the most successful and widely-adopted next-generation sequencing platform worldwide for miRNAs discovery. It supports massively parallel sequencing using a proprietary reversible terminator-based method that enables detection of single bases as they are incorporated into growing DNA strands. A fluorescently-labeled terminator is imaged as each dNTP is added and then cleaved to allow incorporation of the next base. The Illumina/Solexa utilizes a unique ''bridged'' amplification reaction that occurs on the surface of the flow cell. And then, genome analyzer is capable of generating 26-50 bases reads and producing at least 1 Gb of sequence per run in 2-3 days [15]. The Illumina/Solexa technology was recently used to sequence small RNA libraries from human embryonic stem cells before and after their differentiation into embryonic bodies [16]. The results generated more than six million short sequence reads from each library and identified 334 known and 104 novel miRNA genes in one of the most comprehensive miRNA profiling exercises to date [1,16]. The production of billions of NGS reads has also challenged the infrastructure of existing information technology systems in terms of data transfer, storage and quality control, computational analysis to align or assembly read data, and laboratory information management systems for sample tracking and process management.

## 2) Computational Approaches

### MiRNA Discovery Tools

Computational approaches have been developed to complement experimental methods in discovery of miRNA genes that express restrictively in specific environmental conditions or cell types using methods based on sequence conservation and/or structural similarity [17-19]. The most frequently used bioinformatic tools are listed in Table 3.1. Examples include: MiRscan using seven miRNA features with associated weights to build a computational tool which assigns scores to hairpin candidates and reaches 70% specificity at a sensitivity of 50% [20], miRank - novel ranking algorithm based on a random walk through a graph consisting of known miRNA examples and unknown candidate sequences [21]; miRseeker - the first attempt to identify conserved stem-loops due to selection, and not as an artefact of considering genomes that are not sufficiently distant [18]; miRnalyzer, in turn, implements all necessary methods for a comprehensive analysis of deep-sequencing experiments of small RNA molecules [22].

In practice, all these prediction methods require a sufficient number of characterized miRNAs as training samples and rely on genome annotation to reduce the number of predicted putative miRNAs. Although each of these methods has its own unique advantages, they have not been perfected yet. No consensus has been reached on the problem of verification. Each miRNA prediction program has sought to verify its computational conclusions by differently methods of experimental detection.

**Table 3.1. Computational resources for miRNA predictions**

| Algorithm | Web link | References |
|---|---|---|
| MiRscan | http://genes.mit.edu/mirscan/ | [20] |
| miRank | MiRank is programmed in MATLAB | [21] |
| MiRseeker | online not available | [18] |
| proMiR II | http://cbit.snu.ac.kr/~ProMiR2/ | [23] |
| mir-abela | http://www.mirz.unibas.ch/cgi/pred_miRNA_genes.cgi | [24] |
| triplet-SVM | http://bioinfo.au.tsinghua.edu.cn/mirnasvm/ | [21] |
| RNA micro | http://www.bioinf.uni-leipzig.de/*jana/software/index.html | [25] |
| BayesMiRNAFind | https://bioinfo.wistar.upenn.edu/miRNA/miRNA/login.php | [26] |
| One-ClassMirnaFind | http://wotan.wistar.upenn.edu/OneClassmiRNA/ | [27] |
| miPred | http://www.bioinf.seu.edu.cn/miRNA/ | [28] |
| findMiRNA | http://sundarlab.ucdavis.edu/mirna/ | [29] |

## MiRNA Target Identification

Sequencing data from several different species further led to the discovery of many miRNAs which in turn spurred the development of computational techniques to identify targets.

The mechanisms behind miRNA action have not been revealed completely which pose a challenge in identifying true targets. Some of the earliest data in flies showed regulatory motifs on the 3' UTRs of mRNAs that were complementary to the 5' end of miRNAs [18]. It soon became clear that a short region (6-8 nt) on the 5' end of the mature miRNA called the 'seed' was the primary participant in Watson-Crick base-pairing with the 3' UTR of mRNAs and contributed to efficient repression [30].

Considering the short length (6-8 nt) of a match, this is a source for many false-positive predictions. To counter this problem most programs employ a combination of two or more of three major criteria to identify miRNA targets: 1) seed-match between miRNA and target 3' UTR – while some programs require or prefer perfect seed-matches [31,32], others allow imperfect base-pairing [33,34], 2) free energy of binding between the miRNA and target site, and 3) cross-species conservation of miRNAs and/or target sites – all programs use *a priori* conservation information across two or more species based on the idea that evolutionary constraint could signify function. Available bioinformatic tools for miRNA targets prediction are summarized in Table 3.2, the most popular are characterized in detail below.

PicTar utilizes the sequence complementarity to target sites, emphasizing perfect base pairing in the seed region [31,35], while TargetScan, one of more established computational tools, accounts for both complementarity as well as evolutionary conservation to provide the relative likelihood that a given sequence is an miRNA target [32,36].

Another general framework for predicting miRNA targets involves energetic calculations. DIANA-microT, developed by Kiriakidou and co-workers, is an algorithm that identifies miRNA targets based on the binding energies between two imperfectly paired RNAs [34,37], and RNAHybrid predicts miRNA targets by finding the most energetically favorable hybridization sites of a small RNA in a larger RNA sequence [38,39]. The miRanda prediction algorithm includes contributions from the interaction binding energy, sequence complementarity between a set of mature miRNAs and a given mRNA, and also weights the conservation of the target site across various species [40,41]. In contrast to other energetic calculations, STarMIR models the secondary structure of mRNA to determine the likelihood of miRNA binding [42].

The past few years have seen incredible growth in the area of the computational prediction of miRNA targets.

However, continued progress remains to be achieved, as many of the aforementioned tools offer too many false-positive target sites. Furthermore, many of the approaches have been developed using experimentally validated miRNA:mRNA systems, therefore introducing bias against miRNAs with an unusual or uncommon sequence. Nonetheless, the continued evolution of miRNA target prediction methodologies will, along with emerging detection methods, play a key role in fully elucidating the mechanisms by which miRNAs regulate normal and potentiate abnormal organismal function, providing a link between diagnostic insight and potential therapeutic opportunities [43].

**Table 3.2. MiRNA target prediction tools**

| Algorithm | Web link | References |
|---|---|---|
| TargetScan | http://genes.mit.edu/targetscan | [30] |
| miRanda | http://www.microma.org | [40] |
| PicTar | http://pictar.bio.nyu.edu | [31] |
| RNAhybrid | http://bibiserv.techfak.uni-bielefeld.de/rnahybrid | [38] |
| Diana-microT | http://www.diana.pcbi.upenn.edu/cgi-bin/micro_t.cgi | [37] |
| MicroTar | http://tiger.dbs.nus.edu.sg/microtar/ | [44] |
| STarMIR | http://sfold.wadsworth.org/cgi-bin/starmir.pl | [42] |
| NBmiRTar | http://wotan.wistar.upenn.edu/NBmiRTar | [26] |

*Databases for miRNAs and Targets*

There is a variety of very useful databases that provide a significant amount of information on miRNA and Target predictions (Table 3.3). The most extensive database for both miRNA and target sequences is miRBase [45]. MiRBase contains miRNA mature sequences, hairpin sequences of precursors and associated annotation. Release 16.0 of the database contains 15172 entries representing hairpin precursor miRNAs, responsible for the production of 17341 mature miRNA products, in primates, rodents, birds, fish, worms, flies, plants and viruses. MiRBase also contains predicted miRNA target genes in miRBase Targets, and provides a gene naming and nomenclature function in the miRBase Registry. The miRNA target genes are predicted using the miRanda tool [34] and are not necessarily experimentally validated [2]. MiRecords depository offers miRNA targets divided according to their experimental validation status [46].

**Table 3.3. Web databases for miRNA and targets**

| Database | Web link |
|---|---|
| MiRBase | http://microrna.sanger.ac.uk/ |
| TarBase | http://diana.cslab.ece.ntua.gr/tarbase/ |
| miRWalk | http://www.ma.uni-heidelberg.de/apps/zmf/mirwalk/ |
| miRecords | http://mirecords.biolead.org/ |

# 3.2. MiRNA Detection

Experimental detection of miRNAs is technically challenging because of their small size, sequence similarity among various members, high-level dynamic range, and tissue-specific or developmental stage-specific expression. Standard methods widely used for miRNA detection include northern blotting, *in situ* hybridization, and the most precise and frequently used QRT-PCR based methods. Each technique has its advantages along with some limitations over its application at the moment. A suitable method should be chosen based on the requirements of the investigation and the experimental conditions in order to get accurate information on miRNA expression.

## Northern Blotting

The most standard method for the detection of miRNAs is northern blotting. Northern blotting offers a number of advantages for miRNA analysis, including a number of well-established protocols and amenability to equipment readily available in most molecular biology laboratories [47,48]. Additionally, since northern blotting involves a size-based separation step, it can be used to detect both mature and precursor forms of a miRNA, which is appealing for studies which focus on the mechanisms of miRNA processing [43]. Common protocols for northern blotting involve miRNA isolation, polyacrylamide gel electrophoresis, transfer of the separated sample to the blotting membrane, and visualization via hybridization with a radioactively labeled DNA strand complementary to the miRNA of interest. Despite its widespread use, traditional northern blotting is, in general, plagued by a lack of sensitivity (up to 20 μg of total RNA are required per blot) and a laborious and time-consuming protocol (often taking several days for complete analysis), which limits its utility in a clinical setting [49]. Furthermore, the technique often displays a limited dynamic range (2-3 orders of magnitude, depending on the visualization method), and its reliance on a radioactive tag (typically $^{32}$P) can be disadvantageous in some settings [43].

Locked nucleic acid (LNA)-modified oligonucleotide probes were used to enhance the efficiency of hybridization for solving the sensitivity problem of miRNA northern blotting technology [50,51]. The technique can be extremely beneficial when small amounts of samples are available, expression levels of target miRNAs are low, or subtle discrimination of related miRNAs (differing only by a few nucleotides) is necessary. LNA probes exhibit unprecedented thermal stability and show improved hybridization properties against complementary RNA targets [1].

## In Situ Hybridization

*In situ* hybridization (IHS) for miRNA detection has been developed recently [52]. The main advantage of ISH is that it may be used to locate the cellular and subcellular distribution and determine the spatio-temporal expression patterns of candidate miRNAs. However, the normal DNA or RNA probes may not work well in this method owing to their poor binding affinity to target miRNA. To increase the affinity, two approaches for detection of miRNAs by ISH have been developed recently. Kloosterman and co-workers [53] introduced LNA into the ISH probes and successfully observed the expression of 115 conserved vertebrate miRNAs in zebrafish embryos by ISH. By use of these probes were detected also conserved vertebrate miRNAs in zebrafish, mice, and frog embryos [54]. On the other hand, Deo and co-workers [55] have recently improved the specificity by using RNA oligonucleotide probes linked to a fluorescein hapten and highly specific washing conditions with tetra-methyl ammonium chloride (TMAC).

The method could directly detect mature miRNAs in tissue sections from developing mouse embryos, adult brain, and the eye. ISH can precisely locate a specific miRNA within tissue, but it is not suitable for high-throughput profiling [56].

## QRT-PCR

Similar to its use in conventional studies of gene expression, qRT-PCR can also be applied to the analysis of miRNAs. Reverse transcription (RT) is first utilized to convert the target RNA into its cDNA, which is then subsequently amplified and quantified via one of several conventional PCR methods. However, the simple translation of these methods to miRNAs is complicated by the short size of the target, as the length of the primers normally used in the PCR step are as long as mature miRNAs themselves. Shorter primers are typically not useful, as their low duplex melting temperature with the miRNA can introduce signal bias. To avoid these challenges, researchers have developed several of creative approaches based upon the enzymatic modification of conventional primers or altogether new primers for mature miRNAs. Currently, there are three methods for quantitative PCR of miRNAs. One of the advantages of three type of detection is that it can verify miRNAs that are expressed at low levels, but it is limited by high cost [43].

The first method is primer-extension (PE), qRT-PCR [57]. The miRNA template is converted to cDNA with a gene-specific primer (GSP) that includes a tail sequence. The resulting cDNA-GSP chimera is quantified by qRT-PCR. In the first cycle, the reverse primer (RP) containing LNA directs synthesis of the strand complementary to the cDNA. In subsequent cycles, the universal primer (UP) and LNA-R primer amplify a short sequence that can be monitored in real time by SYBR green fluorescence (see Figure 3.2). The assay has a high dynamic range and provides linear readout over differences in miRNA concentrations that span 6-7 orders of magnitude. It is capable of discriminating between related miRNA family members that differ by subtle sequence differences. The author used the method for quantitative analysis of six miRNAs across 12 tissue samples. The data confirm striking variation in the patterns of expression of these noncoding regulatory RNAs [57]. This approach was formerly used by Exiqon.

Life Technologies (Applied Biosystems) offers a commercial miRNA analysis method based upon stem-loop primer RT-PCR with TaqMan quantification. First, the stem-loop RT primer is hybridized to a miRNA molecule and then reverse transcribed with a multiscribe reverse transcriptase (Figure 3.3). Next, the RT products are quantified using conventional TaqMan PCR. The assays method was specific for mature miRNAs and discriminated among related miRNAs that differ by as little as one nucleotide. Furthermore, they are not affected by genomic DNA contamination. The assay is achieved routinely with as little as 25 pg of total RNA for precise quantification of most miRNAs [58].

The third and most frequently used method on the market is based on miRNA polyadenylation prior to RT reaction (Agilent, Invitrogen, Exiqon, Qiagen). Total RNA is polyadenylated by poly-(A)-polymerase and then cDNA synthesized by an RT primer and reverse transcriptase using the 3'-tailed total RNA as templates [59]. The cDNAs of miRNAs are quantified in qRT-PCR, with miRNA-specific forward primer and reverse primer complementary to 3' adaptor (see Figure 3.4). It was demonstrated that this method can readily discriminate the expression of miRNAs having as few as one nucleotide sequence difference using as little as 100 pg total RNA for miRNAs sequence [59]. However, the main advantage of poly-(A)-polymerase is that the enzyme shows no sequence preference in its activity, so it should be a useful tool for high-throughput miRNA analysis applications.

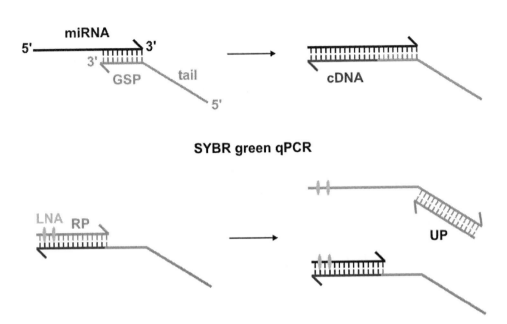

Figure 3.2. Schematic overview of primer-extension based qRT-PCR.

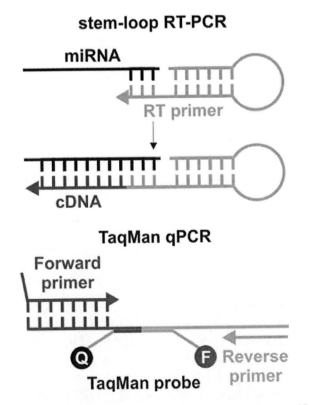

Figure 3.3. Schematic description of miRNA stem-loop RT-PCR with TaqMan quantification.

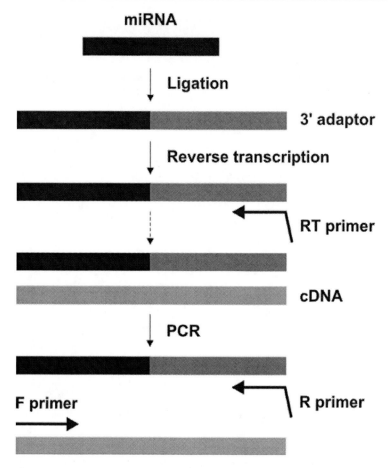

Figure 3.4. QRT-PCR of miRNAs with 3' adaptor.

## High-Troughput Analysis

Although qRT-PCR based methods for individual miRNA expression analysis reached high-level of accuracy and precision, significant progress in the miRNAs field, mainly in translational cancer research, required the development of new methods for the rapid, and high-troughput multiplexed detection of all miRNAs that are present in a particular cell or tissue sample. In general, all high-throughput methods can be separated into two categories – one that utilizes direct oligo hybridization without sample RNA amplification (miRNA microarrays) and the other requiring sample amplification (qPCR arrays) (see Figure 3.5).

## Challenges in miRNA Profiling

The challenges associated with detecting miRNAs by microarray technologies are associated with the inherent nature of miRNA sequences. It has been proven that the mature sequences are involved in hybridizing with the designed probes and not their hairpin precursors [60]. This means that probes designed to hybridize with the mature miRNAs are, in essence, reverse complementary to the candidate miRNAs. Since there is only one candidate sequence for a probe, there are at least three main challenges to overcome:

1. Cross-hybridization with closely-related sequences – many miRNAs constitute families based on the sequence homology. One of such family is the human let-7 group of miRNAs (see Figure 3.6). It is evident that these miRNAs share extensive similarity and are different only by one or two nucleotides.
2. Non-uniform melting temperatures – the base compositions of all mature sequences are fairly varied which results in a diverse range of melting temperatures. Finding a suitable experimental condition to assay for all miRNAs is therefore not a trivial task.
3. Probe secondary structure –probes may fold upon themselves to form secondary structures rendering them unable to bind to target sequences.

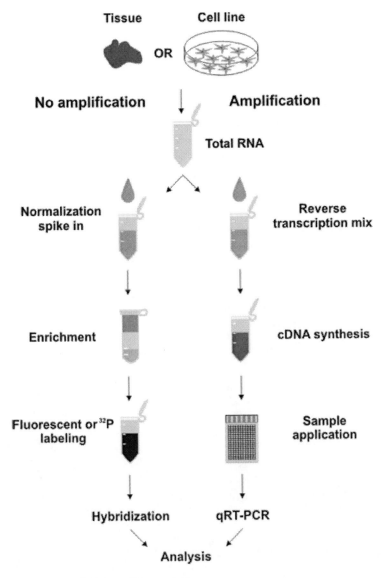

Figure 3.5. Classification of miRNA profiling methods.

| | |
|---|---|
| hsa-let-7a | ugagguaguagguuguauaguu |
| hsa-let-7b | ugagguaguagguugugugguu |
| hsa-let-7c | ugagguaguagguuguaugguu |
| hsa-let-7d | agagguaguagguugcauaguu |
| hsa-let-7e | ugagguaggagguuguauaguu |
| hsa-let-7f | ugagguaguagauuguauaguu |
| hsa-let-7g | ugagguaguaguuuguacaguu |
| hsa-let-7i | ugagguaguaguuugugcuguu |
| hsa-miR-98 | ugagguaguaaguuguauuguu |

Figure 3.6. Sequence homology of human let-7 family.

The approaches taken to increase specificity of hybridization or to balance melting temperatures of sequences either use modified nucleotides [61] or linker sequences [62].

## Microarrays

MiRNA microarray technology is actually based on nucleic acid hybridization (Watson-Crick base pairing nature of nucleic acids) between target molecules and their corresponding complementary probes [11,63]. A schematic flow chart of the miRNA profiling microarray is shown in Figure 3.7.

MiRNA oligonucleotide probes that usually have amine-modified 5' termini are immobilized onto glass slides through covalent crosslinking between the amino groups and the SAM (self-assembling monolayer), forming a ready-to-use miRNA microarray. The isolated miRNAs are labeled with fluorescent dye and then hybridized with the miRNA microarray, resulting in specific binding of the labeled miRNAs to the corresponding probes.

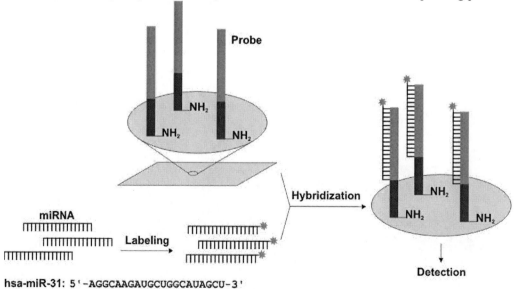

Figure 3.7. The principle of the miRNA profiling microarray.

The fluorescence emission from labeled miRNAs bound at different positions on the slides can be detected. Consequently, the kinds of miRNAs and their relative quantities in the studied sample can be evaluated by analyzing the fluorescence signal data [64,65]. The design of the miRNA probes, the preparation of miRNA samples, and the labeling of miRNAs are considered the most important procedures in the miRNA microarray platform. There is a plenty of miRNA microrray technological platforms available on the biotechnology market represented by Agilent, Exiqon, Affymetrix, Ambion and Invitrogen.

## QRT-PCR Arrays

Direct hybridization of miRNA samples onto a microarray may require a large amount of total RNA; and according to lower dynamic range and potential cross-reactivity caused by high-level sequence homology in miRNA families, need validation by independent method, mostly qRT-PCR.

Some research protocols might have access only to a small and limited amount of RNA, such as needle biopsies. A qRT-PCR based approach address this issue. In principal, there are two main technological approaches in the field of qRT-PCR arrays. The first is multiplexed qRT-PCR of miRNAs with 3' adaptor, LNA modified primers and SYBR green detection. A kit that applies this technology into a high-throughput format is now commercially available in the 384-well plate set-up (Exiqon).

The second approach is miRNA stem-loop RT-PCR with TaqMan quantification in pre-configured microfluidic card (TaqMan low density arrays – TLDA), minimizing the experimental variability and effort required to run 384 TaqMan miRNA assays in parallel (Applied Biosystems). The commercial products are composed of two 384-well plates or two TLDAs enabling together detection of expression levels of about 700 miRNAs with no need for further technical validation.

## Bead Based Arrays

Bead based profiling method involves both amplification and hybridization, and requires flow cytometry for analysis. Capture probes for a specific miRNA are synthesized and attached to a bead that is uniquely coded by a mixture of two fluorescent dyes for identification. Total RNA is enriched for short RNAs. Adapter oligos are then ligated to both the 3' and 5' ends of enriched RNAs. Primers with sequence specificity to adapters are used to create a library of cDNAs through reverse transcription. Finally, a PCR reaction using primers antisense to the adaptors is performed to amplify the population of cDNAs. An important feature of this step is the use of biotinylated PCR forward primers to tag each PCR duplex with a biotin molecule, which can enzymatically react with streptavidin–phycoerythrin to emit a colored reaction that can be registered by a flow cytometer. The resulting PCR product is hybridized to a mix of fluorescent beads that make up a miRNA library. This mixture is then run through a flow cytometer to analyze both fluorescent and streptavidin–phycoerythrin intensity. The fluorescent bead will indicate the specific miRNA probe, whereas the streptavidin–phycoerythrin intensity will indicate quantity of a specific miRNA [65,66].

## Cloning miRAGE

The methods described above can only profile known miRNAs. MiRAGE-miRNA serial analysis of gene expression uses an amplification based method not only profile but also potentially identify new miRNAs. The first half of this protocol resembles the bead based method in that linkers are ligated to both 5' and 3' ends of enriched small RNAs for reverse transcription. A PCR reaction is carried out on the resulting cDNA mix, also with the help of biotinylated primers. This method deviates from the bead based method here. The linkers which now contain biotins are cleaved from the PCR products. The mixture containing amplified small RNA sequence and biotinylated linkers are run through a column of streptavidin-coated beads for purification. Streptavidin acts as magnets to bind the biotin tagged linkers. The eluted product, at least in theory, is purified small RNAs. The small RNAs are concatenated, cloned, and sequenced for analysis [67]. However, this technique is extremely labor intensive, requires hundreds of μg of total RNA, and only provides information on the presence or absence of a particular miRNA from within a sample.

## Acknowledgment

This work was supported by grants NS 10361-3/2009, NR/9814-4/2008, NS 10352-3/2009, NT/11214-4/2010 of Czech Ministry of Health, Project No. MZ0MOU2005 of the Czech Ministry of Health and by the project "CEITEC – Central European Institute of Technology" (CZ.1.05/1.1.00/02.0068).

## References

[1] Huang Y, Zou Q, Wang SP, Tang SM, Zhang GZ, Shen XJ: The discovery approaches and detection methods of microRNAs. *Mol. Biol. Rep.* 2010 DOI:10.1007/s11033-010-0532-1.

[2] Yousef M, Showe L, Showe M: A study of microRNAs in silico and in vivo: bioinformatics approaches to microRNA discovery and target identification. *FEBS J.* 2009 276:2150-6.

[3] Lee RC, Feinbaum RL, Ambros V: The C. elegans heterochronic gene lin-4 encodes small RNAs with antisense complementarity to lin-14. *Cell* 1993 75:843-54.

[4] Reinhart BJ, Slack FJ, Basson M, Pasquinelli AE, Bettinger JC, Rougvie AE, Horvitz HR, Ruvkun G: The 21-nucleotide let-7 RNA regulates developmental timing in Caenorhabditis elegans. *Nature* 2000 403:901-6.

[5] Peters JL, Cnudde F, Gerats T: Forward genetics and map-based cloning approaches. *Trends Plant Sci.* 2003 8:484-91.

[6] Ambros V, Lee RC: Identification of microRNAs and other tiny noncoding RNAs by cDNA cloning. *Methods Mol. Biol.* 2004 265:131-58.

[7] Long JE, Chen HX: Identification and characteristics of cattle microRNAs by homology searching and small RNA cloning. *Biochem. Genet.* 2009 47:329-43.

[8] He X, Zhang Q, Liu Y, Pan X: Cloning and identification of novel microRNAs from rat hippocampus. *Acta Biochim Biophys Sin (Shanghai)* 2007 39:708-14.

[9] Pfeffer S, Lagos-Quintana M, Tuschl T: Cloning of small RNA molecules. *Curr. Protoc. Mol. Biol.* 2005 Chapter 26:Unit 26 24.

[10] Bentwich I, Avniel A, Karov Y, Aharonov R, Gilad S, Barad O, Barzilai A, Einat P, Einav U, Meiri E, Sharon E, Spector Y, Bentwich Z: Identification of hundreds of conserved and nonconserved human microRNAs. *Nat. Genet.* 2005 37:766-70.

[11] Li W, Ruan K: MicroRNA detection by microarray. *Anal. Bioanal. Chem.* 2009 394:1117-24.

[12] Lee LW, Zhang S, Etheridge A, Ma L, Martin D, Galas D, Wang K: Complexity of the microRNA repertoire revealed by next-generation sequencing. *RNA* 2010 16:2170-80.

[13] Buermans HP, Ariyurek Y, van Ommen G, den Dunnen JT, t Hoen PA: New methods for next generation sequencing based microRNA expression profiling. *BMC Genomics* 2010 11:716.

[14] Git A, Dvinge H, Salmon-Divon M, Osborne M, Kutter C, Hadfield J, Bertone P, Caldas C: Systematic comparison of microarray profiling, real-time PCR, and next-generation sequencing technologies for measuring differential microRNA expression. *RNA* 2010 16:991-1006.

[15] Metzker ML: Sequencing technologies - the next generation. *Nat. Rev. Genet.* 2010 11:31-46.

[16] Morin RD, O'Connor MD, Griffith M, Kuchenbauer F, Delaney A, Prabhu AL, Zhao Y, McDonald H, Zeng T, Hirst M, Eaves CJ, Marra MA: Application of massively parallel sequencing to microRNA profiling and discovery in human embryonic stem cells. *Genome Res.* 2008 18:610-21.

[17] Weber MJ: New human and mouse microRNA genes found by homology search. *FEBS J.* 2005 272:59-73.

[18] Lai EC, Tomancak P, Williams RW, Rubin GM: Computational identification of Drosophila microRNA genes. *Genome Biol.* 2003 4:R42.

[19] Grad Y, Aach J, Hayes GD, Reinhart BJ, Church GM, Ruvkun G, Kim J: Computational and experimental identification of C. elegans microRNAs. *Mol. Cell* 2003 11:1253-63.

[20] Lim LP, Lau NC, Weinstein EG, Abdelhakim A, Yekta S, Rhoades MW, Burge CB, Bartel DP: The microRNAs of Caenorhabditis elegans. *Genes Dev* 2003 17:991-1008.

[21] Xue C, Li F, He T, Liu GP, Li Y, Zhang X: Classification of real and pseudo microRNA precursors using local structure-sequence features and support vector machine. *BMC Bioinformatics* 2005 6:310.

[22] Hackenberg M, Sturm M, Langenberger D, Falcon-Perez JM, Aransay AM: miRanalyzer: a microRNA detection and analysis tool for next-generation sequencing experiments. *Nucleic. Acids Res.* 2009 37:W68-76.

[23] Nam JW, Shin KR, Han J, Lee Y, Kim VN, Zhang BT: Human microRNA prediction through a probabilistic co-learning model of sequence and structure. *Nucleic. Acids Res.* 2005 33:3570-81.

[24] Sewer A, Paul N, Landgraf P, Aravin A, Pfeffer S, Brownstein MJ, Tuschl T, van Nimwegen E, Zavolan M: Identification of clustered microRNAs using an ab initio prediction method. *BMC Bioinformatics* 2005 6:267.

[25] Hertel J, Stadler PF: Hairpins in a Haystack: recognizing microRNA precursors in comparative genomics data. *Bioinformatics* 2006 22:e197-202.
[26] Yousef M, Nebozhyn M, Shatkay H, Kanterakis S, Showe LC, Showe MK: Combining multi-species genomic data for microRNA identification using a Naive Bayes classifier. *Bioinformatics* 2006 22:1325-34.
[27] Yousef M, Jung S, Showe LC, Showe MK: Learning from positive examples when the negative class is undetermined--microRNA gene identification. *Algorithms Mol. Biol.* 2008 3:2.
[28] Jiang P, Wu H, Wang W, Ma W, Sun X, Lu Z: MiPred: classification of real and pseudo microRNA precursors using random forest prediction model with combined features. *Nucleic. Acids Res.* 2007 35:W339-44.
[29] Adai A, Johnson C, Mlotshwa S, Archer-Evans S, Manocha V, Vance V, Sundaresan V: Computational prediction of miRNAs in Arabidopsis thaliana. *Genome Res.* 2005 15:78-91.
[30] Lewis BP, Shih IH, Jones-Rhoades MW, Bartel DP, Burge CB: Prediction of mammalian microRNA targets. *Cell* 2003 115:787-98.
[31] Krek A, Grun D, Poy MN, Wolf R, Rosenberg L, Epstein EJ, MacMenamin P, da Piedade I, Gunsalus KC, Stoffel M, Rajewsky N: Combinatorial microRNA target predictions. *Nat. Genet.* 2005 37:495-500.
[32] Lewis BP, Burge CB, Bartel DP: Conserved seed pairing, often flanked by adenosines, indicates that thousands of human genes are microRNA targets. *Cell* 2005 120:15-20.
[33] Enright AJ, John B, Gaul U, Tuschl T, Sander C, Marks DS: MicroRNA targets in Drosophila. *Genome Biol.* 2003 5:R1.
[34] Kiriakidou M, Nelson PT, Kouranov A, Fitziev P, Bouyioukos C, Mourelatos Z, Hatzigeorgiou A: A combined computational-experimental approach predicts human microRNA targets. *Genes Dev.* 2004 18:1165-78.
[35] Grun D, Wang YL, Langenberger D, Gunsalus KC, Rajewsky N: microRNA target predictions across seven Drosophila species and comparison to mammalian targets. *PLoS Comput. Biol.* 2005 1:e13.
[36] Friedman RC, Farh KK, Burge CB, Bartel DP: Most mammalian mRNAs are conserved targets of microRNAs. *Genome Res.* 2009 19:92-105.
[37] Maragkakis M, Reczko M, Simossis VA, Alexiou P, Papadopoulos GL, Dalamagas T, Giannopoulos G, Goumas G, Koukis E, Kourtis K, Vergoulis T, Koziris N, Sellis T, Tsanakas P, Hatzigeorgiou AG: DIANA-microT web server: elucidating microRNA functions through target prediction. *Nucleic. Acids Res.* 2009 37:W273-6.
[38] Rehmsmeier M, Steffen P, Hochsmann M, Giegerich R: Fast and effective prediction of microRNA/target duplexes. *RNA* 2004 10:1507-17.
[39] Hammell M, Long D, Zhang L, Lee A, Carmack CS, Han M, Ding Y, Ambros V: mirWIP: microRNA target prediction based on microRNA-containing ribonucleoprotein-enriched transcripts. *Nat. Methods* 2008 5:813-9.
[40] John B, Sander C, Marks DS: Prediction of human microRNA targets. *Methods Mol. Biol.* 2006 342:101-13.
[41] Betel D, Wilson M, Gabow A, Marks DS, Sander C: The microRNA.org resource: targets and expression. *Nucleic. Acids Res.* 2008 36:D149-53.
[42] Long D, Lee R, Williams P, Chan CY, Ambros V, Ding Y: Potent effect of target structure on microRNA function. *Nat. Struct. Mol. Biol.* 2007 14:287-94.

[43] Qavi AJ, Kindt JT, Bailey RC: Sizing up the future of microRNA analysis. *Anal. Bioanal. Chem.* 2010 398:2535-49.

[44] hadani R, Tammi MT: MicroTar: predicting microRNA targets from RNA duplexes. *BMC Bioinformatics* 2006 7 Suppl 5:S20.

[45] Griffiths-Jones S: miRBase: microRNA sequences and annotation. *Curr Protoc Bioinformatics* 2010 Chapter 12:Unit 12 19 11-10.

[46] Xiao F, Zuo Z, Cai G, Kang S, Gao X, Li T: miRecords: an integrated resource for microRNA-target interactions. *Nucleic. Acids Res.* 2009 37:D105-110.

[47] Lagos-Quintana M, Rauhut R, Lendeckel W, Tuschl T: Identification of novel genes coding for small expressed RNAs. *Science* 2001 294:853-8.

[48] Sempere LF, Freemantle S, Pitha-Rowe I, Moss E, Dmitrovsky E, Ambros V: Expression profiling of mammalian microRNAs uncovers a subset of brain-expressed microRNAs with possible roles in murine and human neuronal differentiation. *Genome Biol.* 2004 5:R13.

[49] Streit S, Michalski CW, Erkan M, Kleeff J, Friess H: Northern blot analysis for detection and quantification of RNA in pancreatic cancer cells and tissues. *Nat. Protoc.* 2009 4:37-43.

[50] Varallyay E, Burgyan J, Havelda Z: MicroRNA detection by northern blotting using locked nucleic acid probes. *Nat. Protoc.* 2008 3:190-6.

[51] Valoczi A, Hornyik C, Varga N, Burgyan J, Kauppinen S, Havelda Z: Sensitive and specific detection of microRNAs by northern blot analysis using LNA-modified oligonucleotide probes. *Nucleic. Acids Res.* 2004 32:e175.

[52] Wienholds E, Kloosterman WP, Miska E, Alvarez-Saavedra E, Berezikov E, de Bruijn E, Horvitz HR, Kauppinen S, Plasterk RH: MicroRNA expression in zebrafish embryonic development. *Science* 2005 309:310-1.

[53] Kloosterman WP, Wienholds E, de Bruijn E, Kauppinen S, Plasterk RH: In situ detection of miRNAs in animal embryos using LNA-modified oligonucleotide probes. *Nat. Methods* 2006 3:27-9.

[54] Kloosterman WP, Steiner FA, Berezikov E, de Bruijn E, van de Belt J, Verheul M, Cuppen E, Plasterk RH: Cloning and expression of new microRNAs from zebrafish. *Nucleic. Acids Res.* 2006 34:2558-69.

[55] Deo M, Yu JY, Chung KH, Tippens M, Turner DL: Detection of mammalian microRNA expression by in situ hybridization with RNA oligonucleotides. *Dev. Dyn.* 2006 235:2538-48.

[56] Berezikov E, Cuppen E, Plasterk RH: Approaches to microRNA discovery. *Nat. Genet.* 2006 38 Suppl:S2-7.

[57] Raymond CK, Roberts BS, Garrett-Engele P, Lim LP, Johnson JM: Simple, quantitative primer-extension PCR assay for direct monitoring of microRNAs and short-interfering RNAs. *RNA* 2005 11:1737-44.

[58] Schmittgen TD, Lee EJ, Jiang J, Sarkar A, Yang L, Elton TS, Chen C: Real-time PCR quantification of precursor and mature microRNA. *Methods* 2008 44:31-8.

[59] Shi R, Chiang VL: Facile means for quantifying microRNA expression by real-time PCR. *Biotechniques* 2005 39:519-25.

[60] Barad O, Meiri E, Avniel A, Aharonov R, Barzilai A, Bentwich I, Einav U, Gilad S, Hurban P, Karov Y, Lobenhofer EK, Sharon E, Shiboleth YM, Shtutman M, Bentwich Z, Einat P: MicroRNA expression detected by oligonucleotide microarrays: system

establishment and expression profiling in human tissues. *Genome Res.* 2004 14:2486-94.
[61] Castoldi M, Schmidt S, Benes V, Noerholm M, Kulozik AE, Hentze MW, Muckenthaler MU: A sensitive array for microRNA expression profiling (miChip) based on locked nucleic acids (LNA). *RNA* 2006 12:913-20.
[62] Wang H, Ach RA, Curry B: Direct and sensitive miRNA profiling from low-input total RNA. *RNA* 2007 13:151-9.
[63] Andreasen D, Fog JU, Biggs W, Salomon J, Dahslveen IK, Baker A, Mouritzen P: Improved microRNA quantification in total RNA from clinical samples. *Methods* 2010 50:S6-9.
[64] Sarver AL: Toward understanding the informatics and statistical aspects of micro-RNA profiling. *J. Cardiovasc. Transl. Res.* 2010 3:204-11.
[65] Kong W, Zhao JJ, He L, Cheng JQ: Strategies for profiling microRNA expression. *J. Cell Physiol.* 2009 218:22-5.
[66] Lu J, Getz G, Miska EA, Alvarez-Saavedra E, Lamb J, Peck D, Sweet-Cordero A, Ebert BL, Mak RH, Ferrando AA, Downing JR, Horvitz HR, Golub TR: MicroRNA expression profiles classify human cancers. *Nature* 2005 435:834-8.
[67] Cummins JM, He Y, Leary RJ, Pagliarini R, Diaz LA, Jr., Sjoblom T, Barad O, Bentwich Z, Szafranska AE, Labourier E, Raymond CK, Roberts BS, Juhl H, Kinzler KW, Vogelstein B, Velculescu VE: The colorectal microRNAome. *Proc. Natl. Acad. Sci. USA* 2006 103:3687-92.

In: MicroRNAs in Solid Cancer
Editor: Ondrej Slaby

ISBN: 978-61324-514-9
©2012 Nova Science Publishers, Inc.

*Chapter IV*

# MicroRNAs and the Hallmarks of Cancer

*Ondrej Slaby*
Masaryk Memorial Cancer Institute, Brno, Czech Republic
Central European Institute of Technology, Masaryk University, Brno, Czech Republic

## Abstract

A growing amount of evidences proves that microRNAs (miRNAs) can work as oncogenes (activating the malignant potential) or tumor suppressor genes (blocking the malignant potential) and they can affect all of the six hallmarks of cancer defined by Hanahan and Weinberg (2000) as: self-sufficiency in growth signals, insensitivity to growth inhibitory signals, evasion of apoptosis, limitless replicative potential, sustained angiogenesis and tissue invasion and metastasis. In this chapter we focus on miRNAs significance in these various aspects of cancer biology.

## 4.1. Introduction

Cancer is a multistep process in which normal cells sustain genetic damage over a prolonged period of time, which along with inherited susceptibilities leads to the manifestation of the transformed phenotype. However, emergence of full malignant potential in the form of metastatic behaviour is more than just growth autonomy of the tumor cell. In fact, it involves the acquisition of a set of six characteristics, defined by Hanahan and Weinberg (2000) as: 1) self-sufficiency of tumor cells, 2) insensitivity to antigrowth signals, 3) abnormal apoptosis, 4) limitless replicative potential, 5) induction and sustained angiogenesis, and 6) invasion and metastasis [1]. Most, if not all, of these processes involve changes in the social organization of cells within tissues, whereby tumors recruit and suborn a variety of host stromal cells leading to optimal conditions for rapid growth and dissemination [2]. A growing amount of evidences proves that miRNAs play an important role in different types of cancers and in various aspects of cancer biology [3-5]. Expression of miRNAs and the role of miRNAs in cancer are tissue- and tumor-specific. Abnormal miRNA levels in tumors have important pathogenetic consequences: miRNAs may act as oncogenes or suppressor genes. MiRNAs overexpressed in tumors down-regulate tumor suppressor genes, whereas miRNAs lost by tumors participate in oncogene overexpression (see Figure 4.1). Recent evidence supports the ability of miRNAs to regulate several steps during neoplastic cell transformation and to affect all of the six hallmarks of cancer (summarized in Figure 4.2) [6].

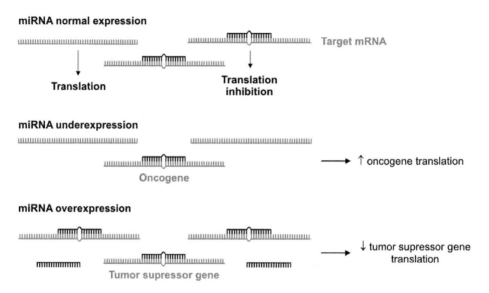

Figure 4.1. MiRNA function in normal cell (a), and in cancer cell as oncogene (b) and tumor suppressor (c).

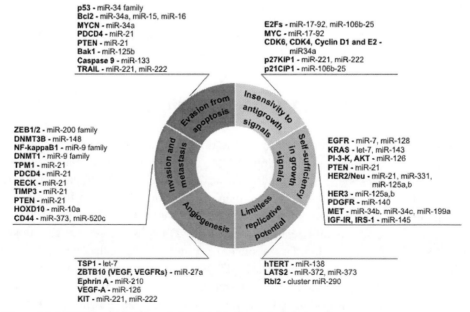

Figure 4.2. MiRNAs and their targets involved in the six hallmarks of cancer.

## 4.2. Self-Sufficiency in Growth Signals

Normal cells require mitogenic signals in order to leave the quiescent state and become actively proliferating cells. These signals are transmitted to the cells by transmembrane receptors that have tyrosine kinase (RTKs) activity. Growth signaling involves interaction of diffusible growth factors or cytokines with transmembrane receptors as well as regulation of growth by components of the surrounding environment, extracellular matrix (ECM), and cell-cell interaction. Many cancer cells can produce their own growth factors in order to succeed at this, a condition known as autocrine regulation. On the other hand, up-regulation of cell surface receptors results in hypersensitivity of cancer cells to low concentrations of growth factors that normally do not trigger proliferation. Overexpression or constitutive activation of RTKs, such as ErbB or epidermal growth factor (EGF) family consisting of EGFR/ErbB1/HER1, ErbB2/HER2Neu and ErbB3/HER3, vascular endothelial growth factor receptor (VEGFR), platelet derived growth factor receptor (PDGFR), and c-Met, is commonly observed in several solid cancers [7]. Deregulation of miRNAs expression in cancer can result in aberrant regulation of these cell surface receptors, and as a consequence induce the self-sufficiency in growth signaling leading to abnormal cell proliferation.

The EGFR pathway contributes to promotion and progression of broad spectrum of solid tumors and it is a promising target for anticancer therapy. Activation of the downstream small GTPase RAS is a common mean by which tumor cells escape growth factor dependency and become oncogene addicted. Two different studies indicated decreased levels of miR-7 and miR-128 that are able to directly down-regulate EGFR and its downstream pathways in breast, glioblastoma and lung cancer cell lines and in lung cancer patients [8,9].

RAS oncogene has been reported to be a direct target of the let-7 miRNA family [10]. When let-7 low-expressing DLD-1 colon cancer cells were transfected with let-7a-1 precursor, significant growth suppression with concurrent decrease of the KRAS protein levels was observed while the levels of both of their mRNAs remained almost unchanged [11]. KRAS expression *in vitro* was significantly abolished also by treatment with miR-143 precursor, whereas miR-143 inhibitor increased the KRAS protein level [12].

Central signaling pathway downstream from EGFR and important in cancer development is the phosphatidylinositol-3-kinase (PI-3-K) pathway. The p85β regulatory subunit involved in stabilizing and propagating the PI-3-K signal was mechanistically proven to be a direct target of miR-126. Furthermore, this p85β reduction mediated by miR-126 was accompanied by a substantial reduction in phosphorylated AKT levels in the cancer cells, suggesting an impairment in PI-3-K signaling [13]. Important regulatory component of the PI-3-K pathway, the tumor suppressor gene PTEN, is strongly repressed by miR-21, which was demonstrated on a hepatocellular carcinoma model [14]. It seems that suppression of PTEN controlled by miR-21 is associated with augmentation of PI-3-K signaling and progression of cancer.

Another recent study showed that the ErbB2 receptor (HER2Neu) regulates the expression of miR-21 via the mitogen-activated protein kinase (MAPK) and extracellular signal-regulated kinase 1/2 (ERK1/2) pathway in breast cancer cell lines, and that miR-21, in turn, was able to regulate the expression of programmed cell death-4 (PDCD4), a tumor suppressor gene that is a new negative regulator of intravasation, and thus revealing a new mechanism for HER2/neu-induced cancer cell proliferation and invasiveness via miRNA deregulation [15]. The ErbB2 RTK is also frequently over-expressed in prostate cancer, and it is associated with disease progression and poor survival. MiR-331 is decreased in prostate cancer, and it targets two specific sites within the 3' UTR of ErbB2 [16]. Reduced expression levels of miR-125a and miR-125b has been reported in breast, ovarian, and prostate cancers [17, 18]. MiR-125a and miR-125b have been proved to directly repress ErbB2/3 and to shut down the downstream phosphorylation of ERK1/2 and AKT; therefore, loss of miR-125a and 125b favors the constitutive activation of the ErbB pro-survival pathway [19].

Platelet-derived growth factor receptor (PDGFR) is known to be an important factor in pathogenesis ovarian cancer. A recent study on PDGFR signaling in organogenesis showed that its correct expression and function depend on miR-140-directed regulation [20], which is among the most significantly down-regulated miRNAs in ovarian cancer [6,18].

c-Met (MET) is a proto-oncogene that encodes a protein known as hepatocyte growth factor receptor (HGFR). Upon HGF stimulation, MET induces several biological responses that collectively give rise to a program known as invasive growth. Three miRNAs miR-34b, miR-34c, and miR-199a have been shown to regulate MET receptor expression. Inhibition of the endogenous miRNAs resulted in increased expression of MET proteins, whereas their exogenous expression in cancer cells blocked MET-induced signal transduction and impaired MET-mediated invasive growth [21].

Insulin receptor substrate-1 (IRS-1) plays an important role in cell growth and cell proliferation. IRS-1, especially when activated by the type 1 insulin-like growth factor receptor (IGF-IR), sends an unambiguous mitogenic, anti-apoptotic, and anti-differentiation signal. IRS-1 levels are often increased in cases of human cancer and are low or even absent in differentiating cells [22]. MiR-145 has been proposed as a tumor suppressor and it has been shown previously that miR-145 targets the 3' UTR of IRS-1 and dramatically inhibits the growth of colon cancer cells [23]. More recently, IGF-IR was proven to be another direct target of miR-145 [24].

The self-sufficiency of tumor cells is also due to their ability to grow in an anchorage-independent manner, and they do not undergo apoptosis following detachment from the basal membrane (a process also termed anoikis). This quality can be achieved by down-modulation of let-7 [25], among other mechanisms, which facilitates anchorage-independent growth. This effect has been linked to de-repression of the pleiotropic architectural transcription factor HMGA2, a major let-7 target [26], serving multiple differentiation programs [6].

## 4.3. Insensitivity to Antigrowth Signals

The tissue homeostasis relies on the appropriate cellular responses to antiproliferative signals, such as cell-cell or cell-ECM contacts and soluble ligands. Cells respond to these signals by entering into either quiescence or a differentiated postmitotic state, both conditions requiring an arrest of and withdrawal from the cell cycle. Becoming insensitive to growth inhibitory signals is common for tumor cells and mainly occurs by dampening the responses to external stimuli in the G1 phase of the cell cycle, during which the cell commits (or not) to duplication. Growth arrest is normally achieved by maintaining the retinoblastoma (Rb) protein and its subunits (Rb1/p105, p107, Rb/p130) in a dephosphorylated state. Hypophoshporylated Rb proteins sequester E2F transcription factors, repressing the expression of genes required for cell cycle progression [27]. Loss of the Rb constraint occurs in tumor cells by many various events (i.e. deletion, mutations, hyperphosphorylation) and enables E2F proteins to induce the transcription of proliferation promoting genes [4].

E2F transcription factor activities are also controlled at the post-transcriptional level by a series of miRNAs. These belong to two highly conserved miRNA families, which are grouped in distinct genomic clusters – the miR-17-92 cluster on chromosome 13q31.1 (miR-17-5p, miR-17-3p, miR-18a, miR-19a, miR-20a, miR-19b, and miR-92) and the miR-106b-25 cluster on chromosome 7q22.1 (miR-106b, miR-93, and miR-25). Specifically, miR-20a inhibits E2F2 and E2F3 [28], whereas miR-17-5p, miR-20a, miR-106b, and miR-92 inhibit E2F1 [29,30]. Unbound E2Fs increase miR-17-92 and miR-106b-25 expression, and in turn these keep in check E2F levels and participate in the delicate equilibrium between cell proliferation and apoptosis, which is affected by alteration of E2F levels. The miR-17-92 cluster is also essential for integrating signals during the G1 phase of the cell cycle and deciding whether a signal should be interpreted as proliferative or apoptotic [31]. In physiological conditions, the miR-17-92 cluster can limit MYC activation by dampening the E2F positive feedback loop. In tumors with MYC activation, miR-17-92 cluster protects cells from MYC induced apoptotic E2F responses, leading to uncontrolled cellular proliferation.

p53-activated G1 cell cycle arrest can also be bypassed through loss of miR-34a response by tumor cells. MiR-34a is transcriptionally induced by p53 and has been proven to directly target CDK6, CDK4, Cyclin D1 and E2, and MET [32,33]. Therefore, miR-34a deficiency increases CDK activity with sequential Rb hyper-phosphorylation in G1, G1-S transition, and initiation of DNA synthesis.

Another crucial cell cycle gatekeeper to which tumor cells can become insensitive is the cyclin-dependent kinase inhibitor (CKI) p27KIP1, the expression of which is frequently lost in cancers [34]. MiR-221 and miR-222, two miRNAs found to be up-regulated in many tumors such as papillary thyroid carcinomas (PTCs), hepatocellular carcinomas, and glioblastomas, directly target p27KIP1, providing cells an additional tool to avoid cell cycle arrest [35,36]. MiR-221 and miR-222 are also able to down-regulate the related CKI p57KIP2, preventing quiescence and favoring S-phase entry [36]. Similarly, the CKI p21CIP1, which is downstream of both TGFβ and the DNA damage induced growth arrest pathways, is repressed by miRNAs up-regulated in tumors from the miR-106b-25 cluster [5,6,37].

## 4.4. Evasion from Apoptosis

Apoptosis is a physiologic cellular self-destruction process, essential for a variety of biologic events (i.e. development, tissue homeostasis, and immune defense in multicellular animals) leading to removal of unwanted cells. Apoptotic stimuli can arise within the cell (e.g. oncogene activation, ROS, DNA damage) and activate the intrinsic apoptotic pathway (based on the Bcl-2 family of mitochondria permeability regulators) or arise from the cell external environment (e.g. death factors such as TNFα, tumor necrosis factor-related apoptosis inducing ligand (TRAIL), FAS ligand, or loss of cell survival signals, cell-cell, and cell-matrix interactions) and trigger the extrinsic apoptotic pathway through the activation of death receptors. In the end, both the intrinsic and extrinsic apoptotic routes converge on the caspase cascade, carries out the cell destruction program, with diffuse proteolysis, endonuclease nucleosomal fragmentation, and cell surface tagging for phagocytosis [38]. Evasion of apoptosis is a one of the six hallmarks of cancer, and plays a role in dictating the evolution of neoplastic cells [1]. The role of miRNAs in apoptotic signaling has yet to be fully determined; however, several studies have indicated a significant regulatory role in this process [4].

Mutations in p53 are found nearly in all types of cancers. Importantly, p53 regulates the expression of the miR-34 family of miRNAs, which consists of three members: miR-34a, which is generated from a transcriptional unit located on chromosome 1p36, and miR-34b and miR-34c, both of which are produced by processing of a bicistronic transcript from chromosome 11q23 [39]. The miR-34 family is down-regulated in cancer cells either due to p53 inactivation by mutations or epigenetically [40]. It is likely that miR-34 family members are necessary mediators of the p53 tumor suppressor activity, since the ectopic expression of miR-34a causes a cell-cycle arrest in G1 phase [32,39,41], as did miR-34b/c [32]. In addition, upon ectopic expression of miR-34a, human colon cancer cell lines showed signs of senescence [42]. Furthermore, direct binding of p53 to a promoter element on the miR-34a gene was demonstrated [41,43]. Inactivation of miR-34a compromises p53-dependent apoptosis, indicating that miR-34a is a proapoptotic transcriptional target of p53 [41]. Indeed, other groups have verified that expression of miR-34a can induce apoptosis [44,45]. In neuroblastoma, loss of miR-34a was observed, which is probably caused by a 1p36 deletion [45], and it synergizes with MYCN amplification. This is in line with the fact that miR-34a is a MYCN negative regulator [46]. Finally, miR-34a-deficient embryonic stem cells showed a slight decrease in spontaneous apoptosis after differentiation, while Bcl2 was identified as one of miR-34a targets [39]. Based on these observations, the miR-34 gene family was suggested as a new tumor suppressor miRNA family.

MiR-21 over-expression is another trait common to several malignancies [47-49]. MiR-21 acts predominantly as an anti-apoptotic protein by blocking the expression of critical apoptosis-related genes [50]. Among miR-21 apoptotic targets are the tumor suppressor PDCD4 in breast cancer cells [51], the tumor suppressor PTEN in hepatocellular cancer (HCC) cells [14] and tumor suppressor gene tropomyosin 1 (TPM1) [52]. MiR-21 favors the transmission of anti-apoptotic survival signals through the PI3K-Akt pathway and indirectly supports Bcl-2 anti-apoptotic activities [53]. Additionally, miR-21 is induced by AP-1 in response to RAS activation. Because PDCD4 is a negative regulator of AP-1, down-regulation of PDCD4 by miR-21 provides an autoregulatory loop that controls RAS-mediated AP-1 activity [54].

MiR-15 and miR-16 have been identified as regulators of the anti-apoptotic factor Bcl-2. Bcl-2 belongs to the Bcl-2 family of apoptotic proteins, which contains pro-apoptotic and anti-apoptotic members, all of which act as pivotal regulators of the intrinsic pathway of apoptosis [55,56]. Endogenous levels of miR-15 and miR-16 were shown to correlate inversely with Bcl-2 protein levels. Importantly, DNA fragmentation, immunoblotting and TUNEL analysis indicated that negative regulation of Bcl-2 by miR-15 and miR-16 resulted in activation of the intrinsic pathway of apoptosis [57]. Taken together these data strongly indicate miR-15 and miR-16 as regulators of Bcl-2, and would explain the mechanism of Bcl-2 over-expression seen in a number of human cancers.

MiR-125b suppresses the expression of the pro-apoptotic gene Bak1 and induces androgen-independent growth of prostate cancer cells [58]. Some cells display a TRAIL-resistant phenotype. Garofalo and co-workers identified miR-221 and miR-222 as regulators of TRAIL sensitivity in non-small cell lung cancer (NSCLC) [59]. TRAIL-resistant (CALU-1) and TRAIL-sensitive (H460) cell lines were identified; differences in sensitivity to TRAIL were not related to differences in endogenous receptor levels, as receptor levels were demonstrated to be comparable in both cell lines. MiRNA expression profiling analysis indicated differential expression of seven miRNAs in TRAIL-resistant cells compared to TRAIL-sensitive H460 cells [59]. Over-expression of two of these miRNAs, miR-221 and miR-222 in TRAIL-sensitive cells increased resistance to TRAIL-induced cell death and reduced activation of caspase-3 and caspase-8. By contrast, inhibition of these miRNAs in TRAIL-resistant cells resulted in a TRAIL-sensitive phenotype, indicating a role in determining cell sensitivity to TRAIL [59]. MiR-133 is the only miRNA that was shown to down-regulate the levels of caspase-9 by direct interaction [60,61].

## 4.5. Limitless Replicative Potential

Cellular senescence is the physiologic withdrawal from the cell cycle in response to a multitude of different stress stimuli. In normal cells, the most important players of the senescent program are p53, p16INK4a, and RB [62]. Intrinsically cells reach senescence when they extinguish the allowed number of doublings, entering a state of permanent proliferative arrest [63]. This is known as replicative senescence, and it is mainly a consequence of telomere attrition. Telomere sequences are located at the end of chromosomes containing the motif (TTAGGG), and in every cell division, telomeres lose 50-150 bp to a certain threshold, at which an irreversible growth arrest called senescence is triggered. Tumor cells may evade replicative senescence and acquire a limitless replicative potential either by abnormal activation of telomerase, which is human telomere reverse transcriptase (hTERT), a reverse transcriptase that synthesizes the telomeres at the ends of the chromosomes or by homologous recombination events at telomeres [64]. Replicative senescence can be accelerated by DNA-damaging agents, ROS, and uncontrolled oncogene activation.

Many miRNAs were predicted to target the mRNA that encodes for hTERT. However, only miR-138 was functionally related to the regulation of hTERT [65]. MiR-138 expression was found to be down-regulated in anaplastic thyroid carcinoma cell lines, leading to over-expression of hTERT. Interestingly, miRNAs may regulate hTERT expression in a subset of osteosarcomas, since in some osteosarcoma cell lines expression of the hTERT mRNA did not correlate with protein levels [66]. MiRNA relevance to oncogene induced premature senescence has been addressed with a genetic miRNA-screening library: miR-373 and miR-372 were identified as capable of allowing transformation of primary cells harboring oncogenic RAS and wild-type p53, by neutralizing p53 mediated CDK inhibition through suppression of LATS2 (Large tumor suppressor homolog 2) [67]. Epigenetic mechanisms are also involved in telomere homeostasis, and recently, they have been shown to be controlled by miR-290 cluster. The miR-290 family is able to target the RbL2 (Retinoblastoma-like protein 2) transcription factor, which in turn controls expression of DNMT3A and DNMT3B methylating enzymes that maintain telomere length [68]. To date, the relevance of this mechanism has not been directly assessed in cancer models. When cells undergo senescence, p53 activated miRNAs are also important: it has been proven that the miR-34 family participates to the senescence program [69] through modulation, at least for miR-34a, of the

E2F signaling pathway [42]. Furthermore, 15 miRNAs were found down-regulated in senescent cells and in breast cancers harboring wild-type p53 and proved that these miRNAs are repressed by p53 in an E2F1-mediated manner [3].

## 4.6. Angiogenesis

Angiogenesis, the growth of new blood vessels from pre-existing vessels, is a process sustained by vasculature endothelial cells under the strict control of pro-angiogenic and anti-angiogenic factors. This delicate balance is subverted by tumors in order to satisfy their growing demand for oxygen and metabolites. Tumor cells turn on the "angiogenic switch," [70] producing high amounts of pro-angiogenic factors and favoring neovascularization. The rapid expansion of tumor cells creates a hypoxic environment, leading to tumor necrosis and inducing cell adaptation responses, such as hypoxia-induced factor (HIF)-dependent survival pathways and angiogenesis. Quiescent endothelial cells are thus activated and recruited by angiogenic factors, and stimulated to proliferate and form new blood vessels. Tumors count on their angiogenic potential to outgrow locally and spread to distant sites, and increased angiogenesis has been correlated with a poor prognostic outcome for patients with many types of tumors [4,71].

The first evidence for the involvement of miRNAs in the regulation of angiogenesis came from Dicer knockout mice carrying a deletion by homologous recombination of the first two exons, which display angiogenic defects during embryogenesis [72]. Further studies based on genetic silencing of Drosha and Dicer1 in human endothelial cells confirmed the involvement of the miRNA processing pathway and consequently of active miRNAs in angiogenesis [73,74]. In particular, in these settings, lef-7f and mir-27b expression was strongly reduced, and the let-7 family was proven to negatively regulate the anti-angiogenic thrombospondin 1 (TSP1) [74].

In tumor progression, hypoxia has been found to contribute to the modulation of miRNA expression, partly by direct HIF-1 transcriptional activation of specific miRNAs (including miR-23, miR-24, miR-26, miR-27, miR-103, miR-107, miR-181, miR-210, and miR-213) [75]. These miRNAs have dual functions: on one hand, they aid the cell in engaging anti-apoptotic programs sustaining cell survival (e.g. miR-26, miR-107, and miR-210), and on the other hand, they participate in the angiogenic process. For example, miR-27a by restraining the zinc finger gene ZBTB10, induces specific protein-dependent transcription of both survival and angiogenic genes, such as survivin, VEGF, and VEGFRs [76]. Furthermore, miR-210, through direct modulation of the tyrosine kinase receptor ligand Ephrin A, represents a component of the circuitry controlling endothelial cell chemotaxis and tubuligenesis. [77]. Recently, it has been shown that VEGF is also restrained at the posttranscriptional level by miRNAs. On one hand, miR-126 was found to directly repress in *in vitro* and *in vivo* lung cancer cell models VEGF-A expression and to induce a G1 cell cycle arrest with an overall reduction of tumor volume [78]. On the other hand, miR-126 expression was found to be enriched in endothelial cells during angiogenesis and to repress negative regulators of the VEGF pathway [79]. Among the miRNAs highly expressed by endothelial cells, attention has been given to miR-221 and miR-222. In endothelial cells, these 2 miRNAs act as negative regulators of the receptor tyrosine kinase KIT, repressing proliferative and angiogenic properties of its ligand stem cell factor and impairing the ability of endothelial cells to form new capillaries [80]. MiR-296 can modulate the expression of VEGF receptor 2 and platelet-derived growth factor (PDGF) receptor β by directly targeting the hepatocyte growth factor-regulated tyrosine kinase substrate (HGS), which mediates degradation of the growth factor receptors [81].

## 4.7. Invasion and Metastasis

Metastasis results from a multi-step cascading process that includes: vascularization of the primary tumor, detachment and invasion of cancer cells, intravasation into lymphatic and blood vessels, survival and arrest in the circulation, extravasation into distant organs, and colonization and growth of metastatic tumors. MiRNAs play critical roles in this multi-step process, both promoting and suppressing metastasis. An increasing number of studies have revealed miRNA signatures of metastasis and have shown that the targets of most of these metastasis-associated miRNAs are proteins involved in the regulation of cell motility, cell-cell adhesion, and cell-matrix interactions [82,83].

Based on available data, there is a number of miRNAs strongly associated with cancer metastasis. In a prototypical mouse model of multistage tumorigenesis that involves the stepwise transformation of pancreatic β cells into pancreatic neuroendocrine carcinomas, down-regulation of the miR-200 family (miR-200a, miR-200b, miR-200c, miR-141, and miR-429) is found to be a metastasis-specific feature [84]. As described in a previous section, the miR-200 family negatively controls expression of ZEB1/2 and inhibits the epithelial-mesenchymal transition (EMT) [85,86], a developmental process through which cells lose their cell-cell and cell-matrix contacts and switch from a collective invasion pattern to a detached and disseminated cell migration phenotype. Recent observations demonstrated that not only miR-200 family regulates ZEB1/2 expression but also ZEB1 regulates miR-200 family transcription [87,88], thus establishing a complex regulatory loop that may ensure the tight control of the EMT process. As such, it makes sense that down-regulation of this family permits cancer cells to acquire aggressive EMT, invasion and metastasis. This finding is further supported by another report that illustrates a metastatic cancer miRNA signature in 43 metastatic lymph nodes of primary tumors (including colon, bladder, breast, and lung cancers) [89]. Down-regulation of miR-148a and miR-148b seems to be a common metastasis feature in HCC and pancreatic cancer [84,90]. This observation is supported by the fact that miR-148 is specifically hyper-methylated in metastatic cancers [91]. MiR-148 is known to target DNMT3B and TGFB-induced factor homeobox 2 (TGIFB, a transcriptional repressor) [91,92]. Down-regulation of the miR-9 family (including miR-9-1, miR-9-2, and miR-9-3) also seems to be a common metastasis feature in a number of solid tumors [89,90,93]. This observation is also supported by the report that the miR-9 family is specifically hyper-methylated in metastatic cancers [91], its down-regulation was shown to activate NF-kappaB1, recruit DNA methyltransferase 1 and increase in DNA methylation [94]. Lastly, expression of the pro-angiogenic miR-210, a hypoxia-induced miRNA [75], has been shown to increase metastatic capability in both breast and pancreatic cancers [84,95]. Taking together, three down-regulated and one up-regulated miRNAs have been confirmed to have a strong association with cancer metastasis (see Table 4.1) [83]. In addition, some miRNAs are reported to link to metastatic cancers at specific organs of origin.

**Table 4.1. MiRNA signature of cancer metastasis**

| miRNAs | Molecular regulation | Deregulation in cancer | Refs |
| --- | --- | --- | --- |
| miR-9 family | ↓NF-kappaB1 ↓DNA methylation | Down-regulated | [91, 94] |
| miR-148a, miR-148b | ↓DNMT3B, ↓TGIFB | Down-regulated | [91, 92] |
| miR-200 family | ↑E-cadherin, ↓EMT, ↓cancer cell migration/ invasion | Down-regulated | [85, 87] |
| miR-210 | hypoxia-induced, ↑angiogenesis | Up-regulated | [77, 95] |

DNMT3B DNA (cytosine-5-)-methyltransferase 3 beta; EMT epithelial-mesenchymal transition; TGIFB TGFB-induced factor homeobox 2.

MiR-21, besides controlling cell survival and proliferation, is also a master regulator of the metastatic process by directly modeling the cell cytoskeleton via tropomyosin 1 (TPM1) suppression [52], and by indirectly regulating the expression of the pro-metastatic uPAR (via maspin and PDCD4 direct suppression) [54] and of matrix metalloproteinases (via RECK, TIMP3 [96], and via PTEN [14] direct suppression).

It was revealed that up-regulation of miR-10b promotes invasion and metastasis. Twist, a metastasis-promoting transcription factor, could induce miR-10b expression, whereas HOXD10, a homeobox transcription factor that promotes or maintains a differentiated phenotype in epithelial cells, was shown to be a target of miR-10b and to be expressed at low level in metastatic tumors. Consequently, the levels of RhoC, a G-protein involved in metastasis that is repressed by HOXD10, increase significantly in response to miR-10b expression [97,98].

MiR-146a, whose expression is lost in metastatic prostate cancer, has been documented to directly inhibit the expression of the Rho target ROCK1 and to affect cell movements [99]. Similarly, down-modulation of the adhesion molecule CD44, induced by miR-373 and miR-520c in a breast cancer model, could explain their effect as metastasis-promoting miRNAs. In fact, CD44 is frequently up-regulated in a wide variety of malignancies [100,101], and CD44 modulates cell adhesiveness, motility, matrix degradation, proliferation, and survival - all traits that allow a tumor cells to progress through the metastatic cascade [102]. Another study reported that miR-122, a marker of hepatocyte differentiation, is specifically repressed in a subset of primary tumors characterized by poor prognosis, and that loss of miR-122 expression in tumor cells segregates with specific gene expression profiles linked to cancer progression and invasion.

Loss of miR-122 resulted in an increase in cell migration and invasion [103]. MiR-155 is another important factor contributing to TGF-induced epithelial cell plasticity and therefore to cell migration and invasiveness. It has been found to be a downstream effector of TGF and SMAD4 and to partially account for TGF-induced RhoA suppression and therefore responsible for the dissolution of cell tight junctions [104]. Consistently, miR-155 has been reported to be up-regulated in invasive breast cancer, supporting its involvement in breast cancer metastasis [17,47].

## Acknowledgment

This work was supported by grants NS 10361-3/2009, NR/9814-4/2008, NS 10352-3/2009, NT/11214-4/2010 of Czech Ministry of Health, Project No. MZ0MOU2005 of the Czech Ministry of Health and by the project "CEITEC – Central European Institute of Technology" (CZ.1.05/1.1.00/02.0068).

## References

[1] Hanahan D, Weinberg RA: The hallmarks of cancer. *Cell* 2000 100:57-70.
[2] Dalmay T, Edwards DR: MicroRNAs and the hallmarks of cancer. *Oncogene* 2006 25:6170-5.
[3] Negrini M, Nicoloso MS, Calin GA: MicroRNAs and cancer--new paradigms in molecular oncology. *Curr. Opin. Cell Biol.* 2009 21:470-9.
[4] Rehman SK, Baldassarre G, Calin GA, Nicoloso MS: MicroRNAs: The Jack of All Trades. *Clinical Leukemia* 2009 3:20-32.
[5] Sotiropoulou G, Pampalakis G, Lianidou E, Mourelatos Z: Emerging roles of microRNAs as molecular switches in the integrated circuit of the cancer cell. *RNA* 2009 15:1443-61.
[6] Santarpia L, Nicoloso M, Calin GA: MicroRNAs: a complex regulatory network drives the acquisition of malignant cell phenotype. *Endocr. Relat. Cancer* 17:F51-75.
[7] Perona R: Cell signalling: growth factors and tyrosine kinase receptors. *Clin. Transl. Oncol.* 2006 8:77-82.
[8] Webster RJ, Giles KM, Price KJ, Zhang PM, Mattick JS, Leedman PJ: Regulation of epidermal growth factor receptor signaling in human cancer cells by microRNA-7. *J. Biol. Chem.* 2009 284:5731-41.
[9] Weiss GJ, Bemis LT, Nakajima E, Sugita M, Birks DK, Robinson WA, Varella-Garcia M, Bunn PA, Jr., Haney J, Helfrich BA, Kato H, Hirsch FR, Franklin WA: EGFR regulation by microRNA in lung cancer: correlation with clinical response and survival to gefitinib and EGFR expression in cell lines. *Ann. Oncol.* 2008 19:1053-9.
[10] Johnson SM, Grosshans H, Shingara J, Byrom M, Jarvis R, Cheng A, Labourier E, Reinert KL, Brown D, Slack FJ: RAS is regulated by the let-7 microRNA family. *Cell* 2005 120:635-47.
[11] Akao Y, Nakagawa Y, Naoe T: let-7 microRNA functions as a potential growth suppressor in human colon cancer cells. *Biol. Pharm. Bull* 2006 29:903-6.
[12] Chen X, Guo X, Zhang H, Xiang Y, Chen J, Yin Y, Cai X, Wang K, Wang G, Ba Y, et al: Role of miR-143 targeting KRAS in colorectal tumorigenesis. *Oncogene* 2009 28:1385-92.
[13] Guo C, Sah JF, Beard L, Willson JK, Markowitz SD, Guda K: The noncoding RNA, miR-126, suppresses the growth of neoplastic cells by targeting phosphatidylinositol 3-kinase signaling and is frequently lost in colon cancers. *Genes Chromosomes Cancer* 2008 47:939-46.

[14] Meng F, Henson R, Wehbe-Janek H, Ghoshal K, Jacob ST, Patel T: MicroRNA-21 regulates expression of the PTEN tumor suppressor gene in human hepatocellular cancer. *Gastroenterology* 2007 133:647-58.

[15] Huang TH, Wu F, Loeb GB, Hsu R, Heidersbach A, Brincat A, Horiuchi D, Lebbink RJ, Mo YY, Goga A, McManus MT: Up-regulation of miR-21 by HER2/neu signaling promotes cell invasion. *J. Biol. Chem.* 2009 284:18515-24.

[16] Epis MR, Giles KM, Barker A, Kendrick TS, Leedman PJ: miR-331-3p regulates ERBB-2 expression and androgen receptor signaling in prostate cancer. *J. Biol. Chem.* 2009 284:24696-704.

[17] Iorio MV, Ferracin M, Liu CG, Veronese A, Spizzo R, Sabbioni S, Magri E, Pedriali M, Fabbri M, Campiglio M, Ménard S, Palazzo JP, Rosenberg A, Musiani P, Volinia S, Nenci I, Calin GA, Querzoli P, Negrini M, Croce CM: MicroRNA gene expression deregulation in human breast cancer. *Cancer Res.* 2005 65:7065-70.

[18] Iorio MV, Visone R, Di Leva G, Donati V, Petrocca F, Casalini P, Taccioli C, Volinia S, Liu CG, Alder H, Calin GA, Ménard S, Croce CM: MicroRNA signatures in human ovarian cancer. *Cancer Res.* 2007 67:8699-707.

[19] Scott GK, Goga A, Bhaumik D, Berger CE, Sullivan CS, Benz CC: Coordinate suppression of ERBB2 and ERBB3 by enforced expression of micro-RNA miR-125a or miR-125b. *J. Biol. Chem.* 2007 282:1479-86.

[20] Eberhart JK, He X, Swartz ME, Yan YL, Song H, Boling TC, Kunerth AK, Walker MB, Kimmel CB, Postlethwait JH: MicroRNA Mirn140 modulates Pdgf signaling during palatogenesis. *Nat Genet* 2008 40:290-8.

[21] Migliore C, Petrelli A, Ghiso E, Corso S, Capparuccia L, Eramo A, Comoglio PM, Giordano S: MicroRNAs impair MET-mediated invasive growth. *Cancer Res.* 2008 68:10128-36.

[22] Pechlivanis S, Pardini B, Bermejo JL, Wagner K, Naccarati A, Vodickova L, Novotny J, Hemminki K, Vodicka P, Forsti A: Insulin pathway related genes and risk of colorectal cancer: INSR promoter polymorphism shows a protective effect. *Endocr. Relat. Cancer* 2007 14:733-40.

[23] Shi B, Sepp-Lorenzino L, Prisco M, Linsley P, deAngelis T, Baserga R: Micro RNA 145 targets the insulin receptor substrate-1 and inhibits the growth of colon cancer cells. *J. Biol. Chem.* 2007 282:32582-90.

[24] La Rocca G, Shi B, Badin M, De Angelis T, Sepp-Lorenzino L, Baserga R: Growth inhibition by microRNAs that target the insulin receptor substrate-1. *Cell Cycle* 2009 8:2255-9.

[25] Mayr C, Hemann MT, Bartel DP: Disrupting the pairing between let-7 and Hmga2 enhances oncogenic transformation. *Science* 2007 315:1576-9.

[26] Lee YS, Dutta A: The tumor suppressor microRNA let-7 represses the HMGA2 oncogene. *Genes Dev.* 2007 21:1025-30.

[27] Iaquinta PJ, Lees JA: Life and death decisions by the E2F transcription factors. *Curr. Opin. Cell Biol.* 2007 19:649-57.

[28] Sylvestre Y, De Guire V, Querido E, Mukhopadhyay UK, Bourdeau V, Major F, Ferbeyre G, Chartrand P: An E2F/miR-20a autoregulatory feedback loop. *J. Biol. Chem.* 2007 282:2135-43.

[29] O'Donnell KA, Wentzel EA, Zeller KI, Dang CV, Mendell JT: c-Myc-regulated microRNAs modulate E2F1 expression. *Nature* 2005 435:839-43.

[30] Petrocca F, Vecchione A, Croce CM: Emerging role of miR-106b-25/miR-17-92 clusters in the control of transforming growth factor beta signaling. *Cancer Res.* 2008 68:8191-4.

[31] Coller HA, Forman JJ, Legesse-Miller A: "Myc'ed messages": myc induces transcription of E2F1 while inhibiting its translation via a microRNA polycistron. *PLoS Genet.* 2007 3:e146.

[32] He L, He X, Lim LP, de Stanchina E, Xuan Z, Liang Y, Xue W, Zender L, Magnus J, Ridzon D, Jackson AL, Linsley PS, Chen C, Lowe SW, Cleary MA, Hannon GJ: A microRNA component of the p53 tumour suppressor network. *Nature* 2007 447:1130-4.

[33] Sun F, Fu H, Liu Q, Tie Y, Zhu J, Xing R, Sun Z, Zheng X: Downregulation of CCND1 and CDK6 by miR-34a induces cell cycle arrest. *FEBS Lett.* 2008 582:1564-8.

[34] Chu IM, Hengst L, Slingerland JM: The Cdk inhibitor p27 in human cancer: prognostic potential and relevance to anticancer therapy. *Nat. Rev. Cancer* 2008 8:253-67.

[35] Visone R, Russo L, Pallante P, De Martino I, Ferraro A, Leone V, Borbone E, Petrocca F, Alder H, Croce CM, Fusco A: MicroRNAs (miR)-221 and miR-222, both overexpressed in human thyroid papillary carcinomas, regulate p27Kip1 protein levels and cell cycle. *Endocr Relat Cancer* 2007 14:791-8.

[36] Fornari F, Gramantieri L, Ferracin M, Veronese A, Sabbioni S, Calin GA, Grazi GL, Giovannini C, Croce CM, Bolondi L, Negrini M: MiR-221 controls CDKN1C/p57 and CDKN1B/p27 expression in human hepatocellular carcinoma. *Oncogene* 2008 27:5651-61.

[37] Petrocca F, Visone R, Onelli MR, Shah MH, Nicoloso MS, de Martino I, Iliopoulos D, Pilozzi E, Liu CG, Negrini M, Cavazzini L, Volinia S, Alder H, Ruco LP, Baldassarre G, Croce CM, Vecchione A: E2F1-regulated microRNAs impair TGFbeta-dependent cell-cycle arrest and apoptosis in gastric cancer. *Cancer Cell* 2008 13:272-86.

[38] Letai AG: Diagnosing and exploiting cancer's addiction to blocks in apoptosis. *Nat. Rev. Cancer* 2008 8:121-32.

[39] Bommer GT, Gerin I, Feng Y, Kaczorowski AJ, Kuick R, Love RE, Zhai Y, Giordano TJ, Qin ZS, Moore BB, MacDougald OA, Cho KR, Fearon ER: p53-mediated activation of miRNA34 candidate tumor-suppressor genes. *Curr. Biol.* 2007 17:1298-1307.

[40] Hermeking H: p53 enters the microRNA world. *Cancer Cell* 2007 12:414-8.

[41] Tarasov V, Jung P, Verdoodt B, Lodygin D, Epanchintsev A, Menssen A, Meister G, Hermeking H: Differential regulation of microRNAs by p53 revealed by massively parallel sequencing: miR-34a is a p53 target that induces apoptosis and G1-arrest. *Cell Cycle* 2007 6:1586-93.

[42] Tazawa H, Tsuchiya N, Izumiya M, Nakagama H: Tumor-suppressive miR-34a induces senescence-like growth arrest through modulation of the E2F pathway in human colon cancer cells. *Proc. Natl. Acad. Sci. USA* 2007 104:15472-7.

[43] Raver-Shapira N, Marciano E, Meiri E, Spector Y, Rosenfeld N, Moskovits N, Bentwich Z, Oren M: Transcriptional activation of miR-34a contributes to p53-mediated apoptosis. *Mol. Cell* 2007 26:731-43.

[44] Chang TC, Wentzel EA, Kent OA, Ramachandran K, Mullendore M, Lee KH, Feldmann G, Yamakuchi M, Ferlito M, Lowenstein CJ, Arking DE, Beer MA, Maitra A, Mendell JT: Transactivation of miR-34a by p53 broadly influences gene expression and promotes apoptosis. *Mol. Cell* 2007 26:745-52.

[45] Welch C, Chen Y, Stallings RL: MicroRNA-34a functions as a potential tumor suppressor by inducing apoptosis in neuroblastoma cells. *Oncogene* 2007 26:5017-22.
[46] Wei JS, Song YK, Durinck S, Chen QR, Cheuk AT, Tsang P, Zhang Q, Thiele CJ, Slack A, Shohet J, Khan J: The MYCN oncogene is a direct target of miR-34a. *Oncogene* 2008 27:5204-13.
[47] Volinia S, Calin GA, Liu CG, Ambs S, Cimmino A, Petrocca F, Visone R, Iorio M, Roldo C, Ferracin M, Prueitt RL, Yanaihara N, Lanza G, Scarpa A, Vecchione A, Negrini M, Harris CC, Croce CM: A microRNA expression signature of human solid tumors defines cancer gene targets. *Proc. Natl. Acad. Sci. USA* 2006 103:2257-61.
[48] Slaby O, Svoboda M, Fabian P, Smerdova T, Knoflickova D, Bednarikova M, Nenutil R, Vyzula R: Altered expression of miR-21, miR-31, miR-143 and miR-145 is related to clinicopathologic features of colorectal cancer. *Oncology* 2007 72:397-402.
[49] Hiyoshi Y, Kamohara H, Karashima R, Sato N, Imamura Y, Nagai Y, Yoshida N, Toyama E, Hayashi N, Watanabe M, Baba H: MicroRNA-21 regulates the proliferation and invasion in esophageal squamous cell carcinoma. *Clin. Cancer Res.* 2009 15:1915-22.
[50] Chan JA, Krichevsky AM, Kosik KS: MicroRNA-21 is an antiapoptotic factor in human glioblastoma cells. *Cancer Res.* 2005 65:6029-33.
[51] Frankel LB, Christoffersen NR, Jacobsen A, Lindow M, Krogh A, Lund AH: Programmed cell death 4 (PDCD4) is an important functional target of the microRNA miR-21 in breast cancer cells. *J. Biol. Chem.* 2008 283:1026-33.
[52] Zhu S, Wu H, Wu F, Nie D, Sheng S, Mo YY: MicroRNA-21 targets tumor suppressor genes in invasion and metastasis. *Cell Res* 2008 18:350-9.
[53] Si ML, Zhu S, Wu H, Lu Z, Wu F, Mo YY: miR-21-mediated tumor growth. *Oncogene* 2007 26:2799-803.
[54] Talotta F, Cimmino A, Matarazzo MR, Casalino L, De Vita G, D'Esposito M, Di Lauro R, Verde P: An autoregulatory loop mediated by miR-21 and PDCD4 controls the AP-1 activity in RAS transformation. *Oncogene* 2009 28:73-84.
[55] Cory S, Adams JM: The Bcl2 family: regulators of the cellular life-or-death switch. *Nat Rev Cancer* 2002 2:647-56.
[56] Danial NN, Korsmeyer SJ: Cell death: critical control points. *Cell* 2004 116:205-19.
[57] Cimmino A, Calin GA, Fabbri M, Iorio MV, Ferracin M, Shimizu M, Wojcik SE, Aqeilan RI, Zupo S, Dono M, Rassenti L, Alder H Volinia S, Liu CG, Kipps TJ, Negrini M, Croce CM: miR-15 and miR-16 induce apoptosis by targeting BCL2. *Proc. Natl. Acad. Sci. USA* 2005 102:13944-9.
[58] Shi XB, Xue L, Yang J, Ma AH, Zhao J, Xu M, Tepper CG, Evans CP, Kung HJ, deVere White RW: An androgen-regulated miRNA suppresses Bak1 expression and induces androgen-independent growth of prostate cancer cells. *Proc. Natl. Acad. Sci. USA* 2007 104:19983-8.
[59] Garofalo M, Quintavalle C, Di Leva G, Zanca C, Romano G, Taccioli C, Liu CG, Croce CM, Condorelli G: MicroRNA signatures of TRAIL resistance in human non-small cell lung cancer. *Oncogene* 2008 27:3845-55.
[60] Xu C, Lu Y, Pan Z, Chu W, Luo X, Lin H, Xiao J, Shan H, Wang Z, Yang B: The muscle-specific microRNAs miR-1 and miR-133 produce opposing effects on apoptosis by targeting HSP60, HSP70 and caspase-9 in cardiomyocytes. *J. Cell Sci.* 2007 120:3045-52.

[61] Lynam-Lennon N, Maher SG, Reynolds JV: The roles of microRNA in cancer and apoptosis. *Biol. Rev. Camb. Philos. Soc.* 2009 84:55-71.

[62] Campisi J: Senescent cells, tumor suppression, and organismal aging: good citizens, bad neighbors. *Cell* 2005 120:513-22.

[63] Zuckerman V, Wolyniec K, Sionov RV, Haupt S, Haupt Y: Tumour suppression by p53: the importance of apoptosis and cellular senescence. *J. Pathol.* 2009 219:3-15.

[64] Campisi J: Suppressing cancer: the importance of being senescent. *Science* 2005 309:886-7.

[65] Mitomo S, Maesawa C, Ogasawara S, Iwaya T, Shibazaki M, Yashima-Abo A, Kotani K, Oikawa H, Sakurai E, Izutsu N, Kato K, Komatsu H, Ikedu K, Wakabayashi G, Masuda T: Downregulation of miR-138 is associated with overexpression of human telomerase reverse transcriptase protein in human anaplastic thyroid carcinoma cell lines. *Cancer Sci.* 2008 99:280-6.

[66] Blackburn EH: Switching and signaling at the telomere. *Cell* 2001 106:661-73.

[67] Voorhoeve PM, le Sage C, Schrier M, Gillis AJ, Stoop H, Nagel R, Liu YP, van Duijse J, Drost J, Griekspoor A, Zlotorynski E, Yabuta N, De Vita G, Nojima H, Looijenga LH, Agami R: A genetic screen implicates miRNA-372 and miRNA-373 as oncogenes in testicular germ cell tumors. *Cell* 2006 124:1169-81.

[68] Benetti R, Gonzalo S, Jaco I, Munoz P, Gonzalez S, Schoeftner S, Murchison E, Andl T, Chen T, Klatt P, Li E, Serrano M, Millar S, Hannon G, Blasco MA: A mammalian microRNA cluster controls DNA methylation and telomere recombination via Rbl2-dependent regulation of DNA methyltransferases. *Nat. Struct. Mol. Biol.* 2008 15:268-79.

[69] Kumamoto K, Spillare EA, Fujita K, Horikawa I, Yamashita T, Appella E, Nagashima M, Takenoshita S, Yokota J, Harris CC: Nutlin-3a activates p53 to both down-regulate inhibitor of growth 2 and up-regulate mir-34a, mir-34b, and mir-34c expression, and induce senescence. *Cancer Res* 2008 68:3193-203.

[70] Tanaka S, Sugimachi K, Yamashita Y, Shirabe K, Shimada M, Wands JR: Angiogenic switch as a molecular target of malignant tumors. *J. Gastroenterol.* 2003 38 Suppl 15:93-7.

[71] Semenza GL: Targeting HIF-1 for cancer therapy. *Nat Rev Cancer* 2003 3:721-32.

[72] Yang WJ, Yang DD, Na S, Sandusky GE, Zhang Q, Zhao G: Dicer is required for embryonic angiogenesis during mouse development. *J. Biol. Chem.* 2005 280:9330-5.

[73] Suarez Y, Fernandez-Hernando C, Pober JS, Sessa WC: Dicer dependent microRNAs regulate gene expression and functions in human endothelial cells. *Circ. Res.* 2007 100:1164-73.

[74] Kuehbacher A, Urbich C, Zeiher AM, Dimmeler S: Role of Dicer and Drosha for endothelial microRNA expression and angiogenesis. *Circ. Res.* 2007 101:59-68.

[75] Kulshreshtha R, Ferracin M, Wojcik SE, Garzon R, Alder H, Agosto-Perez FJ, Davuluri R, Liu CG, Croce CM, Negrini M, Calin GA, Ivan M: A microRNA signature of hypoxia. *Mol. Cell Biol.* 2007 27:1859-67.

[76] Mertens-Talcott SU, Chintharlapalli S, Li X, Safe S: The oncogenic microRNA-27a targets genes that regulate specificity protein transcription factors and the G2-M checkpoint in MDA-MB-231 breast cancer cells. *Cancer Res.* 2007 67:11001-11.

[77] Fasanaro P, D'Alessandra Y, Di Stefano V, Melchionna R, Romani S, Pompilio G, Capogrossi MC, Martelli F: MicroRNA-210 modulates endothelial cell response to

hypoxia and inhibits the receptor tyrosine kinase ligand Ephrin-A3. *J. Biol. Chem.* 2008 283:15878-83.

[78] Liu B, Peng XC, Zheng XL, Wang J, Qin YW: MiR-126 restoration down-regulate VEGF and inhibit the growth of lung cancer cell lines in vitro and in vivo. *Lung Cancer* 2009 66:169-75.

[79] Fish JE, Santoro MM, Morton SU, Yu S, Yeh RF, Wythe JD, Ivey KN, Bruneau BG, Stainier DY, Srivastava D: miR-126 regulates angiogenic signaling and vascular integrity. *Dev Cell* 2008 15:272-84.

[80] Zhang Q, Kandic I, Kutryk MJ: Dysregulation of angiogenesis-related microRNAs in endothelial progenitor cells from patients with coronary artery disease. *Biochem. Biophys. Res. Commun.* 2011 405:42-6.

[81] Wang S, Olson EN: AngiomiRs--key regulators of angiogenesis. *Curr. Opin. Genet. Dev.* 2009 19:205-11.

[82] Pantel K, Brakenhoff RH: Dissecting the metastatic cascade. *Nat. Rev. Cancer* 2004 4:448-56.

[83] Le XF, Merchant O, Bast RC, Calin GA: The Roles of MicroRNAs in the Cancer Invasion-Metastasis Cascade. *Cancer Microenviron* 2010 3:137-47.

[84] Olson P, Lu J, Zhang H, Shai A, Chun MG, Wang Y, Libutti SK, Nakakura EK, Golub TR, Hanahan D: MicroRNA dynamics in the stages of tumorigenesis correlate with hallmark capabilities of cancer. *Genes Dev.* 2009 23:2152-65.

[85] Gregory PA, Bert AG, Paterson EL, Barry SC, Tsykin A, Farshid G, Vadas MA, Khew-Goodall Y, Goodall GJ: The miR-200 family and miR-205 regulate epithelial to mesenchymal transition by targeting ZEB1 and SIP1. *Nat. Cell Biol.* 2008 10:593-601.

[86] Park SM, Gaur AB, Lengyel E, Peter ME: The miR-200 family determines the epithelial phenotype of cancer cells by targeting the E-cadherin repressors ZEB1 and ZEB2. *Genes Dev.* 2008 22:894-907.

[87] Burk U, Schubert J, Wellner U, Schmalhofer O, Vincan E, Spaderna S, Brabletz T: A reciprocal repression between ZEB1 and members of the miR-200 family promotes EMT and invasion in cancer cells. *EMBO Rep.* 2008 9:582-9.

[88] Bracken CP, Gregory PA, Kolesnikoff N, Bert AG, Wang J, Shannon MF, Goodall GJ: A double-negative feedback loop between ZEB1-SIP1 and the microRNA-200 family regulates epithelial-mesenchymal transition. *Cancer Res.* 2008 68:7846-54.

[89] Baffa R, Fassan M, Volinia S, O'Hara B, Liu CG, Palazzo JP, Gardiman M, Rugge M, Gomella LG, Croce CM, Rosenberg A: MicroRNA expression profiling of human metastatic cancers identifies cancer gene targets. *J. Pathol.* 2009 219:214-21.

[90] Budhu A, Jia HL, Forgues M, Liu CG, Goldstein D, Lam A, Zanetti KA, Ye QH, Qin LX, Croce CM, Tang ZY, Wang XW: Identification of metastasis-related microRNAs in hepatocellular carcinoma. *Hepatology* 2008 47:897-907.

[91] Lujambio A, Calin GA, Villanueva A, Ropero S, Sanchez-Cespedes M, Blanco D, Montuenga LM, Rossi S, Nicoloso MS, Faller WJ, Gallagher WM, Eccles SA, Croce CM, Esteller M: A microRNA DNA methylation signature for human cancer metastasis. *Proc. Natl. Acad. Sci. USA* 2008 105:13556-61.

[92] Duursma AM, Kedde M, Schrier M, le Sage C, Agami R: miR-148 targets human DNMT3b protein coding region. *RNA* 2008 14:872-7.

[93] Laios A, O'Toole S, Flavin R, Martin C, Kelly L, Ring M, Finn SP, Barrett C, Loda M, Gleeson N, DArcy T, McGuinness E, Sheils O, Sheppard B, OLeary J: Potential role of miR-9 and miR-223 in recurrent ovarian cancer. *Mol. Cancer* 2008 7:35.

[94] Guo LM, Pu Y, Han Z, Liu T, Li YX, Liu M, Li X, Tang H: MicroRNA-9 inhibits ovarian cancer cell growth through regulation of NF-kappaB1. *FEBS J.* 2009 276:5537-46.

[95] Foekens JA, Sieuwerts AM, Smid M, Look MP, de Weerd V, Boersma AW, Klijn JG, Wiemer EA, Martens JW: Four miRNAs associated with aggressiveness of lymph node-negative, estrogen receptor-positive human breast cancer. *Proc. Natl. Acad. Sci. USA* 2008 105:13021-6.

[96] Gabriely G, Wurdinger T, Kesari S, Esau CC, Burchard J, Linsley PS, Krichevsky AM: MicroRNA 21 promotes glioma invasion by targeting matrix metalloproteinase regulators. *Mol. Cell Biol.* 2008 28:5369-80.

[97] Sasayama T, Nishihara M, Kondoh T, Hosoda K, Kohmura E: MicroRNA-10b is overexpressed in malignant glioma and associated with tumor invasive factors, uPAR and RhoC. *Int. J. Cancer* 2009 125:1407-13.

[98] Ma L, Teruya-Feldstein J, Weinberg RA: Tumour invasion and metastasis initiated by microRNA-10b in breast cancer. *Nature* 2007 449:682-8.

[99] Bhaumik D, Scott GK, Schokrpur S, Patil CK, Campisi J, Benz CC: Expression of microRNA-146 suppresses NF-kappaB activity with reduction of metastatic potential in breast cancer cells. *Oncogene* 2008 27:5643-7.

[100] Ponta H, Sherman L, Herrlich PA: CD44: from adhesion molecules to signalling regulators. *Nat. Rev. Mol. Cell Biol.* 2003 4:33-45.

[101] Marhaba R, Klingbeil P, Nuebel T, Nazarenko I, Buechler MW, Zoeller M: CD44 and EpCAM: cancer-initiating cell markers. *Curr. Mol. Med.* 2008 8:784-804.

[102] Marhaba R, Zoller M: CD44 in cancer progression: adhesion, migration and growth regulation. *J. Mol. Histol.* 2004 35:211-31.

[103] Coulouarn C, Factor VM, Andersen JB, Durkin ME, Thorgeirsson SS: Loss of miR-122 expression in liver cancer correlates with suppression of the hepatic phenotype and gain of metastatic properties. *Oncogene* 2009 28:3526-36.

[104] Kong W, Yang H, He L, Zhao JJ, Coppola D, Dalton WS, Cheng JQ: MicroRNA-155 is regulated by the transforming growth factor beta/Smad pathway and contributes to epithelial cell plasticity by targeting RhoA. *Mol. Cell Biol.* 2008 28:6773-84.

In: MicroRNAs in Solid Cancer
Editor: Ondrej Slaby

ISBN: 978-61324-514-9
©2012 Nova Science Publishers, Inc.

*Chapter V*

# MicroRNAs and Colorectal Cancer

*Ondrej Slaby, Marek Svoboda and Rostislav Vyzula*
Masaryk Memorial Cancer Institute, Brno, Czech Republic
Central European Institute of Technology, Masaryk University, Brno, Czech Republic

## Abstract

Colorectal cancer (CRC) represents one of the most frequent causes of death for cancer. CRC has been recently defined as the third most common cancer. Polymorphisms within microRNAs binding regions have been described as new risk factors for CRC. Several genome-wide profiling studies have identified miRNAs deregulated in CRC tissue. Furthermore, number of experimental studies on these miRNAs revealed insight into miRNA-mediated, regulatory links to well-known oncogenic and tumor suppressor signaling pathways. Several investigations have also described the ability of specific miRNA expression profiles to predict prognosis and therapy response, and potential of selected miRNAs as therapeutical targets in CRC patients.

## 5.1. Introduction

Colorectal cancer (CRC) accounts for 13% of all cancers and is the second most common cause of cancer death in the Western nations. Early detection of CRC provides a marked survival advantage, and many efforts are focused on improving detection rates and screening utilization. Currently, surgery is the only curative approach for early-stage adenocarcinomas, the most common type of CRC, with chemotherapy providing a modest incremental survival benefit at the cost of additional toxic effects. Therefore, the identification of improved diagnostic, prognostic and predictive markers and new therapeutic options for CRC patients is of great and immediate interest [1]. Among the potential markers of interest are also miRNAs. Given the wide impact of miRNAs on gene expression, it is not surprising that a great number of miRNAs have been implicated in cancer [2,3]. Deregulation of miRNAs can influence carcinogenesis if their mRNA targets are encoded by tumor suppressor genes or oncogenes.

Both overexpression and silencing or switching off of specific miRNAs have been described in the carcinogenesis of CRC. Up-regulation of mature miRNA may occur owing to transcriptional activation or amplification of the miRNA encoding gene, whereas silencing or reduced expression may result from deletion of a particular chromosomal region, epigenetic silencing, or defects in their biogenesis [4,5].

Two approaches are applied today to investigate the connection between miRNAs and CRC. On one hand, miRNAs seem to regulate many known oncogenic and tumor suppressor pathways involved in the Vogelstein model of CRC pathogenesis. Many proteins involved in key signaling pathways of CRC, such as members of the Wnt/β-catenin and phosphatidylinositol-3-kinase (PI-3-K) pathways, KRAS, p53, extracellular matrix regulators as well as epithelial-mesenchymal transition (EMT) transcription factors [6], are altered and seem to be affected by miRNA regulation in CRC (summarized in Figure 5.1). Analyses of these miRNAs in mechanistic studies are crucial to better understanding CRC pathogenesis [3,7,8] and may provide exciting therapeutic opportunities [9]. On the other hand, expression profiles of hundreds of miRNAs have been shown to have at least the same potential for identification of biomarkers as profiling of their mRNA or protein counterparts. This enables predicting prognosis and therapy response as well as distinguishing certain disease entities [10].

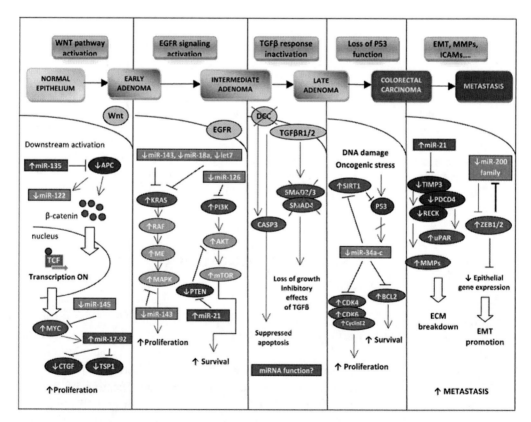

Figure 5.1. MicroRNAs involvement in Vogelstein's model of colorectal cancer development (adapted from Slaby et al. [3]).

Particular signaling pathways affected by miRNAs are described in detail in the review (APC - adenomatous polyposis coli, CTGF - connective tissue growth factor, TSP1 - thrombospondin 1, EGFR - epidermal growth factor receptor, mTOR - mechanistic target of rapamycin, PTEN - phosphatase and tensin homolog, DCC - deleted in colorectal carcinoma, TGFβR1/2 - transforming growth factor, beta receptor 1/2, CASP3 - caspase 3, SIRT1 - sirtuin 1, CDK4,6 - cyclin-dependent kinase 4,6, ECM - extracellular matrix, EMT – epithelial-mesenchymal transition, ICAMs - intercellular adhesive molecules, TIMP3 - tissue inhibitor of metalloproteinase 3, PDCD4 - programmed cell death 4, RECK - reversion-inducing-cysteine-rich protein with kazal motifs, uPAR - plasminogen activator, urokinase receptor, MMPs - matrix metallopeptidases, ZEB1/2 - zinc-finger E-box binding homeobox 1).

## 5.2. Polymorphisms within Mature miRNA Sequence and miRNA Binding Regions and Risk of Cancer

Several genome-wide profiling studies have identified miRNAs deregulated in CRC tissue and blood serum [3]. A number of experimental studies on these miRNAs revealed insight into miRNA-mediated regulatory links to well-known oncogenic and tumor suppressor signaling pathways. Polymorphisms within these miRNA sequences and binding regions within 3' UTRs of their mRNA targets have been described as new risk factors for CRC [11].

By analysing human gene sequences in a public database (http://genome.cse.ucsc.edu/), Kim and co-workers (2010) found that six miRNA regulation genes (AGO1, AGO2, TRBP, TNRC6A, TNRC6C and EXPORTIN5) have mononucleotide repeats with seven or more nucleotides in the coding sequences that could be targets for frameshift mutation in cancers with microsatellite instability (MSI) [12]. Mutations in analyzed genes except the AGO1 were detected in 27% of CRC samples. The significant differences of the mutation frequency between the cancers with MSI-H (19/58), MSI-L (0/32), and MSS (0/90), indicated that association of the mutations with CRC is MSI-H specific. It seems that frameshift mutations of these genes could cause alterations of miRNA regulation and contribute to development of CRC indicating MSI-H phenotype [12].

In the study of Lee and co-workers (2010), 426 consecutive Korean patients with surgically treated CRC were enrolled and forty polymorphisms of miRNA-related genes were determined. In a univariate analysis, the progression-free survival of the patients with the combined miR-492 C/G and G/G genotype was significantly worse than that of the patients with the mir-492 C/C genotype (rs2289030) ($p = 0.0426$), however there was no difference in the overall survival [13].

Pioneering design in the field of miRNAs associated SNPs indicated study of Landi and co-workers (2009) who selected the 3' UTRs of 104 genes candidate for CRC and identified putative miRNA-binding sites by specialized algorithms (PicTar, DianaMicroT, miRBase, miRanda, TargetScan, and microInspector). Fifty-seven SNPs were identified in miRNA-binding sites and evaluated for their ability to affect the binding of the miRNA with its target, by assessing the variation of Gibbs free energy between the two alleles of each SNP. Eight common SNPs were found that were further investigated in a case-control association study. The study was carried out on a series of 968 cases and 697 controls from Czech Republic, a population with the highest worldwide incidence of CRC. Statistically significant associations were found between risk of CRC and variant alleles of CD86 (OR 2.74; 95% CI, 1.24-6.04, for the variant homozygotes) and INSR genes (OR 1.94; 95% CI, 1.03-3.66, for the variant homozygotes). These observations are the first to report positive association between SNPs in miRNA-binding regions and cancer risk [14].

Recent studies have found that KRAS mutations predict resistance to monoclonal antibodies targeting the epidermal growth factor receptor in metastatic colorectal cancer (mCRC). Zhang and co-workers (2010) have tested the hypothesis whether SNP in a let-7 microRNA complementary site (lcs6) in the KRAS 3' UTR may be associated with clinical outcome in 130 KRAS wild-type (KRASwt) mCRC patients enrolled in a phase II study of cetuximab monotherapy (IMCL-0144). KRAS let-7 lcs6 SNP was found to be related to object response rate (ORR) in mCRC patients whose tumors had KRASwt. The 12 KRASwt patients harboring at least a variant G allele (TG or GG) had a 42% ORR compared with a 9% ORR in 55 KRASwt patients with let-7 lcs6 TT genotype ($p = 0.02$). KRASwt patients with TG/GG genotypes also indicated trend of longer median progression-free survival (3.9 versus 1.3 months) and OS (10.7 versus 6.4 months) compared to those with TT genotypes [15].

## 5.3. Serum and Plasma miRNAs: Early Detection of Disease Onset and Progression

Circulating nucleic acids (CNAs) offer unique opportunities for an early diagnosis of CRC. Deregulated expression of miRNAs in various tissues has been associated with a variety of human cancers. More recently, miRNAs' occurrence in the serum and plasma of humans has been repeatedly observed. The levels of miRNAs in serum are more stable, reproducible, and consistent among individuals of the same species than are other CNAs [3].

In a study by Chen and co-workers (2008), CRC patients had a significantly different serum miRNA profile compared to healthy subjects (HS). In all cases, 69 miRNAs were detected in the CRC serum but not in HS. It is of interest to note that CRC patients shared a large number of serum miRNAs (e.g. miR-134, miR-146a, miR-221, miR-222, miR-23a, etc.) with lung cancer patients. Pearson correlation further indicated that the levels of miRNAs in serum from lung cancer patients and CRC patients were consistent, suggesting that there are some "common" tumor-related miRNAs in serum [16]. Differentially expressed miRNAs in the plasma of patients with CRC have been also reported [17]. Expression pattern of 30 miRNAs (miR-17-3p, miR-92, miR-135b, miR-222, miR-95, etc.) in the plasma of patients with CRC were analyzed by qRT-PCR expression profiling. Both miR-17-3p and miR-92 were significantly elevated ($p < 0.0005$). The plasma levels of these miRNAs were significantly reduced after surgery in 10 patients with CRC ($p < 0.05$). Further validation with an independent set of plasma samples (n=180) indicated that miR-92 differentiates CRC not only from normal subjects but also from gastric cancer and inflammatory bowel disease. This marker yielded an ROC (receiver operating characteristic) curve area of 88.5%. In discriminating CRC from control subjects, the sensitivity was 89% and the specificity was

70%. MiR-92 has reasonable sensitivity for CRC detection and compares favorably with the fecal occult blood test [17]. Huang and co-workers (2010) measured the levels of 12 miRNAs (miR-134, -146a, -17-3p, -181d, -191, -221, -222, -223, -25, -29a, -320a, and -92a) in plasma samples from patients with advanced colorectal neoplasia (carcinomas and advanced adenomas) and healthy controls using real-time RT-PCR. Authors found that plasma miR-29a and miR-92a have significant diagnostic value for advanced neoplasia. MiR-29a yielded an AUC (the areas under the ROC curve) of 0.844 and miR-92a yielded an AUC of 0.838 in discriminating CRC from controls. More importantly, these 2 miRNAs also could discriminate advanced adenomas from controls and yielded an AUC of 0.769 for miR-29a and 0.749 for miR-92a. Combined ROC analyses using these 2 miRNAs revealed an elevated AUC of 0.883 with 83.0% sensitivity and 84.7% specificity in discriminating CRC, and AUC of 0.773 with 73.0% sensitivity and 79.7% specificity in discriminating advanced adenomas. These data suggest that plasma miR-29a and miR-92a have a strong potential as novel noninvasive biomarkers for early detection of CRC [18].

More recently, feasibility of fecal miRNAs as biomarkers for colorectal neoplasia screening was evaluated. MiRNA expression profiles from stool of 29 patients showed higher expression of miR-21 and miR-106a in patients with adenomas and CRCs compared with individuals free of colorectal neoplasia [19].

## 5.4. Tissue miRNA Signatures: Implications for Diagnostic Oncology

Alterations in miRNA expression profiles have been successively detected in many types of human tumors [5]. The causes of the widespread differential expression of miRNA genes between malignant and normal cells can be explained by the gene location in cancer-associated regions, alterations in the miRNA processing machinery, and epigenetic mechanisms [20]. In reports on various cancer samples, generally lower miRNA levels were identified in tumors in comparison with normal tissue and, lower miRNA levels in poorly differentiated tumors compared to well-differentiated tumors in tissue samples [21] as well as in cell lines [22]. MiRNAs indicating altered expression in at least two profiling studies in CRC tissue are summarized in Table 5.1.

In 2003, Michael and co-workers published the first such study. Using cloning technology followed by northern blotting, they observed consistently reduced accumulation of the specific mature miR-143 and miR-145 in the adenomatous and carcinoma stages of colorectal neoplasia. The same blots, however, displayed consistent levels of the ~70-bp pre-miR-143 in each of the cell lines. The authors concluded that the levels of mature miR-143 in these cells were controlled post-transcriptionally. These data suggested that abnormal processing might affect miRNAs expression in colon cancer cells [23].

Bandres and co-workers (2006) examined by qRT-PCR the expression of 156 mature miRNAs in colorectal tumors and adjacent non-neoplastic tissues from patients and CRC cell lines. This permitted them to identify a group of 13 miRNAs whose expression is significantly altered in this type of tumor. The most significantly deregulated miRNAs were miR-31, miR-96, miR-135b, miR-183 (up-regulated in tumors and CRC cell-lines) and miR-133b, miR-145 (down-regulated). In addition, the expression level of miR-31 was positively correlated with the stage of CRC tumor. These results, achieved through a standardized qRT-PCR method, suggest that miRNA expression profile could have relevance to the biological and clinical behavior of colorectal neoplasia [24]. MiR-31 expression was positively associated to advanced TNM stage ($p = 0.026$) and deeper invasion of tumors ($p = 0.024$) also in independent study based on 98 primary CRC specimens, along with the corresponding normal mucosa specimens [25].

**Table 5.1. List of representative miRNAs differentially expressed in CRC observed in at least two microRNA profiling studies (N – number of studies; * value is not available)**

| miRNA up-regulated in CRC | | | miRNA down-regulated in CRC | | |
|---|---|---|---|---|---|
| miRNA | N | Refs. + p-value (fold change) | miRNA | N | Refs. + p-value (fold change) |
| miR-21 | 7 | [23]*, [27]*, [26] <0.00001, [38]<0.0001, [32] (1.8), [40]<0.001, [24] (6.0) | miR-145 | 7 | [23]*, [38] 0.003, [32] (0.5), [30]*, [41] (0.3), [24] (0.1), [28]<0.05 |
| miR-20a | 6 | [27]*, [40]<0.001, [41] (1.6), [28]<0.05 (4.4), [17]<0.05 (2.6), [25] (2.4) | miR-143 | 5 | [23]*, [26]<0.00001, [38] 0.01, [30]*, [28]<0.05 |
| miR-31 | 5 | [38] 0.0006, [32] (2.8), [30]*, [24] (2.4), [28]<0.05 (179.3) | | | |
| miR-92 | 5 | [32] (1.5), [30]*, [41] (1.7), [28]<0.05, [17] (2.4) | | | |
| miR-106a | 4 | [27]*, [32] (1.8), [40]<0.001, [17] (2.8) | | | |
| miR-191 | 3 | [27]*, [30]*, [36] 0.03 | | | |
| miR-200c | 3 | [32] (3.0), [42]<0.0001, [36] 0.002 | | | |
| miR-181b | 3 | [40]<0.001, [42] 0.0005, [36] 0.0002 (2.5) | | | |
| miR-135b | 3 | [24] (39.8), [17] (3.1), [25] (5.1) | | | |
| miR-183 | 3 | [30]*, [24] (7.6), [28]<0.05 (18.9) | | | |
| miR-18a | 3 | [28]<0.05 (10.5), [17] (4.2), [25] (2.5) | | | |
| miR-203 | 3 | [27]*, [40]<0.001, [30]* | | | |
| miR-223 | 3 | [27]*, [32] (1.3), [30]* | | | |
| miR-17-5p | 2 | [27]*, [32] (1.8) | | | |
| miR-221 | 2 | [27]*, [17] (2.2) | | | |
| miR-15b | 2 | [32] (1.3), [36] 0.03 | | | |
| let-7g | 2 | [32] (1.2), [42] 0.03 | | | |

Velculescu's group developed an experimental approach called miRNA serial analysis of gene expression (miRAGE) and used it to perform one of the largest experimental analyses of human miRNAs. Sequence analysis of 273,966 small RNA tags from human colorectal cells allowed them to identify 200 known mature miRNAs, 133 novel miRNA candidates, and 112 previously uncharacterized miRNA forms. To aid in evaluating the candidate miRNAs, they disrupted the Dicer locus in three human CRC cell lines and examined known and novel miRNAs in these cells. This study indicates that the human genome contains many more miRNAs than currently identified [26].

From a large-scale analysis of miRNA expression profiles on 540 samples of solid cancers, including CRC, Volinia and co-workers (2006) identified a solid cancer miRNA signature composed by a large portion of overexpressed miRNAs. Among these miRNAs were some with well characterized cancer associations, such as miR-17-5p, miR-20a, miR-21, miR-92, miR-106a, and miR-155 [27]. A microarray-based approach for analysis of miRNA expression profiles in CRC was successfully applied also by Motoyama and co-workers [28].

In another profiling study, Lanza and co-workers (2007) evaluated the expression of miRNAs and mRNAs in CRC samples characterized by microsatellite stability (MSS) or by high levels of microsatellite instability (MSI-H). Their analysis of miRNA expression profiles of MSI-H (n = 16) and MSS CRCs (n = 23) identified 14 differentially expressed miRNAs, while their analysis of messenger RNA expression profiles in these tumors identified 451 differentially expressed genes. Consequently, a smaller selected signature of best predictors of microsatellite status was generated: 27 genes, including 8 miRNAs, were identified as predictors. Further cluster analysis using just these 27 miRNAs and mRNAs also perfectly separated the two tumor classes. Cluster analyses run using either the mRNAs or the miRNAs independently did not perform as well in discriminating the tumor types. Therefore, the combined miRNA/mRNA fingerprint worked as the best discriminator for MSS versus MSI-H [29]. In the study of Earle and co-workers (2010), relative expression levels of miR-92, miR-223, miR-155, miR-196a, miR-31, and miR-26b were significantly different among MSI subgroups (including low MSI and hereditary non-polyposis colorectal cancer (HNPCC) syndrome), and miR-31 and miR-223 were overexpressed in CRC of patients with HNPCC-associated cancer [30]. To identify miRNAs that are differentially expressed in CRC and CRC subtypes, Sarverand co-workers (2009) carried out highly expression profiling of 735 miRNAs on samples obtained from a statistically powerful set of tumors (n = 80) and normal colon tissue (n = 28). Tumor specimens showed highly significant and large fold change differential expression of the levels of 39 miRNAs including miR-135b, miR-96, miR-182, miR-183, miR-1, and miR-133a, relative to normal colon tissue. Significant differences were observed in 6 miRNAs: decreased levels in MSS relative to MSI-H tumors included miR-552, miR-592, miR-181c and miR-196. MiR-625 and miR-31 exhibited increased levels in MSI-H relative to MSS tumors [31].

Monzo and co-workers (2008) assessed the expression of mature miRNAs in human embryonic colon tissue, as well as in CRC and paired normal colon tissue. Overlapping miRNA expression was detected between embryonic colonic mucosa and CRC. The miR-17-92 cluster and its target, E2F1, exhibit a similar pattern of expression in human colon development and in colonic carcinogenesis – regulating cell proliferation in both cases. Authors of this study conclude that miRNA pathways play a major role in both embryonic development and neoplastic transformation of the colonic epithelium [32].

From a diagnostic point of view, miRNA expression profiles might also contribute significantly to the further determination of the tissue origin of the cancer of unknown primary sites. Cancer of unknown primary sites (CUP) is usually a very aggressive disease with a poor prognosis. Identifying of CRC among adenocarcinoma of unknown primary site may improve prognosis of these patients by giving them a chance for modern anticancer targeted therapy. Two recent studies examined metastases of unknown primary tumors with miRNA microarrays for their potential to identify the tissue of origin. After establishing a miRNA classifier (n = 68, 11 tumor types, 217 miRNAs), 12 out of 17 poorly differentiated tumors were accurately classified by miRNA profiling [21]. A second publication reported an overall accuracy of 90% in classifying more than 400 malignant tumor samples of 22 tissue origins based on a set of 48 miRNAs [33]. A recent study on lymph node metastases of several malignant tumors, including CRC, identified three specific miRNAs (miR-148a, miR-34b/c, and miR-9), specifically down-regulated by CpG island hyper-methylation [34].

To offer a new approach for preventing and controlling lymphatic metastasis in colon cancer, Huang and co-workers (2009) compared the miRNA expression profiles (723 human microRNA probes) of normal colonic epithelium from the two CRC patient groups; those with confirmed lymph node metastasis (n = 3), and those without detectable lymph node metastasis (n = 3). Two microRNA (hsa-miR-129* and hsa-miR-137) were differentially expressed in the lymph node positive group compared with the lymph node negative group. After validation through qRT-PCR method, hsa-miR-137 expression was significantly up-regulated nearly 6.6-fold in lymph node positive specimens ($p = 0.036$) [35].

## 5.5. MiRNAs Expression in Prognosis and Response Prediction

Accumulating evidence shows that miRNA expression patterns are unique to certain cancers and have potential to be used as prognostic and predictive factors in clinical routine. Xi and co-workers (2007) performed Kaplan-Meier analysis for CRC patients with International Union Against Cancer (UICC) stages I-IV and found that tumors expressing high levels of miR-200c, recently connected to EMT, are correlated with poorer prognosis, regardless of tumor stage. These investigators also found that p53 mutation, commonly found in CRC, is strongly associated with greater than twofold miR-200c over-expression [36]. Chen and co-workers (2010) identified siginificant decrease of miR-148a and miR-152 expression levels in CRC (both $p < 0.001$) tissue in comparison to their matched non-tumoral tissues. Authors further observed correlation of low expression levels of miR-152 and miR-148a with increased tumor size ($p = 0.004$ and $0.018$, respectively), and advanced pT stage ($p = 0.002$ and $0.023$, respectively) [37].

MiR-21 is up-regulated in many solid tumors, including CRC [52]. Recently, we have found that miR-21 over-expression shows a strong correlation with the established prognostic factors as nodal stage, metastatic disease and UICC stage [38]. Kulda and co-workers (2010) correlated miR-21 and miR-143 expression to disease-free interval (DFI) ($p = 0.0026$ and $0.0191$, respectively). There was shorter DFI in patients with a higher expression of miR-21 and, surprisingly, also in patients with a higher expression of miR-143, which is a putative tumor suppressor [39]. Using class comparison analysis, Shetter eand co-workers (2008) later found that 37 miRNAs were differentially expressed in tumors of CRC patients. From this group, miR-20a, miR-21, miR-106a, miR-181b, and miR-203 were found by Cox regression analysis to be associated also with poor survival and were selected for validation. Validation was performed by measuring miRNAs' expression using qRT-PCR in tumor and paired non-tumor tissues in the validation cohort. In the validation set, only high expression of miR-21 was significantly associated with poor prognosis, and this association was independent of age, sex, and tumor location. Multivariate analysis further revealed that high miR-21 expression in tumors was associated with poor survival, independent of the tumor stage. In patients who received adjuvant therapy, high miR-21 expression indicated a poor response to therapy [40].

Schepeler and co-workers (2008) found that miRNAs were associated with tumor microsatellite status in stage II colon cancer. The predictive molecular signature was composed of only four miRNAs (miR-142-3p, miR-212, miR-151, and miR-144). Furthermore, a biomarker based on miRNA expression profiles could predict recurrence of disease with an overall performance accuracy of 81%, thus, indicating a potential role for miRNAs in determining tumor aggressiveness. Kaplan-Meier survival curves showed that patients who had stage II CRC tumors with high expression of miR-320 or miR-498 had significantly shorter progression-free survival than did patients whose tumors showed low expression. These miRNAs were correlated with the probability of progression-free survival also by multivariate analysis. Although these results are promising, larger studies will be needed to prove whether miRNAs really have significant potential to extend prognostic information based on the recent standard diagnostic procedures [41].

Another important question for management of CRC patients is the possibility of predicting therapy response. Nakajima and co-workers (2006) evaluated the significance of five mature miRNAs in tumors of CRC patients treated with 5-fluorouracil-based antimetabolite S-1. They identified let-7g and miR-181b as significant indicators for chemoresponse to S-1-based chemotherapy [42].

A study published by Rossi and co-workers (2007) reported a suggestive pattern of miRNAs rearrangement in HT-29 and HCT-116 human colon cancer cell lines after exposure to 5-fluorouracil (5-FU), a classical antimetabolite in broad clinical use. At clinically relevant concentrations, the drug up-regulated or down-regulated *in vitro* the expression of 19 and 3 miRNAs, respectively, by a factor of not less than two-fold. In some instances, 5-FU upregulated miRNAs that are already over-expressed in tumor tissue, including, for example, miR-21 [43].

In other instances, by contrast, the drug influenced the expression of miRNAs in a direction that is opposite to that induced by neoplastic transformation. A typical example is provided by miR-200b, which is up-regulated in various tumors but down-regulated by treatment with 5-FU. Interestingly, it is known that miR-200b targets mRNA that codes for a protein tyrosine phosphatase (PTPN12) which inactivates products of oncogenes, such as ABL, SRC or KRAS [41].

Another study evaluated changes in miRNA expression profiles as a response to therapy, focusing on the effects of capecitabine chemoradiotherapy on rectal tumors *in vivo* [44]. Tumor microexcisions were taken before starting a therapy and, again, after a two-week therapy. The extent of tumor response to the therapy was investigated microscopically by an experienced pathologist according to Mandard's tumor regression criteria. In this study, many miRNAs (miR-10a, miR-21, miR-145, miR-212, miR-339, and miR-361) responded to capecitabine chemoradiotherapy in individual tumor samples. In most samples, however, only two miRNAs, miR-125b and miR-137, showed significant increase in expression levels after two-week therapy [44].

Zhou and co-workers (2010) determined how 5-FU and oxaliplatin (L-OHP) modify the expression profiles (856 human miRNA probes) of miRNAs in HCT-8 and HCT-116 colon cancer cells. Fifty-six up- and 50 down-regulations of miRNA expression with statistical significance were identified in colon cancer cells following exposure to 5-FU or L-OHP compared to matched control cells. Expression levels of miR-197, miR-191, miR-92a, miR-93, miR-222, and miR-1826 were significantly down-regulated in both cell lines after the treatment of one drug or in one cell line following exposure to either drug [45].

HCT116 human colorectal cancer cells were used to investigate the biological and potential chemosensitizing role of miR-143 in the study of Borralho and co-workers (2009). Transient miR-143 over-expression resulted in an approximate 60% reduction in cell viability. In addition, stable miR-143 over-expressing cells were selected with G418 and exposed to 5-FU. Increased stable expression of miR-143 was associated with decreased viability and increased cell death after exposure to 5-FU. These changes were associated with increased nuclear fragmentation and caspase -3, -8, and -9 activities. In addition, extracellular-regulated protein kinase 5, NF-kappaB and Bcl-2 protein expression were down-regulated by miR-143, and further reduced by exposure to 5-FU [46].

MiR-215, through the suppression of denticleless protein homolog (DTL), a cell cycle-regulated nuclear and centrosome protein, induces decreased colon cancer cell proliferation by causing G2-arrest, thereby leading to an increase in their chemoresistance to the chemotherapeutic agents, methotrexate and Tomudex [47].

Boni and co-workers (2010) investigated associations between 18 polymorphisms in both miRNA-containing genomic regions (primary and precursor miRNA) and in genes related to miRNA biogenesis with clinical outcome in 61 metastatic colorectal cancer (mCRC) patients treated with 5-FU and irinotecan (CPT-11). A significant association with tumor response and time to progression (TTP) was found for SNP rs7372209 in pri-miR26a-1 ($p = 0.041$ and *0.017*, respectively). The genotypes CC and CT were favorable when compared with the TT variant genotype. SNP rs1834306, located in the pri-miR-100 gene, significantly correlated with a longer TTP ($p = 0.04$). In the miRNA-biogenesis pathway, a trend was identified between SNP rs11077 in the exportin-5 gene and disease control rate ($p = 0.076$) [48].

Despite these results, more studies that will examine the effects of chemotherapeutic agents on the miRNA expression profiles and their possible usage for predicting therapy response in CRC patients are needed.

## 5.6. MiRNAs as Potential Therapeutic Targets

Since miRNAs constitute a robust network for gene regulation, they possess a great potential, as both a novel class of therapeutic targets and a powerful intervention tool. The biosynthesis, maturation and activity of miRNAs can be manipulated with various oligonucleotides that encode the sequences complementary to mature miRNAs [8]. Overexpression of miRNAs can be induced either by using synthetic miRNA mimics or chemically modified oligonucleotides. Conversely, miRNAs can be silenced by antisense oligonucleotides and "antagomirs" (synthetic analogues of miRNAs). Cross-sensitivity with endogenous miRNAs and lack of specificity for cancer cells can cause non-specific side effects during miRNA modulation therapy. However, the use of an effective delivery system and less toxic synthetic anti-miRNA oligonucleotides may minimize such side effects [49,50]. Gene therapies may be designed to treat CRC and to block the progression of precursor lesions by manipulating the tumor suppressive or oncogenic miRNAs. Such manipulation may control the tumor growth rate and have potential as a new therapy for both early and advanced cancers [51].

Studies have revealed that inhibition of miR-21 and miR-17-92 activity is associated with reduced tumor growth, invasion, angiogenesis and metastasis [52,53]. Moreover, overexpression of miR-21 is associated with low sensitivity and poor response to chemotherapy, and its inhibition may improve the response to chemotherapy [52]. On the other hand, restoration of miR-145 expression has been associated with inhibition of tumor cells growth via downregulation of IRS-1. Expression levels of miR-145, down-regulated in tumor tissues of CRC patients, were increased *in vitro* and caused reduced cell proliferation and increased sensitivity to radiotherapy [54]. These miRNAs present only examples of miRNAs validated as oncogenes or tumor suppressors in CRC and thus of potential candidates for miRNA-based targeted CRC therapy. Targeting such miRNAs may help to not only prevent the recurrence of disease in high-risk tumors in UICC stage II and control the growth of advanced metastatic tumors, but they also could provide another possibility for chemo- and radio-resistant cancer patients. Although experimental miRNA therapy results look promising, only a limited number of studies have been conducted under *in vivo* conditions in animal models. There is still a long way to go to reach clinical testing of the first miRNA-based therapy for CRC in the future.

## Acknowledgment

This work was supported by grants NS 10361-3/2009, NR/9814-4/2008, NS 10352-3/2009, NT/11214-4/2010 of Czech Ministry of Health, Project No. MZ0MOU2005 of the Czech Ministry of Health and by the project "CEITEC – Central European Institute of Technology" (CZ.1.05/1.1.00/02.0068).

## References

[1] Benson AB, 3rd: Epidemiology, disease progression, and economic burden of colorectal cancer. *J. Manag. Care Pharm.* 2007 13:S5-18.

[2] Rossi S, Kopetz S, Davuluri R, Hamilton SR, Calin GA: MicroRNAs, ultraconserved genes and colorectal cancers. *Int. J. Biochem. Cell Biol.* 2010 42:1291-7.

[3] Slaby O, Svoboda M, Michalek J, Vyzula R: MicroRNAs in colorectal cancer: translation of molecular biology into clinical application. *Mol. Cancer* 2009 8:102.

[4] Grady WM, Tewari M: The next thing in prognostic molecular markers: microRNA signatures of cancer. *Gut* 2010 59:706-8.

[5] Croce CM: Causes and consequences of microRNA dysregulation in cancer. *Nat. Rev. Genet* 2009 10:704-14.

[6] Fearon ER, Vogelstein B: A genetic model for colorectal tumorigenesis. *Cell* 1990 61:759-67.
[7] Faber C, Kirchner T, Hlubek F: The impact of microRNAs on colorectal cancer. *Virchows Arch.* 2009 454:359-67.
[8] Aslam MI, Taylor K, Pringle JH, Jameson JS: MicroRNAs are novel biomarkers of colorectal cancer. *Br. J. Surg.* 2009 96:702-10.
[9] Cho WC: MicroRNAs in cancer - from research to therapy. *Biochim. Biophys. Acta* 1805:209-17.
[10] Cho WC: MicroRNAs: potential biomarkers for cancer diagnosis, prognosis and targets for therapy. *Int. J. Biochem. Cell Biol.* 2010 42:1273-81.
[11] Ryan BM, Robles AI, Harris CC: Genetic variation in microRNA networks: the implications for cancer research. *Nat. Rev. Cancer* 2010 10:389-402.
[12] Kim MS, Oh JE, Kim YR, Park SW, Kang MR, Kim SS, Ahn CH, Yoo NJ, Lee SH: Somatic mutations and losses of expression of microRNA regulation-related genes AGO2 and TNRC6A in gastric and colorectal cancers. *J. Pathol.* 2010 221:139-46.
[13] Lee HC, Kim JG, Chae YS, Sohn SK, Kang BW, Moon JH, Jeon SW, Lee MH, Lim KH, Park JY, Choi GS, Jun SH: Prognostic impact of microRNA-related gene polymorphisms on survival of patients with colorectal cancer. *J. Cancer Res. Clin. Oncol.* 2010 136:1073-8.
[14] Landi D, Gemignani F, Naccarati A, Pardini B, Vodicka P, Vodickova L, Novotny J, Forsti A, Hemminki K, Canzian F, Landi S: Polymorphisms within micro-RNA-binding sites and risk of sporadic colorectal cancer. *Carcinogenesis* 2008 29:579-84.
[15] Zhang W, Winder T, Ning Y, Pohl A, Yang D, Kahn M, Lurje G, Labonte MJ, Wilson PM, Gordon MA, Hu-Lieskovan S, Mauro DJ, Langer C, Rowinsky EK, Lenz HJ: A let-7 microRNA-binding site polymorphism in 3'-untranslated region of KRAS gene predicts response in wild-type KRAS patients with metastatic colorectal cancer treated with cetuximab monotherapy. *Ann. Oncol.* 2011 22:104-9.
[16] Chen X, Ba Y, Ma L, Cai X, Yin Y, Wang K, Guo J, Zhang Y, Chen J, Guo X, Li Q, Li X, Wang W, Zhang Y, Wang J, Jiang X, Xiang Y, Xu C, Zheng P, Zhang J, Li R, Zhang H, Shang X, Gong T, Ning G, Wang J, Zen K, Zhang J, Zhang CY: Characterization of microRNAs in serum: a novel class of biomarkers for diagnosis of cancer and other diseases. *Cell Res.* 2008 18:997-1006.
[17] Ng EK, Chong WW, Jin H, Lam EK, Shin VY, Yu J, Poon TC, Ng SS, Sung JJ: Differential expression of microRNAs in plasma of patients with colorectal cancer: a potential marker for colorectal cancer screening. *Gut* 2009 58:1375-81.
[18] Huang Z, Huang D, Ni S, Peng Z, Sheng W, Du X: Plasma microRNAs are promising novel biomarkers for early detection of colorectal cancer. *Int. J. Cancer* 2010 127:118-26.
[19] Link A, Balaguer F, Shen Y, Nagasaka T, Lozano JJ, Boland CR, Goel A: Fecal MicroRNAs as novel biomarkers for colon cancer screening. *Cancer Epidemiol. Biomarkers Prev.* 2010 19:1766-74.
[20] Garzon R, Fabbri M, Cimmino A, Calin GA, Croce CM: MicroRNA expression and function in cancer. *Trends Mol. Med.* 2006 12:580-7.
[21] Lu J, Getz G, Miska EA, Alvarez-Saavedra E, Lamb J, Peck D, Sweet-Cordero A, Ebert BL, Mak RH, Ferrando AA, Downing JR, Jacks T, Horvitz HR, Golub TR: MicroRNA expression profiles classify human cancers. *Nature* 2005 435:834-8.

[22] Gaur A, Jewell DA, Liang Y, Ridzon D, Moore JH, Chen C, Ambros VR, Israel MA: Characterization of microRNA expression levels and their biological correlates in human cancer cell lines. *Cancer Res.* 2007 67:2456-68.

[23] Michael MZ, SM OC, van Holst Pellekaan NG, Young GP, James RJ: Reduced accumulation of specific microRNAs in colorectal neoplasia. *Mol. Cancer Res.* 2003 1:882-91.

[24] Bandres E, Cubedo E, Agirre X, Malumbres R, Zarate R, Ramirez N, Abajo A, Navarro A, Moreno I, Monzo M, Garcia-Foncillas J: Identification by Real-time PCR of 13 mature microRNAs differentially expressed in colorectal cancer and non-tumoral tissues. *Mol. Cancer* 2006 5:29.

[25] Wang CJ, Zhou ZG, Wang L, Yang L, Zhou B, Gu J, Chen HY, Sun XF: Clinicopathological significance of microRNA-31, -143 and -145 expression in colorectal cancer. *Dis. Markers* 2009 26:27-34.

[26] Cummins JM, He Y, Leary RJ, Pagliarini R, Diaz LA, Jr., Sjoblom T, Barad O, Bentwich Z, Szafranska AE, Labourier E, Raymond CK, Roberts BS, Juhl H, Kinzler KW, Vogelstein B, Velculescu VE: The colorectal microRNAome. *Proc. Natl. Acad. Sci. USA* 2006 103:3687-92.

[27] Volinia S, Calin GA, Liu CG, Ambs S, Cimmino A, Petrocca F, Visone R, Iorio M, Roldo C, Ferracin M, Prueitt Rl, Yanaihara N, Lanza G, Scarpa A, Vecchione A, Negrini M, Harris CC, Croce CM: A microRNA expression signature of human solid tumors defines cancer gene targets. *Proc. Natl. Acad. Sci. USA* 2006 103:2257-61.

[28] Motoyama K, Inoue H, Takatsuno Y, Tanaka F, Mimori K, Uetake H, Sugihara K, Mori M: Over- and under-expressed microRNAs in human colorectal cancer. *Int. J. Oncol.* 2009 34:1069-75.

[29] Lanza G, Ferracin M, Gafa R, Veronese A, Spizzo R, Pichiorri F, Liu CG, Calin GA, Croce CM, Negrini M: mRNA/microRNA gene expression profile in microsatellite unstable colorectal cancer. *Mol. Cancer* 2007 6:54.

[30] Earle JS, Luthra R, Romans A, Abraham R, Ensor J, Yao H, Hamilton SR: Association of microRNA expression with microsatellite instability status in colorectal adenocarcinoma. *J. Mol. Diagn* 2010 12:433-40.

[31] Sarver AL, French AJ, Borralho PM, Thayanithy V, Oberg AL, Silverstein KA, Morlan BW, Riska SM, Boardman LA, Cunningham JM, Subramanian S, Wang L, Smyrk TC, Rodrigues CM, Thibodeau SN, Steer CJ: Human colon cancer profiles show differential microRNA expression depending on mismatch repair status and are characteristic of undifferentiated proliferative states. *BMC Cancer* 2009 9:401.

[32] Monzo M, Navarro A, Bandres E, Artells R, Moreno I, Gel B, Ibeas R, Moreno J, Martinez F, Diaz T, Martinez A, Balagué O, Garcia-Foncillas J: Overlapping expression of microRNAs in human embryonic colon and colorectal cancer. *Cell Res.* 2008 18:823-33.

[33] Rosenfeld N, Aharonov R, Meiri E, Rosenwald S, Spector Y, Zepeniuk M, Benjamin H, Shabes N, Tabak S, Levy A, Lebanony D, Goren Y, Silberschein E, Targan N, Ben-Ari A, Gilad S, Sion-Vardy N, Tobar A, Feinmesser M, Kharenko O, Nativ O, Nass D, Perelman M, Yosepovich A, Shalmon B, Polak-Charcon S, Fridman A, Avniel A, Bentwich I, Cohen D, Chajut A, Barshack I: MicroRNAs accurately identify cancer tissue origin. *Nat. Biotechnol.* 2008 26:462-9.

[34] Lujambio A, Calin GA, Villanueva A, Ropero S, Sanchez-Cespedes M, Blanco D, Montuenga LM, Rossi S, Nicoloso MS, Faller WJ, Gallagher WM, Eccles SA,, Croce CM, Esteller M: A microRNA DNA methylation signature for human cancer metastasis. *Proc. Natl. Acad. Sci. USA* 2008 105:13556-61.

[35] Huang ZM, Yang J, Shen XY, Zhang XY, Meng FS, Xu JT, Zhang BF, Gao HJ: MicroRNA expression profile in non-cancerous colonic tissue associated with lymph node metastasis of colon cancer. *J. Dig. Dis.* 2009 10:188-94.

[36] Xi Y, Formentini A, Chien M, Weir DB, Russo JJ, Ju J, Kornmann M: Prognostic Values of microRNAs in Colorectal Cancer. *Biomark Insights* 2006 2:113-21.

[37] Chen Y, Song Y, Wang Z, Yue Z, Xu H, Xing C, Liu Z: Altered expression of MiR-148a and MiR-152 in gastrointestinal cancers and its clinical significance. *J. Gastrointest Surg.* 14:1170-9.

[38] Slaby O, Svoboda M, Fabian P, Smerdova T, Knoflickova D, Bednarikova M, Nenutil R, Vyzula R: Altered expression of miR-21, miR-31, miR-143 and miR-145 is related to clinicopathologic features of colorectal cancer. *Oncology* 2007 72:397-402.

[39] Kulda V, Pesta M, Topolcan O, Liska V, Treska V, Sutnar A, Rupert K, Ludvikova M, Babuska V, Holubec L, Jr., Cerny R: Relevance of miR-21 and miR-143 expression in tissue samples of colorectal carcinoma and its liver metastases. *Cancer Genet. Cytogenet.* 2010 200:154-60.

[40] Schetter AJ, Leung SY, Sohn JJ, Zanetti KA, Bowman ED, Yanaihara N, Yuen ST, Chan TL, Kwong DL, Au GK, Liu CG, Calin GA, Croce CM, Harris CG: MicroRNA expression profiles associated with prognosis and therapeutic outcome in colon adenocarcinoma. *JAMA* 2008 299:425-36.

[41] Schepeler T, Reinert JT, Ostenfeld MS, Christensen LL, Silahtaroglu AN, Dyrskjot L, Wiuf C, Sorensen FJ, Kruhoffer M, Laurberg S, Kauppinen S, Orntoft TF, Andersen CL: Diagnostic and prognostic microRNAs in stage II colon cancer. *Cancer Res.* 2008 68:6416-24.

[42] Nakajima G, Hayashi K, Xi Y, Kudo K, Uchida K, Takasaki K, Yamamoto M, Ju J: Non-coding MicroRNAs hsa-let-7g and hsa-miR-181b are Associated with Chemoresponse to S-1 in Colon Cancer. *Cancer Genomics Proteomics* 2006 3:317-24.

[43] Rossi L, Bonmassar E, Faraoni I: Modification of miR gene expression pattern in human colon cancer cells following exposure to 5-fluorouracil in vitro. *Pharmacol Res* 2007 56:248-53.

[44] Svoboda M, Izakovicova Holla L, Sefr R, Vrtkova I, Kocakova I, Tichy B, Dvorak J: Micro-RNAs miR125b and miR137 are frequently upregulated in response to capecitabine chemoradiotherapy of rectal cancer. *Int. J. Oncol.* 2008 33:541-7.

[45] Zhou J, Zhou Y, Yin B, Hao W, Zhao L, Ju W, Bai C: 5-Fluorouracil and oxaliplatin modify the expression profiles of microRNAs in human colon cancer cells in vitro. *Oncol. Rep.* 2010 23:121-8.

[46] Borralho PM, Kren BT, Castro RE, da Silva IB, Steer CJ, Rodrigues CM: MicroRNA-143 reduces viability and increases sensitivity to 5-fluorouracil in HCT116 human colorectal cancer cells. *FEBS J.* 2009 276:6689-700.

[47] Song B, Wang Y, Titmus MA, Botchkina G, Formentini A, Kornmann M, Ju J: Molecular mechanism of chemoresistance by miR-215 in osteosarcoma and colon cancer cells. *Mol. Cancer* 2010 9:96.

[48] Boni V, Zarate R, Villa JC, Bandres E, Gomez MA, Maiello E, Garcia-Foncillas J, Aranda E: Role of primary miRNA polymorphic variants in metastatic colon cancer patients treated with 5-fluorouracil and irinotecan. *Pharmacogenomics J.* 2010 DOI:10.1038/tpj.2010.58

[49] Krutzfeldt J, Rajewsky N, Braich R, Rajeev KG, Tuschl T, Manoharan M, Stoffel M: Silencing of microRNAs in vivo with 'antagomirs'. *Nature* 2005 438:685-9.

[50] Zhang B, Farwell MA: microRNAs: a new emerging class of players for disease diagnostics and gene therapy. *J. Cell Mol. Med.* 2008 12:3-21.

[51] Tong AW, Nemunaitis J: Modulation of miRNA activity in human cancer: a new paradigm for cancer gene therapy? *Cancer Gene Ther.* 2008 15:341-55.

[52] 52. Krichevsky AM, Gabriely G: miR-21: a small multi-faceted RNA. *J. Cell Mol. Med.* 2009 13:39-53.

[53] Dews M, Homayouni A, Yu D, Murphy D, Sevignani C, Wentzel E, Furth EE, Lee WM, Enders GH, Mendell JT, Thomas-Tikhonenko A: Augmentation of tumor angiogenesis by a Myc-activated microRNA cluster. *Nat. Genet.* 2006 38:1060-5.

[54] La Rocca G, Badin M, Shi B, Xu SQ, Deangelis T, Sepp-Lorenzinoi L, Baserga R: Mechanism of growth inhibition by MicroRNA 145: the role of the IGF-I receptor signaling pathway. *J. Cell Physiol.* 2009 220:485-91.

In: MicroRNAs in Solid Cancer
Editor: Ondrej Slaby

ISBN: 978-61324-514-9
©2012 Nova Science Publishers, Inc.

*Chapter VI*

# MicroRNAs and Breast Cancer

*Martina Redova, Marek Svoboda and Rostislav Vyzula*
Masaryk Memorial Cancer Institute, Brno, Czech Republic

## Abstract

Breast cancer is a heterogeneous disease, comprising multiple entities associated with distinctive histological and biological features, clinical presentations and behaviours and responses to therapy. It is the second leading cause of cancer death in women. Despite improvement in treatment over the past few decades, there is an urgent need for development of targeted therapies. MicroRNAs (miRNAs) regulate diverse cellular processes and play an integral role in cancer pathogenesis. Emerging evidences suggest the involvement of altered regulation of miRNAs in the pathogenesis of breast cancer. MiRNAs are therefore thought to be functional as tumor suppressors or oncogenes, and as a consequence not only potential effective biomarkers, but also novel class of therapeutic targets.

## 6.1. Introduction

Breast cancer is the second leading cause of death in women (after lung cancer) and accounts for approximately 15% of female deaths. Male breast cancer accounts for < 1% of total cases. The incidence of this malignancy is highest in developed countries in North America and Western Europe, lowest incidence is, on the contrary, seen in South America, Africa and parts of Asia. The 5-year breast cancer survival rate ranges from 98% for stage I cancer to approximately 16% for stage IV cancer. Death rates from breast cancer have steadily declined since the early 1990s, with the largest decreases among younger women [1].

Most breast cancers are of epithelial origin developing from cells that line ducts or lobules. Cancers are divided into carcinoma in situ which is in fact proliferation of cancer cells within ducts or lobules and without invasion of stromal tissue, and invasive cancer which is a primarily adenocarcinoma accounting 80% of an infiltrating ductal type. As mentioned, the most common type of breast carcinoma is the so-called invasive ductal carcinomas not otherwise specified (IDC-NOS) or of no special type (IDC-NST), which is a diagnosis of exclusion and comprises adenocarcinomas that fail to exhibit sufficient characteristics to warrant their classification in one of the special types [2, 3].

From the molecular point of view, breast cancer is a heterogeneous disease and different subgroups can be recognized on the basis of the steroid receptors, HER2, cytokeratin expression and proliferation patterns. As a result of gene expression profiling studies, five major groups can be recognized, of which the triple-negative and basal-like tumors have the poorest prognosis. Many of these tumors have a high proliferation that has the strongest prognostic value in node negative breast cancer [4].

Despite advances in early detection and the understanding of the molecular bases of breast cancer biology, about 30% of patients with early-stage breast cancer have recurrent disease. To offer more effective and less toxic treatment, selecting therapies requires considering the patient and the clinical and molecular characteristics of the tumor. Systemic treatment of breast cancer includes cytotoxic, hormonal, and immunotherapeutic agents. These medications are used in the adjuvant, neoadjuvant, and palliative settings. However, after a variable period of time, progression occurs. The rates of local and systemic recurrence vary within different series, but in general, distant recurrences are dominant, strengthening the hypothesis that breast cancer is a systemic disease from presentation [5].

To offer better treatment with increased efficacy and lower toxicity, individualized therapies based on the patient and the clinical and molecular characteristics of the tumor is necessary. A rapidly growing number of studied focusing miRNAs significance not only in basic, but also in translational breast cancer research, indicates that miRNAs might fulfill such demands.

## 6.2. Polymorphisms within Mature miRNA Sequence and miRNA Binding Regions and Risk of Cancer

MiRNAs regulate pathways involved in cell differentiation, proliferation, development, and apoptosis by degradation of target mRNAs and/or repression of their translation. Although the single nucleotide polymorphisms (SNPs) in miRNAs target sites have been studied, the effects of SNPs in miRNA itself are largely unknown. Common SNPs in miRNAs may change their property through altering miRNA expression and/or maturation, and thus they may have an effect on thousands of target mRNAs, resulting in diverse functional consequences.

Shen et al. (2008) focused on miR-146a and its predicted target genes BRCA1 and BRCA2, in concrete on a G to C polymorphism (rs2910164) located within the sequence of miR-146a precursor, which leads to a change from a G:U pair to a C:U mismatch in its stem region. They found out that breast cancer patients who had at least one miR-146a variant allele were diagnosed at an earlier age than those with no variant alleles (median age 45 versus 56, $p = 0.029$), in other words, that breast cancer patients with variant C allele miR-146a may have high levels of mature miR-146 and that these variants predispose them to an earlier age of onset of familial breast and ovarian cancers [6]. These findings were further confirmed by Pastrello et al. (2010) also on BRCA1/BRCA2-negative familial breast cancer patients [7]. Also Song et al. (2009) paid attention to early age of breast cancer onset and their data suggest that the miR-502-binding site SNP in the 3' UTR of SET8, which methylates p53 and regulates genome stability, modulates SET8 expression and contributes to the early development of breast cancer, either independently or together with the the SNP in codon 72 of p53 gene [8].

Common sequence variant rs11614913 (C to T) in miR-196a-2 was found to be significantly associated with decreased breast cancer risk (for homozygous variant: OR 0.44; 95% CI 0.28-0.70). It might have a potentially oncogenic role in breast tumorigenesis, and the functional genetic variant in its mature region could serve as a novel biomarker for breast cancer susceptibility [9]. Furthermore, SNPs inside miRNA target sites of miR-187 and miR-138 (rs1982073-TGFB1 and rs1799782-XRCC1, respectively) may alter miRNA gene regulation and, consequently, protein expression, contributing to the likelihood of cancer susceptibility, by a novel mechanism of subtle gene regulation [10].

In premenopausal women, who are not typical breast cancer patients, a variant affecting a putative miRNA target site in estrogen receptor 1 (ESR1) was found to be associated with breast cancer risk. According to *in silico* analysis, ESR1 rs2747648 affects the binding capacity of miR-453, which is stronger when the C allele is present. In contrast, the T allele attenuates the binding of miR-453, which might lead to a reduced miRNA-mediated ESR1 repression, in consequence higher ESR1 protein levels and an increased breast cancer risk. Thus, the breast cancer protective effect observed for the C allele in premenopausal women is biologically reasonable [11]. In the same-aged women, Yang et al. (2010) described the SNP rs895819, located in the terminal loop of pre-miRNA-27a, showing a protective effect. In a large familial breast cancer study cohort, age stratification revealed that the protective effect of the rare G allele of rs895819 was mainly observed in the age group < 50 years of age (G versus A: OR 0.83; 95% CI 0.70-0.98; p = 0.0314), whereas no significant effect was observed in the age group > or =50 years of age, indicating a possible hormone-related effect. It has been shown that artificial mutations in the terminal loop of miR-27a can block the maturation process of the miRNA and on the basis of these findings they hypothesize that the G-variant of rs895819 might impair the maturation of the oncogenic miR-27a and thus, is associated with familial breast cancer risk [12].

## 6.3. Serum and Plasma miRNAs: Early Detection of Disease Onset and Progression

As the presence of malignant tumors are clinically determined and/or confirmed upon biopsy examination - which in itself may have detrimental effects in terms of stimulating cancer progression/metastases - the search for sensitive, non-invasive markers that represent tumor-associated changes in the peripheral blood would be highly advantageous and might facilitate early detection of breast cancer as well as monitoring of tumor progression and treatment responses. Routine laboratory tests (CA15.3, CEA, TPA) lack the sensitivity to be of major clinical value. Recent blood-based miRNA profiling studies, reporting their presence in serum and plasma, have generated the concept that circulating miRNAs remain much potential as novel non-invasive biomarkers for cancer and other disease processes.

There is a number of studies focusing on serum/plasma miRNA and their possible deregulation. For example, Roth et al. (2010) dealt with miRNAs associated with tumor progression. They have found that relative concentrations of total RNA (p = 0.0001) and miR-155 (p = 0.0001) in serum significantly discriminated non-metastatic primary breast cancer patients (M0) from healthy women, whereas miR-10b (p = 0.005), miR-34a (p = 0.001) and miR-155 (p = 0.008) discriminated patients suffering from metastatic disease (M1) from healthy controls. In breast cancer patients, the changes in the levels of total RNA (p =0.0001), miR-10b (p = 0.01), miR-34a (p = 0.003), and miR-155 (p = 0.002) correlated with the presence of overt metastases. Furthermore, they described that within the M0-cohort, patients at advanced tumor stages (pT3 to 4) had significantly more total RNA (p = 0.0001) and miR-34a (p = 0.01) in their blood than patients at early tumor stages (pT1 to 2) [13].

Regarding correlation and quantification of miRNA aberrant expression in tissues and sera from patients with breast tumor Wang et al. (2010) focused on miR-21, miR-126, miR-155, miR-199a, and miR-335 relative expression which was closely associated with clinicopathologic features of breast cancer (p < 0.05), such as histological tumor grades and hormone receptor expression. They found miR-21, miR-106a, and miR-155 significantly over-expressed in the tumor specimens compared with those in normal controls (p < 0.05), and miR-126, miR-199a and miR-335 significantly under-expressed (p < 0.05) [14]. Diagnostic and prognostic potential of circulating miR-21 in breast cancer was confirmed also by Asaga et al. (2011) who also described that high circulating miR-21 levels were significantly correlated (p < 0.001) with visceral metastasis [15].

According to the clinical management during the perioperative period, Heneghan et al. (2010) confirmed that circulating levels of miR-195 and let-7a decreased in cancer patients postoperatively to levels comparable with control subjects, following curative tumor resection. Furthermore, they found that specific circulating miRNAs correlated with certain clinicopathological variables, namely nodal status and estrogen receptor status [16].

Concerning hormone sensitivity in breast cancer, findings of Zhu et al. (2009) who revealed that miR-155 may be differentially expressed in the serum of women with hormone sensitive compared to women with hormone insensitive breast cancer, are very interesting with an important clinical impact [17].

## 6.4. Tissue miRNA Signatures: Implications for Diagnostic Oncology

In various profiling studies which provide information on both the developmental lineage and the differentiation state of tumor samples, breast cancer clinico-pathological features, such as estrogen and progesterone receptor status, proliferation index, vascular invasion and tumor stage, have been revealed to correlate also with miRNA expression profiles [18-21].

According to the particular breast cancer subtypes, Blenkiron et al. (2007), on the basis of integrated analysis of miRNA expression, mRNA expression and genomic changes, found that many miRNAs were differentially expressed among basal-like, luminal A, luminal B, HER2+ and normal-like subtypes. They recognised a miRNA signature that differentiated basal from luminal subtypes in their samples, and they identified nine miRNAs that were differentially expressed between luminal A and luminal B tumors (miR-100, miR-99a, miR-130a, miR-126, miR-136, miR-146b, miR-15b, miR-107, and miR-103) [20,22].

As it has been previously described, in cancer cell, miRNAs may function as tumor suppressors and oncogenes. For example, miR-206 which has been described to be more strongly expressed in estrogen-receptor-α-negative (ERα) breast tumors, suggesting a role of miR-206 in regulation of the estrogen receptor gene ERα (ESR1) [19,22]. Furthemore, ESR1 mRNA was confirmed as a direct target of miR-18a, miR-18b, miR-193b, and miR-302c in breast cancer cells, and moreover, these miRNAs were shown to induce cell cycle arrest and to inhibit estrogen-induced proliferation [24,25].

Another miRNA recognized as a putative tumor suppressor, is miR-17-5p, member of the cluster miR-17-92, also known as miR-91, which is located on chromosome 13q31, a genomic region that undergoes loss of heterozygosity in multiple cancers, including breast cancer. MiR-17-5p was shown to be expressed in very low concentrations in breast cancer and was also shown to down-regulate the oncogene AIB1 (amplified in breast cancer 1) [26].

Tumor suppressor miRNA associated also with cancer cells proliferation is let-7 family which is conserved throughout the animal phyla and is poorly expressed or even deleted in many human cancers [25]. As for breast cancer, the expression of let-7 is lost in an early stage in development of this malignity [27].

MiR-125a and miR-125b, down-regulated in HER2-amplified and HER2-over-expressing breast cancers, suppress cell growth and favors apoptosis in breast cancer cell lines via targeting the mRNA encoding the RNA-stabilizing protein HuR, and moreover, their artificial over-expression in SKBR3 cells (a HER2-dependent human breast cancer cell line) suppresses HER2 and HER3 mRNA and protein levels, leading to a reduction in anchorage-dependent growth, cell motility, and invasiveness [28,29].

Regarding the metastatic potential of breast cancer cells, the process of epithelial-mesenchymal transition (EMT) and consequently EMT inducers ZEB1 and ZEB2, which has been described as direct targets of miR-200 family, play a crucial role. It has been postulated that a decrease in miR-200 family miRNAs was associated with highly aggressive, metastatic breast tumors and that regulation of these miRNAs is an essential step in tumor metastasis [25].

According to metastatic process, miR-31 was recently shown to prevent metastasis at multiple steps by inhibiting the expression of prometastatic genes [30]. The abundance of miR-31 was shown to be dependent on the metastatic state of the tumor. It is moderately decreased in non-metastatic breast cancer cell lines and is almost undetectable in metastatic mouse and human breast cancer cell lines [25].

The set of miRNAs with tumor suppressor role could be supplemented by miR-335, one of the most down-regulated miRNA in metastatic breast cancer [31], miR-27b which is included in the modulation of the tumor response to anti-cancer drugs [32], miR-34a which has been described as beeing transcriptionally regulated by p53 [33], and miR-126 which might inhibit cell cycle progression from G1/G0 to S [34].

To complete the list of miRNAs involved in breast cancer tumorigenesis, miR-21, which plays a key role in tumor growth, invasion and metastasis by targeting multiple anti-metastatic genes, has to be mentioned. MiR-21 was one of the first identified oncogenic miRNAs, being over-expressed in both male and female breast tumors compared with normal breast tissue, and has been associated with advanced stage, lymph node positivity, and reduced survival time [35]. Confirmed targets of miR-21 – TPM1 (tropomyosin 1), PDCD4 (programmed cell death-4), and Maspin were shown to reduce invasiveness of a metastatic breast cancer cell line [36].

Other important dysregulated oncogenic miRNA is miR-155. This miRNA is highly expressed in invasive tumors but not in non-invasive cancer tissues enabling their discrimination, and furthermore, direct inhibition of the RhoA expression, which is a gene that regulates many cellular processes, including cell adhesion, motility, and polarity, and is an important modulator of cell junction formation and stability [25]. Moreover, miR-10b, member of a miR-10 family, was the first miRNA found to influence the metastatic potential of human cancer cells, and described as highly expressed only in metastatic cancer cells, promoting cell migration and invasion *in vitro* and initiate tumor invasion and metastasis *in vivo* [37]. Controversial role plays miR-17-92 cluster – as it tends to be deleted in breast tumors, a simplistic picture of this cluster as an oncogenic group of miRNAs is inadequate, it is more likely that some members are oncogenic and some are tumor-suppressive in a context-dependent manner [38,39].

While individual miRNAs are capable of distinguishing between different breast tumors, multiple miRNAs in combination significantly enhance the predictive power of these models. The study of Lowery et al. (2009) demonstrates that ANN analysis (artificial neural networks) reliably identifies biologically relevant miRNAs associated with specific breast cancer phenotypes [40]. The association of specific miRNAs with ER (estrogen receptor), PR (progesterone) and HER2/neu status indicates a role for these miRNAs in disease classification of breast cancer. The ER signature consisted of six miRNA transcripts (miR-342, miR-299, miR-217, miR-190, miR-135b, miR-218), and discriminated cases correctly with a median accuracy of 100% when classifying between ER-positive and ER-negative phenotypes. Similarly, four miRNA transcripts (miR-520g, miR-377, miR-527-518a, miR-520f-520c) were identified that predicted tumor PR status with 100% accuracy, and HER2/neu status was predicted with 100% accuracy by a signature of five miRNAs (miR-520d, miR-181c, miR-302c, miR-376b, miR-30e) [40].

**Table 6.1. List of representative miRNAs differentially expressed in breast cancer mentioned in at least two miRNA profiling studies**

| Up-regulated miRNAs in breast cancer | | Down-regulated miRNAs in breast cancer | |
|---|---|---|---|
| miRNA | Reference, Fold Change (FC), p-value | miRNA | Reference, Fold Change (FC), p-value |
| miR-21 | [19] p = 4.67E-03 [44] FC = 2.84 | miR-335 | [31] p □ 0.0022 [44] FC = 0.29 |
| miR-155 | [19] p = 1.24E-03 [44] FC = 2.29 | miR-320 | [21] FC = -7.0 [44] FC = 0.29 |
| let-7f | [19] p = 6.57E-03 [44] FC = 2.39 | | |
| let-7a | [19] p = 1.49E-02 [21] FC = 23 | | |

Used methods: [19] miRNA microarrays; [21] Serial Analysis of Gene Expression (SAGE) with a False Discovery Rate of 0.05; [44] miRNA microarray + Real Time PCR.

Regarding the therapeutically challenging triple-negative (ER, PR and Her2/neu) breast tumors, Janssen et al. (2010) observed the presence of miR-532-5p, miR-500, miR-362-5p, and miR-502-3p located at Xp11.23 in these tumors [18], and Radojicic et al. (2011) found miR-21, miR-210, and miR-221 being significantly over-expressed, whereas miR-10b, miR-145, miR-205, and miR-122a significantly under-expressed [41]. Additionally, the supervised analysis performed by Foekens et al. significantly linked miR-210 to metastatic capability (p = 0.05), and bioinformatic analysis coupled this miRNA to hypoxia/VEGF signaling [42].

## 6.5. MiRNAs Expression in Prognosis and Response Prediction

There is an urgent need of specific and reliable prognostic and predictive biomarkers that enable the application of more individualized therapies to different molecular subgroups of breast cancer and that enable to quantify the residual risk of patients and indicate the potential value of additional treatment strategies. These subgroups show specific differences regarding biological clinical behavior. In addition to the classical clinical prognostic factors of breast cancer, established molecular biomarkers such as estrogen receptor and progesterone receptor have played a significant role in the selection of patients benefiting from endocrine therapy for many years. Furthermore, the human epidermal growth factor receptor 2 (HER2) has been validated to serve as both prognostic and also predictive marker of response to HER2 targeting therapy. Moreover, as the combination of biomarkers seem to be of clinical importance, the marker of proliferation Ki67 has recently emerged as an important marker due to several applications in neoadjuvant therapy in addition to its moderate prognostic value. With the introduction of high-throughput technologies, numerous multigene signatures (OncoTypeDX, Agendia MammaPrint) have been identified that aim to outperform traditional markers. From this point of view, miRNA become relevant. Careful randomized prospective testing and comparison with existing established factors will be required to justify their routine use for breast cancer therapy decision-making [43].

Yan et al. (2008) identified the differentiated miRNAs expression profile in breast cancer patients and revealed that miR-21 over-expression was correlated with specific breast cancer clinico-pathologic features, such as advanced tumor stage, lymph node metastasis, and poor survival of the patients, indicating that miR-21 may serve as a molecular prognostic marker for breast cancer and disease progression. Furthermore, as miR-21 was up-regulated in tumors presenting lymph node metastases, it could be concluded that its up-regulation was acquired in the course of tumor progression and, in particular, during the acquisition of metastatic potential [44]. Such a prognostic potential of miR-21 was also confirmed by other groups [45,46].

Also members of let-7 family might serve as prognostic markers. Iorio et al. (2008) found that the expression of several members of the let-7 family was down-modulated in breast cancer samples with either lymph node metastasis or higher proliferation index, suggesting that low levels of this miRNA could be associated with poor prognosis. They also found another miRNA which was potentially involved in cancer progression - miR-9-3, which was down-regulated in breast cancers with either high vascular invasion or presence of lymph node metastasis, suggesting that its down-regulation could be acquired in the course of tumor progression and acquisition of cancer metastatic potential [45].

Furthermore, Foekens et al. (2008) identified four miRNAs (miR-7, miR-128a, miR-210, and miR-516–3p) associated with tumor aggressiveness in ER+/LNN (lymph node negative) and miR-210 linked with early relapse in ER-/LNN breast cancer. MiR-210 was also significantly associated with poor outcome in triple-negative breast cancer patients, and this miRNA may prove to be a valuable marker. Moreover, miR-7 and miR-516-3p, which both were associated with pathological grade, were linked to cell cycle deregulation, the pathway currently most frequently linked to prognosis, particularly in ER+ breast cancer [42,47,48].

Other miRNAs with prognostic value for breast cancer include miR-10b and miR-145, expression levels of which correlate with tumor grade, degree of vascular invasion, lymph node metastases, or metastatic potential [45,49]. Also decreased expression of Dicer, a ribonuclease which process the precursor miRNAs to mature miRNAs after their export to cytoplasm, was recently observed in breast cancer, where loss of expression represented an independent prognostic factor in the metastatic disease, and reduced expression of Dicer was associated with the highly aggressive mesenchymal phenotype [50,51].

## 6.6. MiRNAs as Potential Therapeutic Targets

The targeted therapies currently used in the management of breast cancer are directed at HER2/neu and ER receptors; ER-positive tumors are treated with endocrine therapy in the form of selective ER modulators, pure anti-estrogens such as tamoxifen or fulvestrant that completely inhibits ER signaling, or aromatase inhibitors that deplete extragonadal estrogen synthesis. The monoclonal antibody trastuzumab has been developed to target the HER2/neu, while lapatinib inhibits HER2/neu-associated tyrosine kinase activity. The specific combination of receptor status has a significant impact on the outcome of these targeted therapies, for example, the subset of patients who are HER2/neu-negative and ER-negative (basal like/triple negative) are a particular therapeutic challenge as they typically exhibit aggressive clinical behaviour and poor prognosis [40].

As many studies have documented that miRNAs may play important roles in tumorigenesis, the identification of miRNAs with regulatory roles in clinically distinct breast tumor samples could identify novel targets for therapeutic manipulation. There are basically two possible approaches for their use as cancer therapeutic modalities, in concordance to their dual role in carcinogenesis; firstly through antisense-mediated inhibition of oncogenic miRNAs, and secondly through „restoration" of under-expressed tumor suppressor miRNAs with either miRNA mimetics or viral vector-encoded miRNAs [49].

As it has been previously mentioned, miR-21 might serve as a novel therapeutic target. To confirm miR-21 potential, Si et al. (2007) showed that administration of synthetic 2`-O-methyl anti-miRNA oligonucleotides (AMOs) targeting the oncogenic miR-21 potently inhibited breast cancer cell growth *in vitro*, and reduced tumor growth in an MCF-7 breast cancer xenograft mouse model. Additionally, patients indicating resistance to chemotherapeutic agents may profit from findings, that tumor growth reduction capacity of topotecan (a topoisomerase I inhibitor chemotherapeutic agent) can be increased, if administered after anti-miR-21, indicating that suppression of the oncogenic miR-21 can sensitise cancer cells to chemotherapy [52]. The fact that down-regulation of miR-21 enhances chemotherapeutic effect of taxol in breast carcinoma cells is another proof of miR-21 inhibitor gene therapy combined with taxol chemotherapy potential to represent a promising novel therapeutic approach for the treatment of breast malignancies [53].

Regarding ERα, miR-145 was confirmed to down-regulate ERα protein expression expression through direct interaction with two complementary sites within its coding sequence. It was also demonstrated that miR-145 exhibited a pro-apoptotic effect, which is dependent on p53 activation, and that p53 activation can, in turn, stimulate miR-145 expression, thus establishing a death-promoting loop between miR-145 and p53. Such findings support a view that miR-145 re-expression therapy could be mainly envisioned in the specific group of patients with ERα-positive and/or p53 wild-type tumors [54]. Also Xiong et al. (2010) focused on ERα-positive human breast cancer and found out that miR-22 was frequently downregulated in ERα-positive human breast cancer cell lines and clinical samples. Direct involvement in the regulation of ERalpha may be one of the mechanisms through which miR-22 could play a pivotal role in the pathogenesis of breast cancer [55].

In the field of the development of miRNA-based therapeutic strategies aiming to overcome cancer cell resistance, it has been shown that expression of miR-451 is inversely correlated with MDR1 (multidrug resistance 1 gene) expression in breast cancer drug-resistant cells. Furthermore, the enforced increase of miR-451 levels in the MCF-7/DOX (doxorubicin resistant) cells down-regulates expression of MDR1 and increases sensitivity of the MCF-7-resistant cancer cells to doxorubicin [56]. Concerning chemosensitivity, miR-155 was also proved to have therapeutic potential - Kong et al. (2010) showed that ectopic expression of miR-155 induces cell survival and chemoresistance to multiple agents, whereas knockdown of miR-155 renders cells to apoptosis and enhances chemosensitivity [57]. Beside chemosensitivity and chemoresistance of breast cancer cells, miR-34a, in more concrete - its antagonizing, increases the sensitivity of breast cancer cells towards radiation therapy, thus proving the indispensable therapeutic potential of miR-34a [25].

Metastatic potential of breast cancer cells is critical in breast cancer patients management. From this point of view, miR-205, miR-10b, miR-31, and miR-335 are worth noting.

It was observed that ectopic expression of miR-205 significantly inhibits cell proliferation and anchorage-independent growth as well as cell invasion. These findings establish the tumor suppressive role of miR-205, which is probably through direct targeting of oncogenes such as ERBB3 and ZEB1. Therefore, miR-205 may serve as a unique therapeutic target for breast cancer [59].

In a mouse mammary tumor model it was demonstrated that systemic treatment of tumor-bearing mice with miR-10b antagomirs - a class of chemically modified anti-miRNA oligonucleotide -suppresses breast cancer metastasis. According to these results, the miR-10b antagomir, which is well tolerated by normal animals, appears to be a promising candidate for the development of new anti-metastasis agents [59]. Moreover, miR-31 was shown to inhibit metastasis in the early stages of the metastatic cascade. Introducing miR-31 in metastatic breast cancer cells suppressed metastasis-related functions such as motility, invasion and resistance to anoikis *in vitro* and metastasis *in vivo* [25]. Also the restoration of function of miR-335, which is one of the mostly down-regulated miRNAs in metastatic breast cancer cells, through retroviral transduction significantly suppressed metastatic potential of LM2 cells (MDA-MB-231 human breast cancer cell derivatives that are highly metastatic to lung) [31].

## Acknowledgment

This work was supported by grants NS 10361-3/2009, NR/9814-4/2008, NS 10352-3/2009, NT/11214-4/2010 of Czech Ministry of Health, Project No. MZ0MOU2005 of the Czech Ministry of Health.

## References

[1] Weigelt B, Geyer FC, Reis-Filho JS: Histological types of breast cancer: how special are they? *Mol. Oncol.* 2010 4:192-208.

[2] Ellis P, Schnitt SJ, Sastre-Garau X, Bussolati G, Tavassoli FA, Eusebi V, Peterse JL, Mukai K, Tabar L, Jacquemier J, Cornelisse CJ, Sasco AJ, Kaaks R, Pisani P, Goldgar DE, Devilee P, Cleton-Jansen MJ, Borresen-Dale AL, van't Veer L, Sapino A: Invasive breast carcinoma. In: Tavassoli FA, Devilee P (Eds.), WHO Classification of Tumours Pathology and Genetics of Tumours of the Breast and Female Genital Organs. Lyon Press, Lyon. 2003

[3] Narod SA: BRCA mutations in the management of breast cancer: the state of the art. *Nat. Rev. Clin. Oncol.* 2010 7:702-7.

[4] Weigelt B, Reis-Filho JS: Histological and molecular types of breast cancer: is there a unifying taxonomy? *Nat. Rev. Clin. Oncol.* 2009, 6:718-730.

[5] Gonzalez-Angulo AM, Morales-Vasquez F, Hortobagyi GN: Overview of resistance to systemic therapy in patients with breast cancer. *Adv. Exp. Med. Biol.* 2007 608:1-22.

[6] Shen J, Ambrosone CB, DiCioccio RA, Odunsi K, Lele SB, Zhao H: A functional polymorphism in the miR-146a gene and age of familial breast/ovarian cancer diagnosis. *Carcinogenesis* 2008 29:1963-66.

[7] Pastrello C, Polesel J, Della Puppa L, Viel A, Maestro R: Association between hsa-mir-146a genotype and tumor age-of-onset in BRCA1/BRCA2-negative familial breast and ovarian cancer patients. *Carcinogenesis* 2010 31:2124-26.

[8] Song F, Zheng H, Liu B, Wei S, Dai H, Zhang L, Calin GA, Hao X, Wei Q, Zhang W, Chen K: An miR-502-binding site single-nucleotide polymorphism in the 3'-untranslated region of the SET8 gene is associated with early age of breast cancer onset. *Clin. Cancer Res.* 2009 15:6292-300.

[9] Hoffman AE, Zheng T, Yi C, Leaderer D, Weidhaas J, Slack F, Zhang Y, Paranjape T, Zhu Y: microRNA miR-196a-2 and breast cancer: a genetic and epigenetic association study and functional analysis. *Cancer Res.* 2009 69:5970-77.

[10] Nicoloso MS, Sun H, Spizzo R, Kim H, Wickramasinghe P, Shimizu M, Wojcik SE, Ferdin J, Kunej T, Xiao L, Manoukian S, Secreto G, Ravagnani F, Wang X, Radice P, Croce CM, Davuluri RV, Calin GA: Single-nucleotide polymorphisms inside microRNA target sites influence tumor susceptibility. *Cancer Res.* 2010 70:2789-98.

[11] Tchatchou S, Jung A, Hemminki K, Sutter C, Wappenschmidt B, Bugert P, Weber BH, Niederacher D, Arnold N, Varon-Mateeva R, Ditsch N, Meindl A, Schmutzler RK, Bartram CR, Burwinkel B: A variant affecting a putative miRNA target site in estrogen receptor (ESR) 1 is associated with breast cancer risk in premenopausal women. *Carcinogenesis* 2009 30:59-64.

[12] Yang R, Schlehe B, Hemminki K, Sutter C, Bugert P, Wappenschmidt B, Volkmann J, Varon R, Weber BH, Niederacher D, Arnold N, Meindl A, Bartram CR, Schmutzler RK, Burwinkel B: A genetic variant in the pre-miR-27a oncogene is associated with a reduced familial breast cancer risk. *Breast Cancer Res. Treat.* 2010 121:693-702.

[13] Roth C, Rack B, Muller V, Janni W, Pantel K, Schwarzenbach H: Circulating microRNAs as blood-based markers for patients with primary and metastatic breast cancer. *Breast Cancer Res.* 2010 12:R90.

[14] Wang F, Zheng Z, Guo J, Ding X: Correlation and quantitation of microRNA aberrant expression in tissues and sera from patients with breast tumor. *Gynecol. Oncol.* 2010 119:586-93.

[15] Asaga S, Kuo C, Nguyen T, Terpenning M, Giuliano AE, Hoon DS: Direct serum assay for microRNA-21 concentrations in early and advanced breast cancer. *Clin. Chem.* 2011 57:84-91.

[16] Heneghan HM, Miller N, Lowery AJ, Sweeney KJ, Newell J, Kerin MJ: Circulating microRNAs as novel minimally invasive biomarkers for breast cancer. *Ann. Surg.* 2010 251:499-505.

[17] Zhu W, Qin W, Atasoy U, Sauter ER: Circulating microRNAs in breast cancer and healthy subjects. *BMC Res. Notes* 2009 2:89.

[18] Janssen EA, Slewa A, Gudlaugsson E, Jonsdottir K, Skaland I, Soiland H, Baak JP: Biologic profiling of lymph node negative breast cancers by means of microRNA expression. *Mod. Pathol.* 2010 23:1567-76.

[19] Iorio MV, Ferracin M, Liu ChG, Veronese A, Spizzo R, Sabbioni S, Magri E, Pedriali M, Fabbri M, Campiglio M, Ménard S, Palazzo JP, Rosenberg A, Musiani P, Volinia S, Nenci I, Calin GA, Querzoli P, Negrini M, Croce CM: MicroRNA gene expression deregulation in human breast cancer. *Cancer Res.* 2005 65:7065-70.

[20] Khoshnaw SM, Green AR, Powe DG, Ellis IO: MicroRNA involvement in the pathogenesis and management of breast cancer. *J. Clin. Pathol.* 2009 62:422-8.

[21] Nygaard S, Jacobsen A, Lindow M, Eriksen J, Balslev E, Flyger H, Tolstrup N, Møller S, Krogh A, Litman T: Identification and analysis of miRNAs in human breast cancer and teratoma samples using deep sequencing. *BMC Med. Genomics* 2009 2:35.

[22] Blenkiron C, Goldstein LD, Thorne NP, Spiteri I, Chin SF, Dunning MJ, Barbosa-Morais NL, Teschendorff AE, Green AR, Ellis IO, Tavaré S, Caldas C, Miska EA: MicroRNA expression profiling of human breast cancer identifies new markers of tumor subtype. *Genome Biol.* 2007 8:R214.

[23] Kondo N, Toyama T, Sugiura H, Fujii Y, Yamashita H: miR-206 expression is down-regulated in estrogen receptor α-positive human breast cancer. *Cancer Res.* 2008 68:5004-8.

[24] Leivonen SK, Makela R, Ostling P, Kohonen P, Haapa-Paananen S, Kleivi K, Enerly E, Aakula A, Hellstrom K, Sahlberg N, Kristensen VN, Børresen-Dale AL, Saviranta P, Perälä M, Kallioniemi O: Protein lysate microarray analysis to identify microRNAs

regulating estrogen receptor signaling in breast cancer cell lines. *Oncogene* 2009 28:3926-36.

[25] O'Day E, Lal A: MicroRNAs and their target networks in breast cancer. *Breast Cancer Res* 2010 12:201.

[26] Hossain A, Kuo MT, Saunders GF. Mir-17-5p regulates breast cancer cell proliferation by inhibiting translation of AIB1 mRNA. *Mol. Cell Biol.* 2006 26:8191-201.

[27] Sempere LF, Christensen M, Silahtaroglu A, Bak M, Heath CV, Schwartz G, Wells W, Kauppinen S, Cole CN: Altered microRNA expression confined to specific epithelial cell subpopulations in breast cancer. *Cancer Res.* 2007 67:11612-20.

[28] Guo X, Wu Y, Hartley RS: MicroRNA-125a represses cell growth by targeting HuR in breast cancer. *RNA Biol.* 2009 6:575-83.

[29] Scott GK, Goga A, Bhaumik D, Berger CE, Sullivan CS, Benz CC: Coordinate suppression of ERBB2 and ERBB3 by enforced expression of micro-RNA miR-125a or miR-125b. *J. Biol. Chem.* 2007 282:1479-1486.

[30] Valastyan S, Reinhardt F, Benaich N, Calogrias D, Szasz AM, Wang ZC, Brock JE, Richardson AL, Weinberg RA: A pleiotropically acting microRNA, miR-31, inhibits breast cancer metastasis. *Cell* 2009 137:1032-46.

[31] Tavazoie SF, Alarcon C, Oskarsson T, Padua D, Wang Q, Bos PD, Gerald WL, Massagué J: Endogenous human microRNAs that suppress breast cancer metastasis. *Nature* 2008 451:147-52.

[32] Tsuchiya Y, Nakajima M, Takagi S, Taniya T, Yokoi T: MicroRNA regulates the expression of human cytochrome P450 1B1. *Cancer Res.* 2006 66:9090-8.

[33] Kato M, Paranjape T, Muller RU, Ullrich R, Nallur S, Gillespie E, Keane K, Esquela-Kerscher A, Weidhaas JB, Slack FJ: The mir-34 microRNA is required for the DNA damage response in vivo in *C. elegans* and *in vitro* in human breast cancer cells. *Oncogene* 2009 28:2419-24.

[34] Zhang J, Du YY, Lin YF, Chen YT, Yang L, Wang HJ, Ma D: The cell growth suppressor, mir-126, targets IRS-1. *Biochem. Biophys. Res. Commun.* 2008 377:136-40.

[35] Corcoran C, Friel AM, Duffy MJ, Crown J, O'Driscoll L: Intracellular and extracellular microRNAs in breast cancer. *Clin. Chem.* 2011 57:18-32.

[36] Zhu S, Si ML, Wu H, Mo YY: MicroRNA-21 targets the tumor suppressor gene tropomyosin 1 (TPM1). *J. Biol. Chem.* 2007 282:14328-36.

[37] Ma L, Teruya-Feldstein J, Weinberg RA: Tumour invasion and metastasis initiated by microRNA-10b in breast cancer. *Nature* 2007 449:682-8.

[38] Zhang L, Huang J, Yang N, Greshock J, Megraw MS, Giannakakis A, Liang S, Naylor TL, Barchetti A, Ward MR, Yao G, Medina A, O'brien-Jenkins A, Katsaros D, Hatzigeorgiou A, Gimotty PA, Weber BL, Coukos G: MicroRNAs exhibit high frequency genomic alterations in human cancer. *Proc. Natl. Acad. Sci. USA* 2006 103:9136-41.

[39] Le Quesne J, Caldas C: Micro-RNAs and breast cancer. *Mol Oncol* 2010 4:230-41.

[40] Lowery AJ, Miller N, Devaney A, McNeill RE, Davoren PA, Lemetre C, Benes V, Schmidt S, Blake J, Ball G, Kerin MJ: MicroRNA signatures predict oestrogen receptor, progesterone receptor and HER2/neu receptor status in breast cancer. *Breast Cancer Res* 2009 11:R27.

[41] Radojicic J, Zaravinos A, Vrekoussis T, Kafousi M, Spandidos DA, Stathopoulos EN: MicroRNA expression analysis in triple-negative (ER, PR and Her2/neu) breast cancer. *Cell Cycle* 2011 10:507-17.

[42] Foekens JA, Sieuwerts AM, Smid M, Look MP, de Weerd V, Boersma AW, Klijn JG, Wiemer EA, Martens JW: Four miRNAs associated with aggressiveness of lymph node-negative, estrogen receptor-positive human breast cancer. *Proc. Natl. Acad. Sci. USA* 2008 105:13021-6.

[43] Weigel MT, Dowsett M: Current and emerging biomarkers in breast cancer: prognosis and prediction. *Endocr. Relat. Cancer* 2010 17:R245-62.

[44] Yan LX, Huang XF, Shao Q, Huang MY, Deng L, Wu QL, Zeng YX, Shao JY: MicroRNA miR-21 overexpression in human breast cancer is associated with advanced clinical stage, lymph node metastasis and patient poor prognosis. *RNA* 2008 14:2348-60.

[45] Iorio MV, Casalini P, Tagliabue E, Menard S, Croce CM: MicroRNA profiling as a tool to understand prognosis, therapy response and resistance in breast cancer. *Eur. J. Cancer* 2008 44:2753-9.

[46] Wickramasinghe NS, Manavalan TT, Dougherty SM, Riggs KA, Li Y, Klinge CM: Estradiol downregulates miR-21 expression and increases miR-21 target gene expression in MCF-7 breast cancer cells. *Nucleic. Acids Res.* 2009 37:2584-95.

[47] Sotiriou C, Wirapati P, Loi S, Harris A, Fox S, Smeds J, Nordgren H, Farmer P, Praz V, Haibe-Kains B, Desmedt C, Larsimont D, Cardoso F, Peterse H, Nuyten D, Buyse M, Van de Vijver MJ, Bergh J, Piccart M, Delorenzi M: Gene expression profiling in breast cancer: understanding the molecular basis of histologic grade to improve prognosis. *J. Natl. Cancer Inst.* 2006 98:262-72.

[48] Yu JX, Sieuwerts AM, Zhang Y, Martens JW, Smid M, Klijn JG, Wang Y, Foekens JA: Pathway analysis of gene signatures predicting metastasis of node-negative primary breast cancer. *BMC Cancer* 2007 7:182.

[49] Heneghan HM, Miller N, Kerin MJ: MiRNAs as biomarkers and therapeutic targets in cancer. *Curr. Opin. Pharmacol.* 2010 10:543-50.

[50] Grelier G, Voirin N, Ay AS, Cox DG, Chabaud S, Treilleux I, Léon-Goddard S, Rimokh R, Mikaelian I, Venoux C, Puisieux A, Lasset C, Moyret-Lalle C: Prognostic value of Dicer expression in human breast cancers and association with the mesenchymal phenotype. *Br. J. Cancer* 2009 101:673-83.

[51] Veeck J, Esteller M: Breast cancer epigenetics: from DNA methylation to microRNAs. *J Mammary Gland Biol Neoplasia* 2010 15:5-17.

[52] Si ML, Zhu S, Wu H, Lu Z, Wu F, Mo YY: MiR-21-mediated tumor growth. *Oncogene* 2007 26:2799-803.

[53] Mei M, Ren Y, Zhou X, Yuan XB, Han L, Wang GX, Jia Z, Pu PY, Kang CS, Yao Z: Downregulation of miR-21 enhances chemotherapeutic effect of taxol in breast carcinoma cells. *Technol. Cancer Res. Treat.* 2010 9:77-86.

[54] Spizzo R, Nicoloso MS, Lupini L, Lu Y, Fogarty J, Rossi S, Zagatti B, Fabbri M, Veronese A, Liu X, Davuluri R, Croce CM, Mills G, Negrini M, Calin GA: MiR-145 participates with TP53 in a death-promoting regulatory loop and targets estrogen receptor-alpha in human breast cancer cells. *Cell Death Differ.* 2010 17:246-54.

[55] Xiong J, Yu D, Wei N, Fu H, Cai T, Huang Y, Wu C, Zheng X, Du Q, Lin D, Liang Z: An estrogen receptor alpha suppressor, microRNA-22, is downregulated in estrogen

receptor alpha-positive human breast cancer cell lines and clinical samples. *FEBS J.* 2010 277:1684-94.

[56] Kovalchuk O, Filkowski J, Meservy J, Ilnytskyy Y, Tryndyak VP, Chekhun VF, Pogribny IP: Involvement of microRNA-451 in resistance of the MCF-7 breast cancer cells to chemotherapeutic drug doxorubicin. *Mol. Cancer Ther.* 2008 7:2152-9.

[57] Kong W, He L, Coppola M, Guo J, Esposito NN, Coppola D, Cheng JQ: MicroRNA-155 regulates cell survival, growth, and chemosensitivity by targeting FOXO3a in breast cancer. *J. Biol. Chem.* 2010 285:17869-79.

[58] Wu H, Mo YY: Targeting miR-205 in breast cancer. *Expert. Opin. Ther. Targets* 2009 13:1439-48.

[59] Ma L, Reinhardt F, Pan E, Soutschek J, Bhat B, Marcusson EG, Teruya-Feldstein J, Bell GW, Weinberg RA: Therapeutic silencing of miR-10b inhibits metastasis in a mouse mammary tumor model. *Nat. Biotechnol.* 2010 28:341-7.

*Chapter VII*

# MicroRNAs and Lung Cancer

*Jiri Sana and Ondrej Slaby*
Masaryk Memorial Cancer Institute, Brno, Czech Republic
Central European Institute of Technology, Masaryk University, Brno, Czech Republic

## Abstract

Lung cancer is one of the most common cancers in the world. Alterations in microRNA (miRNA) funtionality are frequently found in malignancies, including lung cancer. In this chapter, we summarize the current understanding of miRNAs in lung cancer pathogenesis, and highlight their potential in early diagnosis, in extending histological sub-classification techniques, in overcoming drug resistance, and serving not only as biomarkers for risk stratification and outcome prediction, but also as potential therapeutic targets in lung cancer.

## 7.1. Introduction

Lung cancers represent one of the leading causes of cancer death worldwide with an incidence more than 150,000 new cases diagnosed in Europe every year, and only 15% of all lung cancer patients are alive 5 years or more after diagnosis. Combined treatment regimens, neoadjuvant or adjuvant chemotherapy and combined radiotherapy seem to improve overall survival slightly [1]. The primary risk factor for lung cancer is smoking, which accounts for more than 85% of all lung cancer-related deaths [2].

There are two major forms of lung cancer - small cell lung cancer (SCLC) (about 15% of all lung cancers) and non-small cell lung cancer (NSCLC) (about 85%), the latter one is histopathologically sub-classified as non-squamous carcinoma (including adenocarcinoma, large-cell carcinoma, and other cell types), and squamous cell (epidermoid) carcinoma [2-4]. SCLC is characterized by its rapid doubling time, high rate of dissemination, and increased sensitivity to chemotherapy and radiation. Although the incidence of SCLC has been steadily decreasing over time, it remains a serious public health problem given its aggressive clinical behaviour [5]. Squamous cell carcinoma and adenocarcinoma are two most often diagnosed NSCLC. Squamous cell carcinoma is the most frequently occurring histologic type among men; adenocarcinoma is the more common cell type in women and in non-smokers. Adenocarcinomas are glandular with alveolar, tubular or papillary structures while squamous cell carcinomas are squamous with or without keratin differentiation [6,7]. Lung carcinomas typically display numerical and structural chromosome abberations. Among the most frequent cytogenetic changes belongs deletion in the short arm of chromosome 3. Loss of heterozygosity at chromosome arm 3p is thought to be an early genetic change in the development of both SCLC (>90%) and NSCLC (>50%) [8]. Except well known tumor suppressors, it can be hypothesized that in lung cancer one or more of the miRNAs located at the short arm of chromosome 3 may function as a tumor suppressor.

Studies that both examine global changes in miRNAs within lung tumors as well as those that have focused on the effects of individual miRNAs on lung cancer cell phenotype suggest miRNAs are involved in lung tumor development and progression and may potentially serve as biomarkers for diagnosis and prognosis, and therapeutic targets. Here we provide an overview of emerging roles of miRNA in lung cancer.

## 7.2. Polymorphisms within Mature miRNA Sequence and miRNA Binding Regions and Risk of Cancer

Tian et al. (2009) conducted study focusing on significance of 4 miRNA SNPs (rs2910164 in miR-146a, rs3746444 in miR-499, rs2292832 in miR-149 and rs11614913in miR-196-a2) as a potential risk factors of NSCLC in a case-control study of 1058 sporadic lung cancer patients in Chinese population, as a control group 1035 cancer-free tissue samples were used. CC homozygote of miR-196a2 rs11614913 variant was associated with approximately 25% significantly increased risk of lung cancer compared with their wild-type homozygote TT and heterozygote TC (OR 1.25; 95% CI, 1.01-1.54). However, no significant association was observed between the other three SNPs and lung cancer risk. These findings suggest that functional SNP rs11614913 in miR-196a2 could contribute to lung cancer susceptibility [9]. Same research group evaluated in detail the association of identical SNPs with the survival of patients with NSCLC. When they assumed that disease susceptibility was inherited as a recessive phenotype, they found that the rs11614913 SNP in mir-196a2 was associated with survival in 556 individuals with NSCLC. Specifically, survival was significantly decreased in individuals who were homozygous for CC. Binding assays revealed that this SNP can affect binding of mature mir-196a2 to its target mRNA. This is the first study to describe miRNA SNPs and NSCLC outcome with a relatively large study population size and a high statistical power (if $\alpha = 0.05$, based on the data set for mir-196a2 rs11614913, an 80% power to detect an HR of 1.41 was reached) [10]. Kim et al. (2010) observed that the frequency of the rs11614913C allele was significantly higher in the patients who were diagnosed with primary lung cancer, specifically squamous cell carcinoma (SqCC), adenocarcinoma (AC), large cell carcinoma (LCC), and small cell carcinoma (SCC), than in the controls (0.519 versus 0.477, p = 0.03). The risk of lung cancer increased as the number of C alleles increased (Ptrend = 0.02), and the CC genotype was associated with a significantly increased risk of lung cancer compared with the TT genotype (adjusted OR 1.45, 95% CI 1.07-1.98, p = 0.02). When the lung cancer cases were categorized by tumor histology, the CC genotype was associated with a significantly increased risk of SqCC compared to the TT genotype (adjusted OR 1.86, 95% CI 1.23-2.80, p = 0.003), whereas there was no significant association between the genotypes and the risk of AC or SCC [11].

Further, rs928508 in miR-30c-1 gene was also confirmed as a NSCLC survival predictor and the protective role of rs928508 AG/GG genotypes were more pronounced among early stage (I/II) patients and patients treated with surgery. The area under curve at year 5 was significantly increased from 0.658 to 0.741 after adding the miR-30c-1 rs928508 risk score to the traditional clinical risk score (stage and surgery). Furthermore, in the genotype-phenotype correlation analysis, rs928508 AG/GG genotypes were associated with a significantly decreased expression of precursor and mature miR-30c (p = 0.009 and 0.011), but not with that of its primary miRNA [12].

Let-7 complementary sites (lcs) were sequenced in the KRAS 3' UTR from 74 NSCLC cases to identify mutations and SNPs that correlated with NSCLC. The allele frequency of a previously unidentified SNP at lcs6 was characterized in 2,433 people (representing 46 human populations). The frequency of the variant allele was 18.1% to 20.3% in NSCLC patients and 5.8% in world populations. The association between the SNP and the risk for NSCLC was defined in a case-control study of lung cancer from New Mexico showed a 2.3-fold increased risk (CI, 1.1-4.6; p = 0.02) for NSCLC cancer. Functionally, the variant allele results in KRAS over-expression *in vitro*. The lcs6 variant allele in a KRAS miRNA complementary site is significantly associated with increased risk for NSCLC among moderate smokers and represents a new paradigm for miRNA involvement in cancer susceptibility [13].

## 7.3. Serum and Plasma miRNAs: Early Detection of Disease Onset and Progression

The identification of specific differences of serum-based miRNA expression profiles between patients with NSCLC and controls may promise the ability to detect NSCLC at an early stage. It was found that the expressions of miR-1254 and miR-574-5p were significantly increased in the early-stage NSCLC samples in comparison to the non-cancer controls. Receiver operating characteristic curves plotting these two miRNAs were able to discriminate early-stage NSCLC samples from controls with 82% and 77% of sensitivity and specificity, respectively, in the discovery cohort and with 73% and 71% of sensitivity and specificity, respectively, in the validation cohort [14]. Another research group published eleven serum miRNAs (miR-486, miR-22, miR-30d, miR-21, miR-26b, let-7i, miR-378, miR-1, miR-206, miR-146b, and miR-499) which were altered more than five-fold in the longer-survival NSCLC patients (average 49.54 months; range 34.6 to 61.8 months) compared with shorter-survival group (average 9.54 months; range 2.0 to 22.5 months). Then they performed individual qRT-PCR assay to quantify each of the identified miRNAs. The levels of four miRNAs (miR-486, miR-30d, miR-1 and miR-499; p < 0.001) were significantly different between above mentioned two groups of patients [15]. At last, Chen et al. (2008) identified specific expression patterns of serum miRNAs for NSCLC. Compared to healthy subjects, 28 miRNAs were missing and 63 new miRNA species were detected in the lung cancer patients, 69 miRNAs were detected both in normal serum and lung cancer serum [16].

## 7.4. Tissue miRNA Signatures: Implications for Diagnostic Oncology

MiRNA expression profiles in lung cancer were firstly examined to discriminate tumor from non-tumoral lung tissue. When Yanaihara et al. (2006) realized such comparative study, 43 miRNAs indicated significant differences in expression levels between groups. In the same way, comparison of lung adenocarcinomas versus noncancerous tissues and squamous cell carcinomas versus noncancerous tissues revealed 17 and 16 miRNAs with statistically different expression, respectively. Six miRNAs (miR-21, miR-191, miR-155, miR-210, miR-126*, and miR-224) were shared in both histological types of NSCLC [17]. Davidson et al. (2010) observed the down-regulation of miR-218 expression in 85% (33/39) of NSCLC tumors compared with paired normal lung. Statistically significant decreases were observed in both squamous cell carcinomas ($p < 1.0e-4$) and to a lesser extent adenocarcinomas ($p = 0.001$) [18]. Moreover, Raponi et al. (2009) identified 15 unique miRNAs that were significantly altered in squamous cell carcinomas compared to adjacent normal lung tissue samples. The majority of these miRNAs were over-expressed in tumors including members of the miR-17-92 cluster and its paralogue clusters miR-106a-363 and miR-93-106b. Other miRNAs up-regulated in tumor tissues included the miR-182-183 cluster, whereas the only down-regulated miRNAs were from the miR-125a-let7e cluster [19].

Next, Yanaihara asked whether the microarray data revealed specific molecular signatures for subsets of lung cancer that differ also in clinical behavior. They identified six miRNAs (miR-205, miR-99b, miR-203, miR-202, miR-102, and miR-204-prec) that were expressed differently in the two most common histological types of NSCLC, adenocarcinoma and squamous cell carcinoma. The expression levels of miR-99b and miR-102 were higher in adenocarcinoma. No miRNAs were identified as differently expressed when classified by age, gender, or race [17]. Landi et al. (2010) analysed miRNA expression profiles in 165 adenocarcinoma and 125 squamous cell carcinoma tissue samples using a custom oligo array with 440 human mature antisense miRNAs. The results showed that miRNA expression profiles strongly differentiated adenocarcinoma from squamous cell carcinoma (class comparison global permutation test $p < 0.0001$), with 127 miRNAs differentially expressed at $p < 0.05$ and with 86 of the 127 miRNAs differentially expressed at $p < 0.001$ [20].

Moreover, two studies focused on miR-205 significance in lung carcinoma. Based on sample score, which was obtained using the defined formula, the cut-off at score = 2.5 has a sensitivity of 96% and specificity of 90% for identifying squamous cell carcinomas from nonsquamous NSCLC samples in an independent blinded validation set [21]. In the second study, the reference score of 2.5 was found to have 100% sensitivity and 100% specificity in differentiating squamous cell carcinomas and adenocarcinomas. Therefore, miR-205 was proposed as a highly accurate marker for lung cancer of squamous histology [22].

Dacic et al. (2010) investigated the miRNA expression in lung adenocarcinomas with different oncogenic mutations, including EGFR-positive, KRAS-positive and EGFR/KRAS-negative tumors. Overall, miRNA expression was similar among three mutationally different groups with most up-regulated miRNAs being miR-20a, miR-328, miR-34c, and miR-18b, and most down-regulated miRNAs being miR-32, miR-137, and miR-342. However, four miRNAs (miR-155, miR-25, miR-495, and miR-7g) were expressed differently among these tumors. MiR-155 was up-regulated only in EGFR/KRAS-negative group, miR-25 was up-regulated only in EGFR-positive group, and miR-495 was up-regulated only in KRAS-positive adenocarcinomas. In opposite, let-7g was down-regulated in all three groups, with more significant down-regulation in EGFR/KRAS-negative adenocarcinomas [23]. Interestingly, Rabinowits et al. (2009) suggested exosomal miRNAs as diagnostic marker for lung adenocarcinoma. They evaluated the circulating levels of tumor exosomes, exosomal small RNA, and 12 specific exosomal miRNAs (miR-17-3p, miR-21, miR-106a, miR-146, miR-155, miR-191, miR-192, miR-203, miR-205, miR-210, miR-212, and miR-214) in patients with and without lung adenocarcinoma. The mean exosome concentration was 2.85 mg/mL (95% CI 1.94-3.76) for the lung adenocarcinoma group versus 0.77 mg/mL (95% CI 0.68-0.86) for the control group ($p < 0.001$). The mean miRNA concentration was 158.6 ng/mL (95% CI 145.7-171.5) for the lung adenocarcinoma group versus 68.1 ng/mL (95% CI 57.2-78.9) for the control group ($p < 0.001$). Comparisons between of exosomes-derived miRNAs and tumors-derived miRNAs from peripheral circulation indicated that the miRNA signatures were not significantly different. Therefore, the significant difference in total exosome and miRNA levels between lung cancer patients and controls, and the similarity between the circulating exosomal miRNA and the tumor-derived miRNA patterns, suggest that circulating exosomal miRNA might be useful as a screening test for lung adenocarcinoma. However, no correlation between the exosomal miRNA levels and the stage of disease can be made at this point [24].

New useful and for patients non-invasive approach for the diagnosis of lung cancer could be the measurement of miRNA expression levels in sputum. Jiang's research group examined, for the first time, expression of mature miRNAs, miR-21 and miR-155, in sputum of patients with NSCLC and cancer-free subjects. Means of expression for miR-21 in the specimens of cancer patients and cancer-free individuals were 76.32±9.79 and 62.24±3.82, respectively. Means of expression for miR-155 in the specimens of cancer patients and cancer-free individuals were 88.64±9.01 and 85.18±6.54, respectively. Therefore, expression of miR-21 was significantly higher in cancer patients than in cancer free controls ($p = 0.0001$), while there was not statistically significant difference of miR-155 expression in the specimens between the two groups ($p = 0.1669$). The cut-off normalized miRNA expression value (72.97) for mir-21 was further chosen from the receiver-operator characteristic (ROC) curve in order to maximize sensitivity and specificity. Based on the cut-off, mir-21 over-expression was found in 16 of 23 and 0 of 17 sputum samples from cancer patients and cancer-free subjects, resulting in 69.66% (95% CI, 0.46-0.86) sensitivity and 100.00% (95% CI, 0.77-1.00) specificity in the diagnosis of NSCLC [25].

Moreover, other two studies were focused on the early detection of histological types of NSCLC, adenocarcinoma and squamous cell carcinoma, by panels of miRNA markers. From the adenocarcinoma surgical specimens, seven miRNAs with significantly altered expression were identified, of which four miRNAs (miR-21, miR-182, miR-200b, and miR-375) were over-expressed and three miRNAs (miR-486, miR-126, and miR-145) were under-expressed in all tumors. For the validation analysis with sputum samples of the control cohort, four (miR-21, miR-486, miR-375, and miR-200b) of the seven miRNAs were selected, which in combination produced the best prediction in distinguishing lung adenocarcinoma patients from normal subjects with 80.6% sensitivity and 91.7% specificity [26]. In case of squamous cell carcinoma, three miRNAs were over-expressed (miR-126, miR-139, and miR-429) and three were under-expressed (miR-205, miR-210, and miR-708). For the validation study writh sputum samples, three (miR-205, miR-210 and miR-708) miRNAs were selected, which in combination produced the best prediction in distinguishing lung squamous cell carcinoma patients from normal subjects with 73% sensitivity and 96% specificity. Validation of the marker panels in the independent populations confirmed the sensitivity and specificity in both studies [27].

**Table 7.1. List of representative miRNAs differentially expressed in non-small cell lung cancer mentioned in at least two miRNA profiling studies**

| Up-regulated miRNAs in lung cancer | | Down-regulated miRNAs in lung cancer | |
|---|---|---|---|
| miRNA | Reference + p-value | miRNA | Reference + p-value |
| miR-20a | [19] 5.15e-09 [23] | miR-32 | [17] 0.000458 [23] |
| miR-106a | [17] 6.20e-05 [19] 1.54e-18 | miR-125a | [17] 0.000993 [19] 6.52e-13 |
| miR-203 | [17] 0.000267 [19] 4.39e-09 | | |
| miR-210 | [17] 1.00e-07 [19] 1.28e-10 | | |

Lastly, Barshack et al. (2008) compared miRNA microarray data from samples of either primary lung cancer or metastatis to the lung. They have identified 16 miRNAs expressed differentially between these two groups. MiR-182 was most strongly over-expressed in the lung primary tumors and miR-126 was significantly over-expressed in the metastatic tumors. These data suggest that miRNA expression profiles should be considered as a potential clinical biomarker for surgical pathologists faced with discerning the tumor type of an inscrutable lung neoplasm [28].

# 7.5. MiRNAs Expression in Prognosis and Response Prediction

As in other tumors, specific miRNA expression profiles were identified to correlate with the prognosis of lung cancer patients (summarized in Figure 7.1). Yanaihara et al. (2006) indicated eight miRNAs which were related to the adenocarcinoma patients survival. High expression of miR-155, miR-17-3p, miR-106a, miR-93, or miR-21, and low expression of let-7a-2, let-7b, or miR-145, were linked to a significantly poorer prognosis. In addition, the Kaplan-Meier survival estimates showed that the lung adenocarcinoma patients with either high miR-155 or reduced let-7a-2 expression had a poorer survival than the patients with low miR-155 or high let-7a-2 expression, respectively. The difference in the prognosis of these two groups was statistically significant for miR-155 ($p = 0.006$; log-rank test) and marginally significant for let- 7a-2 (p = 0.033; log-rank test). For the validation of these results, an independent set of 64 adenocarcinoma patients was used. Consistently, these analyses showed the significant prognostic impact of high levels of pre-miR-155 expression (p = 0.002; log-rank test) as well as low precursor let-7a-2 expression (p = 0.003; log-rank test) [17].

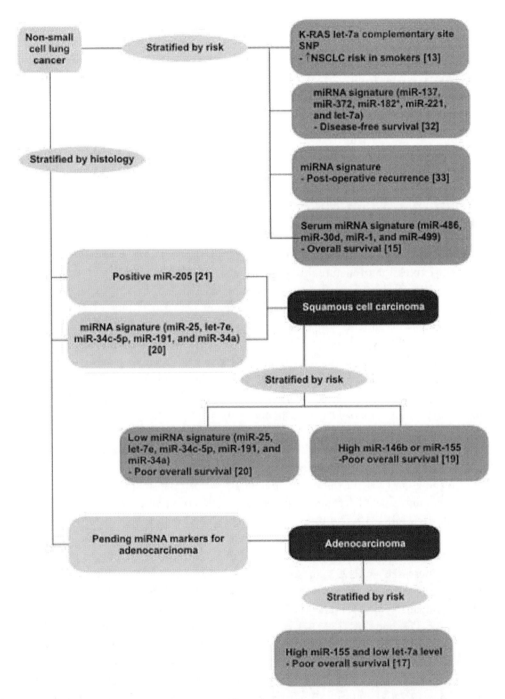

Figure 7.1. Prognostic stratification of lung cancer based on miRNA expression signatures. NSCLC, non-small-cell lung cancer. Modified from [7].

Raponi et al. (2009) identified 20 miRNAs (miR-146b, -191, -206, -299-3p, -155, -15a, -122a, -513, -184, -511, -100, -10a, -453, -379, -202, -21, -126, -494, -432, and -370) that were significantly associated with overall survival in 54 squamous cell lung carcinoma patients. It was found that the highest mean value for predicting overall survival within 3 years was 78% when using miR-146b (AUC = 0.82) alone. The predictive accuracy dropped but stabilized at 68% when three or more miRNAs were added to miR-146b. The group of patients with high miR-146b expression in tumors had significantly worse overall survival compared with the low miR-146b group (HR 2.7, 95% CI 1.4-5.7, p = 0.0035; log-rank test) [19]. Landi et al. (2010) found five other miRNAs (miR-25, miR-34c-5p, miR-191, let-7e, and miR-34a) whose expression strongly predicted squamous cell carcinoma survival for the 107 male smokers with early-stage tumors. Using the cross-validated supervised principal component method, 62 patients (36 lung cancer deaths) were predicted to have high mortality risk and 45 patients (12 lung cancer deaths) were predicted to have low mortality risk. P value for the permutation test comparing the two risk groups was 0.017 based on 10,000 permutations [20]. Markou et al. (2008) investigated the prognostic value of mature miR-21 and miR-205 overexpression in non-small cell lung cancer. MiR-21 was up-regulated in 16 of 29 (55.2%) patients who relapsed and 15 of 23 (65.2%) patients who died. MiR-205 was over-expressed in 19 of 29 patients who relapsed (65.5%) and 15 of 23 patients who died (65.2%). However, only miR-21 over-expression correlated with overall survival of the patients (p = 0.027), whereas over-expression of mature miR-205 did not [29]. The four miRNAs (miR-486, miR-30d, miR-1, and miR-499) from the serum were associated with overall survival of NSCLC. This four-miRNA signature was significantly different between groups of 30 patients with longer survival and 30 patients with shorter survival (p ≤ 0.001 for all) and, moreover, hazard ratios showed that the expression levels of these miRNAs were significantly associated with cancer death in a dose-dependent manner. The difference in the median survival time of lung cancer between different expression levels of the four miRNAs in quartiles were all statistically significant (miR-486, p = 0.009; miR-30d, p < 0.001; miR-1, p < 0.001; and miR-499, p = 0.001; log-rank test). The subsequent results from the analysis of training and testing sets (n = 243) corresponded to those above mentioned [15]. At last, over-expression of miR-130a was also strongly associated with poor prognosis, lymph node metastasis, and stage of tumor node metastasis classification in NSCLC patients [30].

Duncavage et al. (2010) examined patients at risk for relapse after surgical resection. In an exploratory study, they determined whether expression of selected miRNAs (let-7a, miR-7, miR-21, miR-155, miR-210, and miR-221) was associated with tumor recurrence in patients with surgically resected T1 or T2 stage I NSCLC. The data showed that tumors which recurred had 0.14-fold lower miR-221 expression than those which did not recur (p = 0.0036). In addition, increased miR-221 in tumor tissue when compared with adjacent normal appearing lung in the same patient also correlated with nonrecurrence (p = 0.0011) [31]. Yu et al. (2008) confirmed miR-221 and let-7a as protective miRNAs and other three miRNAs (miR-137, miR-372, and miR-182*) as risky in cohorts of NSCLC patients. In training set (n = 56), patients with high-risk five-miRNA signature had shorter median overall survival than patients with low-risk miRNA signature (20 months versus not reached, p < 0.001). Patients with high-risk five-miRNA signature had shorter median relapse-free survival than patients with low-risk miRNA signature (10 months versus not reached, p = 0.002). Using the same five-miRNA signature, similar findings were found in the testing set (n = 56). The median overall survival was significantly shorter in patients with high-risk miRNA signature than in low-risk patients (25 months versus not reached, p = 0.008). Likewise, patients with high-risk miRNA signature had shorter median relapse-free survival than patients with low-risk miRNA signature (14 months versus not reached, p = 0.003). Revalidation study in an independent cohort (n = 62) fully confirmed that patients with high-risk scores in their miRNA signature had poor overall (40 months versus not reached, p = 0.007) and disease-free (20 months versus 48 months, p = 0.037) survivals compared to the low-risk-score patients [32]. Another research group found 130 miRNAs (p ≤ 0.01) which were differentially expressed between recurrence and no recurrence groups. From these, miR-129-5p, miR-194*, miR-631, miR-200b*, miR-585, miR-623, miR-617, miR-622, miR-638, and miRPlus_27560 were most under-expressed, and miR-24, miR-141, miR-27b, miR-16, miR-21, miR-30c, miR-106a, miR-15b, miR-23b, and miR-130a were most over-expressed [33].

In study, which investigated the different miRNA expression profiles of postoperative radiotherapy sensitive and resistant thirty NSCLC patients, Wang et al. (2010) showed five up-regulated (miRNA-126, let-7a, miRNA-495, miRNA-451, and miRNA-128b), and seven greatly down-regulated miRNAs (miRNA-130a, miRNA-106b, miRNA-19b, miRNA-22, miRNA-15b, miRNA-17-5p, and miRNA-21) in the radiotherapy sensitive group [34]. On the other hand, Voortman et al. (2010) accomplished the large randomized study of adjuvant chemotherapy in patients with radically resected NSCLC where an expression of miR-21, miR-29b, miR-34a, miR-34b, miR-34c, miR-155, and let-7a was determined in 639 FFPE tumor specimens. Their results indicate that the seven miRNAs chosen for evaluation were neither predictive nor prognostic in this NSCLC patient cohort [35]. Although the majority of patients with small cell lung cancer (SCLC) respond to initial chemotherapy, those with disease progression at first response assessment (chemoresistance) have inferior outcomes. Therefore, one of very few studies occupying by aforementioned lung cancer subgroup examined miRNA profiles in SCLC specimens. Results indicated that miRNAs significantly associated with chemoresistance were miR-92a-2* (p = 0.010), miR-147 (p = 0.018), and miR-574-5p (p = 0.039). Moreover, higher tumor miR-92a-2* level contributed significantly to decreased survival in patients with SCLC (p = 0.015) [36].

## 7.6. MiRNAs as Potential Therapeutic Targets

The let-7 family is frequently examined miRNA group in NSCLC. Many publications have proposed that its members play important roles in the pathogenesis of lung cancer. Kumar et al. showed (2008) that let-7 functionally inhibited NSCLC development. Ectopic expression of let-7g in KRAS(G12D)-expressing murine lung cancer cells induced cell cycle arrest and apoptosis. Moreover, in tumor xenografts, they showed significant reduction of both murine and human NSCLC when over-expression of let-7g was induced from lentiviral vectors [37]. The similar effect was described in other three publications. In all cases, the authors observed an inhibition of the lung carcinoma cells growth *in vitro* and/or a significant reduction of tumor burden in immunodeficient mice after increasing of let-7 expression [38-40]. Moreover, Wang et al. (2010) found up-regulated let-7a in radiotherapy sensitive patients. This observation suggests that the let-7a could acts in NSCLC resistance to the radiotherapy [34]. Other miRNAs were proposed to be involved in lung cancer resistance. Guo et al. (2010) evaluated the global expression of miRNAs and approximately 20,000 genes in cellular models of SCLC which were widely used as sensitive (NCI-H69) and resistant cell lines (NCI-H69AR) to chemotherapy. On the basis of retrieved results and a subsequent analysis, the sensitivity to anti-cancer drugs cisplatin, etoposide and doxorubicin greatly increased or reduced following transfection of the drug-resistant H69AR cells with the mimics or antagomirs of miR-134, miR-379 and miR-495, respectively. MiR-134 increases the cell survival by inducing G1 arrest in H69AR cells. Multidrug resistance protein 1 (MRP1/ABCC1) is negatively regulated by miR-134 and down-regulation of MRP1/ABCC1 at the protein level largely correlates with elevated levels of miR-134 in H69AR cells [41]. Rui et al. (2010) identified miRNA expression profiles involved in the development of docetaxel resistance in NSCLC. The expression of three miRNAs (miR-200b, miR-194, and miR-212) was significantly down-regulated in docetaxel-resistant human NSCLC cell line (SPC-A1/docetaxel) while the expression of other three miRNAs (miR-192, miR-424, and miR-98) was significantly up-regulated in SPC-A1/docetaxel cells ($p < 0.01$). Potential target genes controlled by six selected miRNAs were divided into four groups according to various functions: apoptosis and proliferation (71 genes), cell cycle (68 genes), DNA damage (26 genes) and DNA repair (59 genes) [42]. Zhang et al. (2010) demonstrated that curcumin, an anticancer agent, significantly down-regulated the expression of miR-186* in A549/DDP cells. In addition, transfection of cells with a miR-186* inhibitor promoted A549/DDP apoptosis, and over-expression of miR-186* significantly inhibited curcumin-induced apoptosis [43]. At last, Garofalo et al. (2008) showed that miR-221 and miR-222 impair TRAIL-dependent apoptosis by inhibiting the expression of key functional proteins. Indeed, transfection with anti-miR-221 and miR-222 rendered CALU-1-resistant cells sensitive to TRAIL. Conversely, H460-sensitive cells treated with pre-miR-221 and pre-miR-222 become resistant to TRAIL. MiR-221 and miR-222 target the 3' UTR of Kit and p27 (kip1) mRNAs, but interfere with TRAIL signaling mainly through p27 (kip1) [44]. Thus, the aforementioned observations suggest that selected miRNAs could serve as promising therapeutic approach to overcome chemoresistace in lung cancer.

MiR-21 is known oncogenic miRNA which was described also as potential therapeutic target in other tumors many times. In NSCLC, decreased expression of this miRNA markedly reduced cell growth and invasiveness, and increased apoptosis. These effects could be caused through modulation of PTEN and/or inhibition of negative regulators of the Ras/MEK/ERK pathway [45,46]. Liu et al. (2010) studied another oncogenic miRNA in human and mouse lung cancers. They revealed that miR-31 targeted tumor-suppressive genes large tumor suppressor 2 (LATS2) and PP2A regulatory subunit B alpha isoform (PPP2R2A), and expression of each was augmented by miR-31 knockdown. Decreasing of miR-31 consequently led to substantial repression of lung cancer cell growth and tumorigenicity in a dose-dependent manner [47]. MiR-145 is another potential therapeutic target. Chen et al. (2010) examined that cell growth was inhibited and the G1/S transition was blocked by miR-145 in A549 and H23 NSCLC cells. They further showed that c-Myc was a direct target for miR-145. Introduction of miR-145 dramatically suppressed the c-Myc/eIF4E pathway, which was demonstrated to be crucial for cell proliferation in NSCLC cells. Furthermore, they found that CDK4 was regulated by miR-145 in cell cycle control [48].

Some other miRNAs were found to be involved in lung cancer biology. MiR-34a is an important component of PRIMA-1-induced apoptotic network in human lung cancer cells harbouring mutant p53, and knockdown of this miRNA decreased the rate of apoptosis caused by PRIMA-1 [49]. MiR-126 altered lung cancer cell phenotype by inhibiting adhesion, migration, and invasion, and these effects seem to be partially mediated through Crk, a member of a family of adaptor proteins [50]. The same authors published that miR-133b in adenocarcinoma (H2009) cell lines reduced expression of MCL-1 and BCL2L2 through directly targeting their 3' UTRs, and over-expression of miR-133b induced apoptosis in these tumor cells [51]. At last, paxillin is a target gene of miR-218 and its gene mutations are associated with lung adenocarcinoma progression. Mir-218 suppression led to the paxillin over-expression following by enhancement of cell proliferation, invasion, and soft agar colony formation in NSCLC cells [52]. Involvement of miRNAs in core signaling pathways of lung cancer pathogenesis make them also promising therapeutic targets in lung cancer.

## Acknowledgment

This work was supported by grants NS 10361-3/2009, NR/9814-4/2008, NS 10352-3/2009, NT/11214-4/2010 of Czech Ministry of Health, Project No. MZ0MOU2005 of the Czech Ministry of Health and by the project "CEITEC – Central European Institute of Technology" (CZ.1.05/1.1.00/02.0068).

## References

[1] Huber RM, Stratakis DF: Molecular oncology--perspectives in lung cancer. *Lung Cancer* 2004 45 Suppl 2:S209-13.

[2] Ettinger DS, Akerley W, Bepler G, Blum MG, Chang A, Cheney RT, Chirieac LR, D'Amico TA, Demmy TL, Ganti AK, et al: Non-small cell lung cancer. *J. Natl. Compr. Canc. Netw.* 2010 8:740-801.

[3] Paggi MG, Vona R, Abbruzzese C, Malorni W: Gender-related disparities in non-small cell lung cancer. *Cancer Lett.* 2010 298:1-8.

[4] Herbst RS, Heymach JV, Lippman SM: Lung cancer. *N. Engl. J. Med.* 2008 359:1367-80.

[5] Rodriguez E, Lilenbaum RC: Small cell lung cancer: past, present, and future. *Curr. Oncol. Rep.* 2010 12:327-34.

[6] Bastide K, Ugolin N, Levalois C, Bernaudin JF, Chevillard S: Are adenosquamous lung carcinomas a simple mix of adenocarcinomas and squamous cell carcinomas, or more complex at the molecular level? *Lung Cancer* 2010 68:1-9.

[7] Lin PY, Yu SL, Yang PC: MicroRNA in lung cancer. *Br. J. Cancer* 2010, 103:1144-1148.

[8] Mitsuuchi Y, Testa JR: Cytogenetics and molecular genetics of lung cancer. *Am. J. Med. Genet.* 2002 115:183-8.

[9] Tian T, Shu Y, Chen J, Hu Z, Xu L, Jin G, Liang J, Liu P, Zhou X, Miao R, Ma H, Chen Y, Shen H: A functional genetic variant in microRNA-196a2 is associated with increased susceptibility of lung cancer in Chinese. *Cancer Epidemiol. Biomarkers Prev.* 2009 18:1183-7.

[10] Hu Z, Chen J, Tian T, Zhou X, Gu H, Xu L, Zeng Y, Miao R, Jin G, Ma H, Chen Y, Shen H: Genetic variants of miRNA sequences and non-small cell lung cancer survival. *J. Clin. Invest.* 2008 118:2600-8.

[11] Kim MJ, Yoo SS, Choi YY, Park JY: A functional polymorphism in the pre-microRNA-196a2 and the risk of lung cancer in a Korean population. *Lung Cancer* 2010 69:127-9.

[12] Hu Z, Shu Y, Chen Y, Chen J, Dong J, Liu Y, Pan S, Xu L, Xu J, Wang Y, Dai J, Ma H, Jin G, Shen H: Genetic Polymorphisms in the pre-MicroRNA Flanking Region and Non-Small-Cell Lung Cancer Survival. *Am. J. Respir. Crit. Care Med.* 2010.

[13] Chin LJ, Ratner E, Leng S, Zhai R, Nallur S, Babar I, Muller RU, Straka E, Su L, Burki EA, Crowell RE, Patel R, Kulkarni T, Homer R, Zelterman D, Kidd KK, Zhu Y, Christiani DC, Belinsky SA, Slack FJ, Weidhaas JB: A SNP in a let-7 microRNA complementary site in the KRAS 3' untranslated region increases non-small cell lung cancer risk. *Cancer Res.* 2008 68:8535-40.

[14] Foss KM, Sima C, Ugolini D, Neri M, Allen KE, Weiss GJ: miR-1254 and miR-574-5p: Serum-Based microRNA Biomarkers for Early-Stage Non-small Cell Lung Cancer. *J. Thorac. Oncol.* 2011.

[15] Hu Z, Chen X, Zhao Y, Tian T, Jin G, Shu Y, Chen Y, Xu L, Zen K, Zhang C, Shen H: Serum microRNA signatures identified in a genome-wide serum microRNA expression profiling predict survival of non-small-cell lung cancer. *J. Clin. Oncol.* 2010 28:1721-6.

[16] Chen X, Ba Y, Ma L, Cai X, Yin Y, Wang K, Guo J, Zhang Y, Chen J, Guo X, Li Q, Li X, Wang W, Zhang Y, Wang J, Jiang X, Xiang Y, Xu C, Zhang J, Li R, Zhang H, Shang X, Gong T, Ning G, Wang J, Zen K, Zhang J, Zhang CY: Characterization of microRNAs in serum: a novel class of biomarkers for diagnosis of cancer and other diseases. *Cell Res.* 2008 18:997-1006.

[17] Yanaihara N, Caplen N, Bowman E, Seike M, Kumamoto K, Yi M, Stephens RM, Okamoto A, Yokota J, Tanaka T, Calin GA, Liu CG, Croce CM, Harris CC: Unique microRNA molecular profiles in lung cancer diagnosis and prognosis. *Cancer Cell* 2006 9:189-98.

[18] Davidson MR, Larsen JE, Yang IA, Hayward NK, Clarke BE, Duhig EE, Passmore LH, Bowman RV, Fong KM: MicroRNA-218 is deleted and downregulated in lung squamous cell carcinoma. *PLoS One* 2010 5:e12560.

[19] Raponi M, Dossey L, Jatkoe T, Wu X, Chen G, Fan H, Beer DG: MicroRNA classifiers for predicting prognosis of squamous cell lung cancer. *Cancer Res.* 2009 69:5776-83.

[20] Landi MT, Zhao Y, Rotunno M, Koshiol J, Liu H, Bergen AW, Rubagotti M, Goldstein AM, Linnoila I, Marincola FM, Tucker MA, Bertazzi PA, Pesatori AC, Caporaso NE, McShane LM, Wang E: MicroRNA expression differentiates histology and predicts survival of lung cancer. *Clin. Cancer Res.* 2010 16:430-41.

[21] Lebanony D, Benjamin H, Gilad S, Ezagouri M, Dov A, Ashkenazi K, Gefen N, Izraeli S, Rechavi G, Pass H, Nonaka D, Li J, Spector Y, Rosenfeld N, Chajut A, Cohen D, Aharonov R, Mansukhani M: Diagnostic assay based on hsa-miR-205 expression distinguishes squamous from nonsquamous non-small-cell lung carcinoma. *J. Clin. Oncol.* 2009 27:2030-7.

[22] Bishop JA, Benjamin H, Cholakh H, Chajut A, Clark DP, Westra WH: Accurate classification of non-small cell lung carcinoma using a novel microRNA-based approach. *Clin. Cancer Res.* 2010 16:610-9.

[23] Dacic S, Kelly L, Shuai Y, Nikiforova MN: miRNA expression profiling of lung adenocarcinomas: correlation with mutational status. *Mod. Pathol.* 2010 23:1577-82.

[24] Rabinowits G, Gercel-Taylor C, Day JM, Taylor DD, Kloecker GH: Exosomal microRNA: a diagnostic marker for lung cancer. *Clin. Lung Cancer* 2009 10:42-6.

[25] Xie Y, Todd NW, Liu Z, Zhan M, Fang H, Peng H, Alattar M, Deepak J, Stass SA, Jiang F: Altered miRNA expression in sputum for diagnosis of non-small cell lung cancer. *Lung Cancer* 2010 67:170-6.

[26] Yu L, Todd NW, Xing L, Xie Y, Zhang H, Liu Z, Fang H, Zhang J, Katz RL, Jiang F: Early detection of lung adenocarcinoma in sputum by a panel of microRNA markers. *Int. J. Cancer* 2010.

[27] Xing L, Todd NW, Yu L, Fang H, Jiang F: Early detection of squamous cell lung cancer in sputum by a panel of microRNA markers. *Mod. Pathol.* 2010 23:1157-64.

[28] Barshack I, Lithwick-Yanai G, Afek A, Rosenblatt K, Tabibian-Keissar H, Zepeniuk M, Cohen L, Dan H, Zion O, Strenov Y, Polak-Charcon S, Perelman M: MicroRNA expression differentiates between primary lung tumors and metastases to the lung. *Pathol. Res. Pract.* 2010 206:578-84.

[29] Markou A, Tsaroucha EG, Kaklamanis L, Fotinou M, Georgoulias V, Lianidou ES: Prognostic value of mature microRNA-21 and microRNA-205 overexpression in non-small cell lung cancer by quantitative real-time RT-PCR. *Clin. Chem.* 2008 54:1696-704.

[30] Wang XC, Tian LL, Wu HL, Jiang XY, Du LQ, Zhang H, Wang YY, Wu HY, Li DG, She Y, Liu QF, Fan FY, Meng AM: Expression of miRNA-130a in nonsmall cell lung cancer. *Am. J. Med. Sci.* 2010 340:385-8.

[31] Duncavage E, Goodgame B, Sezhiyan A, Govindan R, Pfeifer J: Use of microRNA expression levels to predict outcomes in resected stage I non-small cell lung cancer. *J. Thorac. Oncol.* 2010 5:1755-63.

[32] Yu SL, Chen HY, Chang GC, Chen CY, Chen HW, Singh S, Cheng CL, Yu CJ, Lee YC, Chen HS, Su TJ, Chiang CC, Li HN, Hong QS, Su HY, Chen CC, Chen WJ, Liu CC, Chan WK, Chen WJ, Li KC, Chen JJ, Yang PC: MicroRNA signature predicts survival and relapse in lung cancer. *Cancer Cell* 2008 13:48-57.

[33] Patnaik SK, Kannisto E, Knudsen S, Yendamuri S: Evaluation of microRNA expression profiles that may predict recurrence of localized stage I non-small cell lung cancer after surgical resection. *Cancer Res.* 2010 70:36-45.

[34] Wang XC, Du LQ, Tian LL, Wu HL, Jiang XY, Zhang H, Li DG, Wang YY, Wu HY, She Y, Liu QF, Fan FY, Meng AM: Expression and function of miRNA in postoperative radiotherapy sensitive and resistant patients of non-small cell lung cancer. *Lung Cancer* 2010.

[35] Voortman J, Goto A, Mendiboure J, Sohn JJ, Schetter AJ, Saito M, Dunant A, Pham TC, Petrini I, Lee A, Khan MA, Hainaut P, Pignon JP, Brambilla E, Popper HH, Filipits M, Harris CC, Giaccone G: MicroRNA expression and clinical outcomes in patients treated with adjuvant chemotherapy after complete resection of non-small cell lung carcinoma. *Cancer Res.* 2010 70:8288-98.

[36] Ranade AR, Cherba D, Sridhar S, Richardson P, Webb C, Paripati A, Bowles B, Weiss GJ: MicroRNA 92a-2*: a biomarker predictive for chemoresistance and prognostic for survival in patients with small cell lung cancer. *J. Thorac. Oncol.* 2010 5:1273-8.

[37] Kumar MS, Erkeland SJ, Pester RE, Chen CY, Ebert MS, Sharp PA, Jacks T: Suppression of non-small cell lung tumor development by the let-7 microRNA family. *Proc. Natl. Acad. Sci. USA* 2008 105:3903-8.

[38] Trang P, Medina PP, Wiggins JF, Ruffino L, Kelnar K, Omotola M, Homer R, Brown D, Bader AG, Weidhaas JB, Slack FJ: Regression of murine lung tumors by the let-7 microRNA. *Oncogene* 2010 29:1580-7.

[39] He XY, Chen JX, Zhang Z, Li CL, Peng QL, Peng HM: The let-7a microRNA protects from growth of lung carcinoma by suppression of k-Ras and c-Myc in nude mice. *J. Cancer Res. Clin. Oncol.* 2010 136:1023-8.

[40] Esquela-Kerscher A, Trang P, Wiggins JF, Patrawala L, Cheng A, Ford L, Weidhaas JB, Brown D, Bader AG, Slack FJ: The let-7 microRNA reduces tumor growth in mouse models of lung cancer. *Cell Cycle* 2008 7:759-64.

[41] Guo L, Liu Y, Bai Y, Sun Y, Xiao F, Guo Y: Gene expression profiling of drug-resistant small cell lung cancer cells by combining microRNA and cDNA expression analysis. *Eur. J. Cancer* 2010 46:1692-702.

[42] Rui W, Bing F, Hai-Zhu S, Wei D, Long-Bang C: Identification of microRNA profiles in docetaxel-resistant human non-small cell lung carcinoma cells (SPC-A1). *J. Cell Mol. Med* 2010 14:206-14.

[43] Zhang J, Zhang T, Ti X, Shi J, Wu C, Ren X, Yin H: Curcumin promotes apoptosis in A549/DDP multidrug-resistant human lung adenocarcinoma cells through an miRNA signaling pathway. *Biochem. Biophys. Res. Commun.* 2010 399:1-6.

[44] Garofalo M, Quintavalle C, Di Leva G, Zanca C, Romano G, Taccioli C, Liu CG, Croce CM, Condorelli G: MicroRNA signatures of TRAIL resistance in human non-small cell lung cancer. *Oncogene* 2008 27:3845-55.

[45] Hatley ME, Patrick DM, Garcia MR, Richardson JA, Bassel-Duby R, van Rooij E, Olson EN: Modulation of K-Ras-dependent lung tumorigenesis by MicroRNA-21. *Cancer Cell* 2010 18:282-93.

[46] Zhang JG, Wang JJ, Zhao F, Liu Q, Jiang K, Yang GH: MicroRNA-21 (miR-21) represses tumor suppressor PTEN and promotes growth and invasion in non-small cell lung cancer (NSCLC). *Clin. Chim. Acta.* 2010 411:846-52.

[47] Liu X, Sempere LF, Ouyang H, Memoli VA, Andrew AS, Luo Y, Demidenko E, Korc M, Shi W, Preis M, Dragnev KH, Li H, Direnzo J, Bak M, Freemantle SJ, Kauppinen S, Dmitrovsky E: MicroRNA-31 functions as an oncogenic microRNA in mouse and human lung cancer cells by repressing specific tumor suppressors. *J. Clin. Invest.* 2010 120:1298-309.

[48] Chen Z, Zeng H, Guo Y, Liu P, Pan H, Deng A, Hu J: miRNA-145 inhibits non-small cell lung cancer cell proliferation by targeting c-Myc. *J. Exp. Clin. Cancer Res.* 2010 29:151.

[49] Duan W, Gao L, Wu X, Wang L, Nana-Sinkam SP, Otterson GA, Villalona-Calero MA: MicroRNA-34a is an important component of PRIMA-1-induced apoptotic network in human lung cancer cells. *Int. J. Cancer* 2010 127:313-20.

[50] Crawford M, Brawner E, Batte K, Yu L, Hunter MG, Otterson GA, Nuovo G, Marsh CB, Nana-Sinkam SP: MicroRNA-126 inhibits invasion in non-small cell lung carcinoma cell lines. *Biochem. Biophys. Res. Commun.* 2008 373:607-12.

[51] Crawford M, Batte K, Yu L, Wu X, Nuovo GJ, Marsh CB, Otterson GA, Nana-Sinkam SP: MicroRNA 133B targets pro-survival molecules MCL-1 and BCL2L2 in lung cancer. *Biochem. Biophys. Res. Commun.* 2009 388:483-9.

[52] Wu DW, Cheng YW, Wang J, Chen CY, Lee H: Paxillin predicts survival and relapse in non-small cell lung cancer by microRNA-218 targeting. *Cancer Res.* 2010 70:10392-401.

*Chapter VIII*

# MicroRNAs and Prostate Cancer

*Jiri Sana*
Masaryk Memorial Cancer Institute, Brno, Czech Republic

## Abstract

Prostate cancer is the most frequently diagnosed cancer in men in Western countries. The mechanisms initiating and subsequently supporting growth of this cancer remain largely unknown. Results from recent studies indicate that miRNA expression profiles may distinguish prostate carcinoma from non-neoplastic specimens and further classify tumors according to androgen dependence. In addition, a prognostic significance was attributed to specific miRNA patterns as predictors of clinical recurrence following radical prostatectomy. Finally, therapeutic potential of selected miRNAs were tested on *in vitro* and *in vivo* models indicating promising results. This chapter summarizes the current knowledge about miRNA deregulation in prostate cancer disease.

## 8.1. Introduction

In developed western countries, prostate cancer is the most common malignant tumor in men, and is the second highest cause of cancer mortality after lung [1]. The highest prostate cancer incidence rates are in the developed world and the lowest rates in African and Asia. The extremely high rate of prostate cancer is in the USA (125 per 100,000) [2]. To date, the mechanisms that underlie the occurrence and progression of prostate cancer remain largely unknown. Nevertheless, it has been shown that both genetic and environmental factors are involved in the etiology and prognosis of prostate cancer [3]. Some genes have been identified as potentially associated with this cancer. The first gene locus identified was named hereditary prostate cancer locus-1 (HPC1), for which RNASEL is the candidate allele. Further, the genes most plausibly linked to familial prostate cancer are EPAC2, RNASEL, MSR1, CHEK2, CAPZB, vitamin D receptor, and PON1. Moreover, a germline mutation in

BRCA2 can increase the risk of prostate cancer, and could cause about 5% of cases in men younger than 55 years [1].

The most commonly used system for grading carcinoma of the prostate is the Gleason score. The system describes a score between 2 and 10, with 2 being the least aggressive and 10 the most aggressive. This score is the sum of the two most common patterns (grades 1-5) of tumor growth [1]. Mortality rates can vary considerably depending on tumor Gleason score; men with low-grade prostate cancers (Gleason score 2-4) have a minimal risk of dying from prostate cancer during 20 years of follow-up (six deaths per 1,000 person years; 95% CI, 2-11), while men with high-grade prostate cancers (Gleason score 8-10) have a high probability of dying from prostate cancer within 10 years of diagnosis (121 deaths per 1,000 person-years; 95% CI, 90-156) [2].

Introduction of prostate-specific antigen (PSA) testing has resulted in increased detection of early-stage prostate cancer: while some patients are cured of life-threatening disease, there are concerns about over-treatment and related morbidity [2]. In fact, serum PSA level, primary tumor stage and Gleason grade do not reliably predict outcome for individual patients. Therefore, the identification of indicators of aggressiveness would be helpful in guiding therapeutic decisions, by distinguishing individuals with potentially life-threatening disease for whom treatment is actually necessary. The progression of metastatic androgen-independent prostate cancer is the final stage of this disease and constitutes a substantial threat of morbidity and mortality. The regulatory mechanisms that cause this transition remain largely unknown, and to date, no effective therapy for androgen-independent prostate cancer has been developed. Mainly, in this complex scenarios, miRNAs could find their role [2]. This chapter describes involving of miRNAs in prostate cancer biology and, moreover, shows a possible role for miRNAs in the management of prostate cancer as novel biomarkers and new therapeutic targets or intervention tools can be envisioned.

## 8.2. Polymorphisms within Mature miRNA Sequence and miRNA Binding Regions and Risk of Cancer

It is conceivable that miRNAs have a large effect on the physiology of the cells and that common single-nucleotide polymorphisms (SNPs) within their genes could contribute significantly to an individual risk to develop complex diseases. George et al. (2011) genotyped SNPs hsa-mir196a2 (rs11614913), hsa-mir146a (rs2910164), and hsa-mir499 (rs3746444) in prostate cancer patients. Patients with heterozygous genotype in hsa-mir196a2 and hsa-mir499, showed significant risk for developing prostate cancer ($p = 0.01$; OR = 1.70, and $p \leq 0.001$; OR = 2.27, respectively). Similarly, the variant allele carrier was also associated with prostate cancer, ($p = 0.01$; OR = 1.66, and $p \leq 0.001$; OR = 1.97, respectively) whereas, hsa-mir146a revealed no association in prostate cancer. None of the miRNA polymorphisms were associated with Gleason score and bone metastasis [4].

Xu et al. (2010) also analyzed the association between pre-miR-146a polymorphism and risk of prostate cancer. However, they found that individuals carrying CC homozygotes had a 0.65-fold reduced risk (95% CI = 0.43-0.99) than those carrying GG/GC genotypes (p =

0.03), and the C allele displayed a lower prevalence of prostate cancer compared with the G allele (OR = 0.73, 95% CI = 0.57-0.94, p = 0.01). In addition, they also found that the G to C change in the precursor of miR-146a resulted in reduced expression of mature miR-146a in prostate cancer tissues [5].

Bao et al. (2010) systematically evaluated 10 common SNPs inside pre-miRNAs in men with advanced prostate cancer treated with ADT (androgen-deprivation therapy). Only pre-miR-423 (rs6505162) CC>CA/AA had statistically significant effects on prostate cancer-specific mortality (p = 0.037) [6].

## 8.3. Serum and Plasma miRNAs: Early Detection of Disease Onset and Progression

Non-coding miRNAs in the serum and plasma have been shown to have potential as non-invasive biomarkers for physiological and pathological conditions [7]. In prostate cancer, Mitchel et al. (2010) were the first to show a correlation between miRNAs found in plasma and the presence of this cancer type. They established a list of likely blood-based miRNA biomarker candidates for prostate cancer (miR-100, miR-125b, miR-141, miR-143, miR-205, and miR-296). Further investigation showed that miR-141 (p = $1.47 \times 10^{-7}$) was the most highly over-represented miRNA in prostate cancer serum among the miRNA candidates mentioned above. Furthermore, serum levels of miR-141 could detect individuals with cancer with 60% sensitivity at 100% specificity [8]. Moltzahn et al. (2010) profiled sera from healthy men and untreated prostate cancer patients. The global screen analysis of 384 miRNAs identified 12 candidates from which 10 miRNAs were significantly different between the healthy and all malignant samples. From these, 4 miRNAs were down-regulated (miR-223, miR-26b, miR-30c, and miR-24) and 6 were up-regulated in the cancer group (miR-20b, miR-874, miR-1274a, miR-1207-5p, miR-93, and miR-106a). Further, miR-19a and miR-451 were significantly different between healthy versus high-risk [7]. Another study assessed the potential of serum miR-21 for monitoring the progression of prostate cancer. It was observed that serum miR-21 level was the highest in hormone-refractory prostate cancer (HRPC) patients (p = 0.016), while there were no significant differences between benign prostatic hyperplasia patients, localized cancer prostate patients and androgen-dependent prostate cancer patients. Levels of serum miR-21 before docetaxel-based chemotherapy were higher in the patients resistant to this chemotherapy than the sensitive patients (p = 0.032). Therefore, miR-21 may be applicable as a marker indicating the transformation to HRPC, and a potential predictor for the efficacy of docetaxel-based therapy [9].

## 8.4. Tissue miRNA Signatures: Implications for Diagnostic Oncology

Many authors described that various cancers are associated with the aberrant expression patterns of miRNAs. Recent studies, therefore, profiled and subsequently validated expression of the miRNAs also in prostate cancer. Porkka et al. (2007) examined expression profiles of four benign prostatic hyperplasia and nine prostate carcinoma samples. They detected differential expression of 30 individual miRNAs, 22 of them showing down-regulation and 8 showing up-regulation in carcinoma samples [10]. Other two independent studies compared expression profiles of prostate tumor tissues and adjacent non-tumor tissues.

However, the results were very dissimilar and only miR-145 and miR-221 were up-regulated in all three mentioned studies (summarized in Table 8.1) [10,11,12]. Ozen et al. (2008) analysed expression of 328 known and 152 novel human miRNAs in 10 benign peripheral zone tissues and 16 prostate cancer tissues using microarrays and found widespread, but not universal, down-regulation of miRNAs in clinically localized prostate cancer relative to benign peripheral zone tissue. These findings have been verified by qRT-PCR assays on selected miRNAs, including miR-125b, miR-145, and let-7c [13]. Moreover, Sun et al. (2011) published miR-125b, the miR-99 family members miR-99a, miR-99b, and miR-100 as down-regulated in human prostate tumor tissue compared to normal prostate [14]. Lastly, Volinia et al. (2006) analysed miRNA expressions of six solid cancers including also prostate cancer. They found changed expression levels of miR-17-5p, -20a, -21, -25, -29b-2, -30c, -32, -106a, -146, -181b-1, -191, -199a-1, -214, and -223 in prostate tumor tissues [15].

More importantly, Porkka et al. (2007) identified miRNA signature for hormone-refractory carcinomas. In this study, 6 miRNAs were up-regulated (miR-184, miR-198, miR-302c*, miR-345, miR-491, miR-513; p= 0.0028 for all miRNAs), and 15 miRNAs were down-regulated (let-7f, miR-19b, -22, -26b, -27a, -27b, -29a, -29b, -30a-5p, -30b, -30c, -100, -141, -148a, -205; p = 0.0286 for all miRNAs) compared with the benign prostatic hyperplasia (BPH) samples [10].

**Table 8.1. List of representative miRNAs differentially expressed in prostate cancer mentioned in at least two microRNA profiling studies**

| Up-regulated miRNAs in prostate cancer | | Down-regulated miRNAs in prostate cancer | |
|---|---|---|---|
| miRNA | Reference + fold change (p-value) | miRNA | Reference + fold change (p-value) |
| miR-182 | [11] 1.9 [12] 1.49 (0.0001) | let-7b | [11] 0.8 [10] (0.0028) |
| miR-370 | [11] 1.6 [10] (0.0028) | let-7c | [13] (< 0.00001) [10] (0.0028) |
| miR-375 | [11] 1.6 [12] 1.14 (0.012) | miR-16 | [12] -1.16 (0.0003) [10] (0.0028) |
| | | miR-99a | [14] (0.0086) [10] (0.0028) |
| | | miR-125b | [12] -1.29 (<0.0001) [13] (0.02) [14] (0.012) [10] (0.0028) |
| | | miR-145 | [11] 0.8 [12] -1.69 (<0.0001) [13] (0.003) [10] (0.0028) |
| | | miR-205 | [11] 0.8 [12] -2.86 (<0.0001) |
| | | miR-221 | [11] 0.7 [12] -2.04 (<0.0001) [10] (0.0028) |
| | | miR-222 | [12] -2.08 (<0.0001) [10] (0.0028) |

## 8.5. MiRNAs Expression in Prognosis and Response Prediction

Recently, several studies examined miRNAs expressions in relation to the prognosis of prostate cancer patients. Leite et al. (2009) identified miRNAs involved in prostate cancer progression comparing the profile of miRNAs expressed by localized high grade prostate carcinoma and bone metastasis. Let-7c, miR-100, and miR-218 were significantly overexpressed by all localized high Gleason score, pT3 prostate carcinoma in comparison with metastatic carcinoma (35.065 vs. 0.996; p < 0.001), (55.550 vs. 8.314; p = 0.010), and (33.549 vs. 2.748; p = 0.001), respectively. Therefore, they hypothesized that these miRNAs may be involved in the process of metastasization of prostate cancer [16]. MiR-221 and miR-34c were identified as other metastasis hallmarks. MiR-221 was down-regulated in prostate carcinoma metastasis. Moreover, this miRNA was progressively down-regulated in aggressive forms of prostate carcinoma. Down-regulation of miR-221 was associated with the Gleason score and the clinical recurrence during follow up. Kaplan-Meier estimates and Cox proportional hazard models showed that miR-221 down-regulation was linked to tumor progression and recurrence in a high risk prostate cancer cohort [17]. MiR-34c expression was found to inversely correlate to aggressiveness of the tumor, WHO grade, PSA levels and occurrence of metastases. Furthermore, a Kaplan-Meier analysis of patient survival based on miR-34c expression levels divided into low (<50(th) percentile) and high (>50(th) percentile) expression, significantly stratify the patients into high risk and low risk group (p = 0.0003, long-rank test) [18]. MiR-17-3p expression was compared in prostate benign stroma, hyperplastic stroma, glandular epithelium and adenocarcinoma of differing Gleason patterns 3-5. MiR-17-3p levels declined significantly in tumor tissue with increasing Gleason pattern 3-5 compared to hyperplastic epithelium and normal glandular epithelium [19]. Lastly, Pesta et al. (2010) observed that miR-20a expression was significantly higher in the group of patients with a Gleason score of 7-10 in comparison with the group of patients with a Gleason score of 0-6 (p = 0.0082). On the other hand, they found no statistical differences in the miRNA expressions (mir-20a, let-7a, miR-15a, and miR-16) in the prostate carcinoma tissue samples in comparison with the BPH tissue samples [20].

## 8.6. MiRNAs as Potential Therapeutic Targets

Recent studies have shown that miR-21 is up-regulated in many types of cancers including prostate cancer. Moreover, this miRNA plays probably key roles in tumor growth, invasion, metastasis, and drug resistance. Inhibition of miR-21 diminished androgen-induced prostate cancer cell proliferation. Elevated expression of miR-21 enhanced prostate cancer tumor growth *in vivo* and, surprisingly, was sufficient for androgen-dependent tumors to overcome castration-mediated growth arrest [21]. In addition, inactivation of miR-21 in androgen-independent prostate cancer cell lines resulted in sensitivity to apoptosis and inhibition of cell motility and invasion. These effects may be partly due to its regulation of PDCD4, TPM1, and MARCKS [22]. According to this data, gene therapy using miR-21 inhibition strategy may be useful as a prostate cancer therapy. Nevertheless, Folini et al.

(2010) also investigated the role of miR-21 and its potential as a therapeutic target in prostate cancer cell lines, characterized by different miR-21 expression levels and PTEN gene status. Their data suggest that miR-21 is not a central player in the onset of prostate cancer and that its single hitting is not a valuable therapeutic strategy in the disease. This supports the notion that the oncogenic properties of miR-21 could be cell and tissue dependent and that the potential role of a given miRNA as a therapeutic target should be contextualized with respect to the disease [23].

Other miRNAs, which would be potential targets in prostate cancer therapy, are miR-221 and miR-222. An inverse relationship between the expression of miR-221 and miR-222 and the cell cycle inhibitor p27 (Kip1) was described [24]. MiR-221 and miR-222 knock-down directly increases p27 (Kip1) in PC3 cells and strongly reduces their clonogenicity *in vitro*. In addition, these data were subsequently confirmed *in vivo* [24,25]. Moreover, Sun et al. (2009) described that an over-expression of miR-221 or miR-222 in androgen-dependent cell lines (LNCaP) significantly reduced the level of the dihydrotestosterone induced up-regulation of PSA expression and increased androgen-independent growth of examined cells. Knocking down the expression level of these miRNAs restored the response to the dihydrotestosterone induction of PSA transcription and also increased the growth response of the LNCaP-derived cell line LNCaP-Abl to the androgen treatment [26]. Finally, miR-221 and 222 significantly reduce ARHI (tumor suppressor gene) expression by direct targeting of 3' UTR of ARHI. Genistein, a potential nontoxic chemopreventive agent, down-regulates miR-221/222 and, thus, restores expression of ARHI [27].

Zaman et al. (2010) investigated the expression and functional significance of miR-145 in prostate cancer. The expression of miR-145 was low in the three tested prostate cell lines compared with the normal cell line, and in cancerous regions of human prostate tissue when compared with the matched adjacent normal tissue. Analyses of miR-145-over-expressing PC3 cells showed up-regulation of the pro-apoptotic gene TNFSF10. In accordance with this result, over-expression of miR-145 showed an increasing of apoptosis and an increase in cells in the G2/M phase [28]. Further, Clapé et al. (2009) showed in their study that miR-143 levels are inversely correlated with advanced stages of prostate cancer. Rescue of miR-143 expression in cancer cells results in the arrest of cell proliferation and the abrogation of tumor growth in mice. Furthermore, they showed that the effects of miR-143 were mediated, at least in part, by the inhibition of ERK5 activity [29]. Therefore, modulation of miR-143 and miR-145 may be also an important therapeutic approach for the management of prostate cancer.

## Acknowledgment

This work was supported by grants NS 10361-3/2009, NR/9814-4/2008, NS 10352-3/2009, NT/11214-4/2010 of Czech Ministry of Health, Project No. MZ0MOU2005 of the Czech Ministry of Health.

# References

[1] Damber JE, Aus G: Prostate cancer. *Lancet* 2008 371:1710-21.

[2] Coppola V, De Maria R, Bonci D: MicroRNAs and prostate cancer. *Endocr. Relat. Cancer* 2010, 17:F1-17.

[3] Xu B, Feng NH, Li PC, Tao J, Wu D, Zhang ZD, Tong N, Wang JF, Song NH, Zhang W, Hua LX, Wu HF: A functional polymorphism in Pre-miR-146a gene is associated with prostate cancer risk and mature miR-146a expression in vivo. *Prostate* 2010 70:467-72.

[4] George GP, Gangwar R, Mandal RK, Sankhwar SN, Mittal RD: Genetic variation in microRNA genes and prostate cancer risk in North Indian population. *Mol. Biol. Rep.* 2010 [Epub ahead of print].

[5] Xu B, Feng NH, Li PC, Tao J, Wu D, Zhang ZD, Tong N, Wang JF, Song NH, Zhang W, Hua LX, Wu HF: A functional polymorphism in Pre-miR-146a gene is associated with prostate cancer risk and mature miR-146a expression in vivo. *Prostate* 2010 70:467-72.

[6] Bao BY, Pao JB, Huang CN, Pu YS, Chang TY, Lan YH, Lu TL, Lee HZ, Juang SH, Chen LM, Hsieh CJ, Huang SP: Polymorphisms inside MicroRNAs and MicroRNA Target Sites Predict Clinical Outcomes in Prostate Cancer Patients Receiving Androgen-Deprivation Therapy. *Clin Cancer Res* 2010 [Epub ahead of print].

[7] Moltzahn F, Olshen AB, Baehner L, Peek AS, Fong L, Stoppler HJ, Simko J, Hilton JF, Carroll PR, Blelloch R: Microfluidic based multiplex qRT-PCR identifies diagnostic and prognostic microRNA signatures in sera of prostate cancer patients. *Cancer Res.* 2010 [Epub ahead of print].

[8] Mitchell PS, Parkin RK, Kroh EM, Fritz BR, Wyman SK, Pogosova-Agadjanyan EL, Peterson A, Noteboom J, O'Briant KC, Allen A, Lin DW, Urban N, Drescher CW, Knudsen BS, Stirewalt DL, Gentleman R, Vessella RL, Nelson PS, Martin DB, Tewari M: Circulating microRNAs as stable blood-based markers for cancer detection. *Proc. Natl. Acad. Sci. USA* 2008 105:10513-8.

[9] Zhang HL, Yang LF, Zhu Y, Yao XD, Zhang SL, Dai B, Zhu YP, Shen YJ, Shi GH, Ye DW: Serum miRNA-21: Elevated levels in patients with metastatic hormone-refractory prostate cancer and potential predictive factor for the efficacy of docetaxel-based chemotherapy. Prostate 2010 [Epub ahead of print].

[10] Porkka KP, Pfeiffer MJ, Waltering KK, Vessella RL, Tammela TL, Visakorpi T: MicroRNA expression profiling in prostate cancer. *Cancer Res.* 2007 67:6130-5.

[11] Ambs S, Prueitt RL, Yi M, Hudson RS, Howe TM, Petrocca F, Wallace TA, Liu CG, Volinia S, Calin GA, Yfantis HG, Stephens RM, Croce CM: Genomic profiling of microRNA and messenger RNA reveals deregulated microRNA expression in prostate cancer. *Cancer Res.* 2008 68:6162-70.

[12] Schaefer A, Jung M, Mollenkopf HJ, Wagner I, Stephan C, Jentzmik F, Miller K, Lein M, Kristiansen G, Jung K: Diagnostic and prognostic implications of microRNA profiling in prostate carcinoma. *Int. J. Cancer* 2010 126:1166-76.

[13] Ozen M, Creighton CJ, Ozdemir M, Ittmann M: Widespread deregulation of microRNA expression in human prostate cancer. *Oncogene* 2008 27:1788-93.

[14] Sun D, Lee YS, Malhotra A, Kim HK, Matecic M, Evans C, Jensen RV, Moskaluk CA, Dutta A: miR-99 family of microRNAs suppresses the expression of prostate specific antigen and prostate cancer cell proliferation. *Cancer Res.* 2011 [Epub ahead of print].

[15] Volinia S, Calin GA, Liu CG, Ambs S, Cimmino A, Petrocca F, Visone R, Iorio M, Roldo C, Ferracin M, Prueitt RL, Yanaihara N, Lanza G, Scarpa A, Vecchione A, Negrini M, Harris CC, Croce CM: A microRNA expression signature of human solid tumors defines cancer gene targets. *Proc. Natl. Acad. Sci USA* 2006 103:2257-61.

[16] Leite KR, Sousa-Canavez JM, Reis ST, Tomiyama AH, Camara-Lopes LH, Sañudo A, Antunes AA, Srougi M: Change in expression of miR-let7c, miR-100, and miR-218 from high grade localized prostate cancer to metastasis. *Urol. Oncol.* 2009 [Epub ahead of print].

[17] Spahn M, Kneitz S, Scholz CJ, Stenger N, Rüdiger T, Ströbel P, Riedmiller H, Kneitz B: Expression of microRNA-221 is progressively reduced in aggressive prostate cancer and metastasis and predicts clinical recurrence. *Int. J. Cancer* 2010 127:394-403.

[18] Hagman Z, Larne O, Edsjö A, Bjartell A, Ehrnström RA, Ulmert D, Lilja H, Ceder Y: miR-34c is down regulated in prostate cancer and exerts tumor suppressive functions. *Int. J. Cancer* 2010 [Epub ahead of print].

[19] Zhang X, Ladd A, Dragoescu E, Budd WT, Ware JL, Zehner ZE: MicroRNA-17-3p is a prostate tumor suppressor in vitro and in vivo, and is decreased in high grade prostate tumors analyzed by laser capture microdissection. *Clin. Exp. Metastasis* 2009 26:965-79.

[20] Pesta M, Klecka J, Kulda V, Topolcan O, Hora M, Eret V, Ludvikova M, Babjuk M, Novak K, Stolz J, Holubec L: Importance of miR-20a expression in prostate cancer tissue. *Anticancer Res.* 2010 30:3579-83.

[21] Ribas J, Ni X, Haffner M, Wentzel EA, Salmasi AH, Chowdhury WH, Kudrolli TA, Yegnasubramanian S, Luo J, Rodriguez R, Mendell JT, Lupold SE: miR-21: an androgen receptor-regulated microRNA that promotes hormone-dependent and hormone-independent prostate cancer growth. *Cancer Res.* 2009 69:7165-9.

[22] Li T, Li D, Sha J, Sun P, Huang Y: MicroRNA-21 directly targets MARCKS and promotes apoptosis resistance and invasion in prostate cancer cells. *Biochem. Biophys. Res. Commun.* 2009 383:280-5.

[23] Folini M, Gandellini P, Longoni N, Profumo V, Callari M, Pennati M, Colecchia M, Supino R, Veneroni S, Salvioni R, Valdagni R, Daidone MG, Zaffaroni N: miR-21: an oncomir on strike in prostate cancer. *Mol. Cancer* 2010 9:12.

[24] Galardi S, Mercatelli N, Giorda E, Massalini S, Frajese GV, Ciafrè SA, Farace MG: miR-221 and miR-222 expression affects the proliferation potential of human prostate carcinoma cell lines by targeting p27Kip1. *J. Biol. Chem.* 2007 282:23716-24.

[25] Mercatelli N, Coppola V, Bonci D, Miele F, Costantini A, Guadagnoli M, Bonanno E, Muto G, Frajese GV, De Maria R, Spagnoli LG, Farace MG, Ciafrè SA: The inhibition of the highly expressed miR-221 and miR-222 impairs the growth of prostate carcinoma xenografts in mice. *PLoS One* 2008 3:e4029.

[26] Sun T, Wang Q, Balk S, Brown M, Lee GS, Kantoff P: The role of microRNA-221 and microRNA-222 in androgen-independent prostate cancer cell lines. *Cancer Res.* 2009 69:3356-63.

[27] Chen Y, Zaman MS, Deng G, Majid S, Saini S, Liu J, Tanaka Y, Dahiya R: MicroRNAs 221/222 and Genistein-Mediated Regulation of ARHI Tumor Suppressor Gene in Prostate Cancer. *Cancer Prev. Res. (Phila)* 2011 4:76-86.
[28] Zaman MS, Chen Y, Deng G, Shahryari V, Suh SO, Saini S, Majid S, Liu J, Khatri G, Tanaka Y, Dahiya R: The functional significance of microRNA-145 in prostate cancer. *Br. J. Cancer* 2010 103:256-64.
[29] Clapé C, Fritz V, Henriquet C, Apparailly F, Fernandez PL, Iborra F, Avancès C, Villalba M, Culine S, Fajas L: miR-143 interferes with ERK5 signaling, and abrogates prostate cancer progression in mice. *PLoS One* 2009 4:e7542.

In: MicroRNAs in Solid Cancer
Editor: Ondrej Slaby

ISBN: 978-61324-514-9
©2012 Nova Science Publishers, Inc.

*Chapter IX*

# MicroRNAs and Renal Cell Carcinoma

*Martina Redova, Jaroslav Michalek and Ondrej Slaby*

Masaryk Memorial Cancer Institute, Brno, Czech Republic
Advanced Cell Immunotherapy Unit, Masaryk University, Brno, Czech Republic
Central European Institute of Technology, Masaryk University, Brno, Czech Republic

## Abstract

Renal cell carcinoma (RCC) is the most common neoplasm of the adult kidney accounting for about 3 % of adult malignancies. As the role of miRNAs in RCC pathogenesis is emerging, it has been postulated that miRNAs can serve as new potential biomarkers that may improve diagnostic, prognostic and predictive abilities, and consequently, the management of RCC patients.

## 9.1. Introduction

Renal cell carcinoma represents the third leading cause of death among genitourinary malignancies [1-3] with having the highest mortality rate at over 40% [4,5]. RCC originates in the lining of the proximal renal tubule, the very small tubes in the kidney that filter blood and remove waste products [6]. The clear cell histology type, renal cell clear carcinoma (RCCC or ccRCC) represents about 75-85 % of RCC, thus being the most frequent subtype of RCC [7,8].

RCCC is generally characterized by the loss of VHL gene (von Hippel-Lindau), which under normal oxygen pressure, binds to the α subunits of hypoxia inducible factors (HIFs), inducing their poly-ubiquitinylation and subsequent degradation in the proteasome. On the contrary, in hypoxic conditions, or if HIF regulation is lost because of VHL inactivation, HIF accumulates to high levels and promotes the transcription of gene such as VEGF, PDGF-β, TGF-α, EPO, etc., which trigger angiogenesis, cell growth, migration and proliferation, and which are known to be relevant to RCC biology and therapy [9-11]. Among classical symptoms, hematuria, palpable renal mass, fever, loss of weight, varicoceles, etc. could be mentioned [6]. The 5 year cancer-specific survival rates for stages I to IV (according to TNM staging system) are 81, 74, 53 and 8 %, respectively (www.cancer.org – 7.1.2011) whereas the 5-year survival ranging of late stage RCC is limited from 5 to 10 % for lack of efficacy in chemotherapy and radiation therapy [8]. Surgical resection remains the best curative therapy for RCC, although after the curative nephrectomy, 20-40 % patients will develop recurrence because chemo- and radioresistance has been described [7,12,13]. As DNA, RNA and protein profile of carcinoma research has not successfully elucidated the pathogenesis of kidney carcinoma and only few data are available on miRNAs in renal carcinoma, further investigation on miRNAs field may provide a useful clue for the pathophysiology research of RCC. Furthermore, the study of miRNAs as potential diagnostic biomarkers may lead to the improvement in diagnosis, prognosis and reveal their impact on future therapeutic strategies.

## 9.2. Polymorphisms within Mature miRNA Sequence and miRNA Binding Regions and Risk of Cancer

With the increasing choices of treatment modalities it is of great clinical interest to have the posibility to predict clinical outcome for RCC patients. Identification of germ line genetic variants that predict RCC clinical outcome has become an increasingly promising approach that complements to somatic biomarkers.

Lin et al. (2010) tested the hypothesis that common sequence variants in genes of miRNA and of the miRNA biogenesis pathway affect RCC clinical outcome. They evaluated 41 potentially functional miRNA-related single-nucleotide polymorphisms (SNPs) as well as took a polygenic approach to evaluate the cumulative effects of these SNPs on survival and recurrence among RCC patients, and have identified 7 SNPs significantly associated with RCC survival with the most significant SNPs in GEMIN4 (rs7813, rs910925, rs3744741), whose products are involved in pre-mRNA splicing and ribonucleoprotein assembly, and 5 SNPs associated with RCC recurrence, with the borderline significant SNP in Dicer (rs3742330) which encode proteins that are members of the ribonuclease III family of double-stranded RNA endunucleases participating in RNA maturation and decay pathways. Besides GEMIN4 and Dicer, one SNP in miR-608 (rs4919510), predicted by *in silico* algorithms to show differential binding to its target genes, which include INSR (insulin receptor) and p53, was significantly associated with both RCC survival and recurrence [3].

Also in the study of Horikawa and coworkers (2008) the non-synonymous SNPs of the GEMIN4 (rs7813 and rs2740348) were found to be associated with higher RCC risk. Furthermore, they have observed borderline significant associations with RCC risk in XPO5 gene which mediate the nuclear transport of pre-miRNAs, and AGO1 gene which is a component of miRISC together with AGO2 and Dicer1, and is involved in miRNA function leading to target mRNA degradation [14]. Results of these groups imply that individual as well as combined genotypes of miRNA processing pathway genes may influence the RCC tumorigenesis and progression.

## 9.3. Tissue miRNA Signatures: Implications for Diagnostic Oncology

MiRNAs have been shown to be differentially expressed in a variety of cancers, including RCC. Differences in miRNAs expression may potentially serve as a „tissue specific" expression signature to distinguish different types of malignancies, to distinguish between RCC versus normal renal tissue or even among various histological subtypes. Petillo et al. (2009) were able to distinguish between favorable and unfavorable prognostic groups of RCCC, and among clear cell, chromophobe, papillary renal cell carcinoma and oncocytoma on the basis of differently expressed miRNAs [15]. Liu et al. (2010) have developed and validated a simple method to identify miRNA/mRNA pairs which can discriminate normal tissue from cancer tissue, and also dysregulated regulation mechanisms between them, that may initiate and/or drive the disease process [11].

Among commonly dysregulated miRNAs, oncogenic miR-155, miR-21 with a role in promoting tumor growth, cell invasion and metastasis, hypoxia inducible miR-210 with known anti-apoptotic potential, miR-34a associated with cell proliferation in an oxidative stress-induced rat renal carcinogenesis model, and miR-221 known to repress the expression of cell cycle regulator p27 (Kip1) together with miR-222, are known to be significantly up-regulated in RCC.

On the contrary, miR-141 and miR-200c, with possible tumor supressor activity, are the most significantly down-regulated miRNAs in RCC [1,7,16,17]. Other dysregulated miRNAs are listed in Table 9.1, and for detailed information see Figure 9.1.

**Table 9.1. List of representative miRNAs differentially expressed in renal cell carcinoma mentioned in at least two miRNA profiling studies**

| Up-regulated miRNAs in RCC | | Down-regulated miRNAs in RCC | |
|---|---|---|---|
| miRNA | Reference + p-value | miRNA | Reference + p-value |
| miR-210 | [16] 6.36E-05 [23] 0.006 [7] 6.55E-02 [17] □0.0001 | miR-200c | [16] 5.14E-06 [23] 0.002 [7] 1.44E-03 [17] □0.0001 |
| miR-155 | [16] 0.000469 [23] 0.0240 [17] □0.0001 | miR-141 | [16] 6.31E-06 [23] 0.0020 [17] 0.0020 |
| miR-21 | [23] 0.1098 [7] 2.79E-02 | miR-182 | [7] 5.15E-02 [17] 0.9190 |
| miR-106a | [7] 1.46E-02 [17] □0.0001 | miR-199a | [23] 0.0020 [7] 5.15E-02 |
| miR-106b | [7] 9.27E-02 [17] □0.0001 | miR-200b | [23] 0.0040 [7] 3.59E-03 |
| miR-122a | [16] 0.00191 [7] 1.12E-02 | miR-411 | [16] 0.000773 [23] 0.0020 |
| miR-185 | [1] □0.0001 [23] 0.6587 | miR-514 | [16] 8.96E-05 [23] 0.0020 |
| miR-224 | [16] 0.0013 [23] 0.9721 | | |

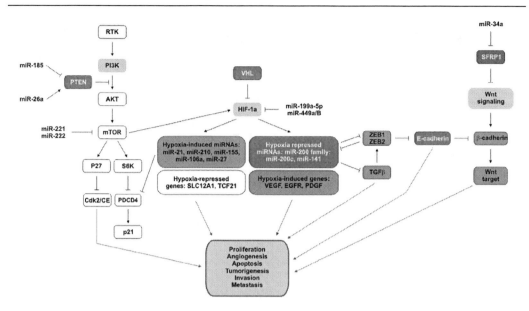

Figure 9.1. Model of dysregulated patways in RCC based on predicted miRNA/mRNA interactions and known signaling pathways. (Modified from [10]).

## 9.4. MiRNAs Expression in Prognosis and Response Prediction

Large-scale profiling of miRNA expressions using microarray or qRT-PCR techniques has revealed significant associations between miRNA expression signatures and the etiology and prognosis of various cancers. Beside an outcome prediction, the most promising application of miRNAs might lie in estimation of response modification in known and well established anti-tumor therapies such as radiation- and chemotherapy. MiRNAs dysregulation may provide an information about sensitivity or resistance to different treatment modalities before starting any therapy („response prediction") or additionally during the therapy it may offer a tool for control of treatment success („response control").

For example, in the study by Neal et al. (2010), miR-210 was shown to be a prognostic marker as its expression correlated with patient survival [18]. Furthermore, they have tested the expression level of CAIX, a transcriptional target of HIF-1, whose expression has been previously shown to be an intrinsic marker of hypoxia/HIF activation and has been reported to be a predictor of outcome in RCC. They have also revealed a striking positive correlation between CAIX and miR-210 expression (r = 0,527, p = 0,002). On the contrary, they have observed no correlation between CAIX levels and other VHL-regulated miRNAs, with the exception of miR-155 which showed only a weak correlation (r = 0,318, p = 0,082). The ability of miR-210 expression levels to provide prognostic information has also been seen in breast cancer [19,20] and head and neck cancers [21].

Because in the case of RCC the current absence of biomarkers for early detection and follow-up may lead to late diagnosis and subsequent poor prognosis, it is of great interest to identify new and powerfull biomarkers enabling prediction of early metastasis after nephrectomy. From these reasons, Slaby et al. (2010) compared the expression levels of individual miRNAs potentially associated with the prognosis of RCC patients in the group of patients who developed metastasis with their levels in the group of patients in remisson. They have observed that metastatic patients tended to have lower levels of miR-155, miR-106a, and miR-106b in tumor tissue, but only miR-106b reached statistical significance (p = 0,03). From this point of view, miRNA-106b might be used for predicting a development of early metastasic disease after nephrectomy in clinical practice, and after validation, this would represent a next step to perform the best treatment modality decisions and, subsequently, to improve the survival rate of RCC patients [17].

## 9.5. MiRNAs as Potential Therapeutic Targets

Apart from response prediction and response control, it has been postulated that modification of miRNAs expression by up- or down-regulation may possibly enhance sensitivity to the applied chemo- or radiotherapy („response modulation"). Furthermore, it has been demonstrated that sensitivity of transformed cells to well known chemotherapeutic agents might be successfully modulated by miRNAs [22]. These data and the growing knowledge about miRNAs impact on several aspects of carcinogenesis indicate that miRNAs may serve as promising candidates for control and modification of conventional and/or new developed anticancer treatments and that the effect of existing therapeutic strategies could be maximised and survival of patients could be improved by combination with miRNAs. MiRNAs based gene therapy is extremely interesting because it allows targeting multiple genes simultaneously, and this is especially exciting in managing RCC as RCC is notorious for being resistant to therapy, especially in the metastatic stage.

MiR-200c and miR-141 have been observed by many authors as being the most significantly down-regulated in RCC tissues [6,16,17,23]. According to the results of Nakada et al. (2008), it is suggested that down-regulated miR-141 and miR-200c in RCC might play a causative role in suppression of CDH1/E-cadherin transcription via up-regulation of their predicted target ZFHX1B (also known as SIP1 and ZEB2; function as a transcriptional repressor for CDH1/E-cadherin) leading to epithelial-mesenchymal transition (EMT) [16]. Park et al. (2008) elucidated this context by co-transfection of cells with ZFHX1B 3'-UTR-luciferase reporter construct and pre-miR-200c which resulted in repressed luciferase activity. These results show that miR-141 and miR-200c may possess a tumor suppressor function in cancer cells and could become a promising anticancer therapeutic modality [24, 25].

Another miRNA with potential therapeutic impact is miR-205 found to be decreased in kidney cancer. In mechanistic study, proliferation of renal cancer cells was suppressed by miR-205, mediated by the pSrc-regulated ERK1/2 pathway. Transient as well as stable over-expression of miR-205 in A498 renal cancer cells resulted suppressed cell proliferation, colony formation, migration, and invasion in renal cancer cells. MiR-205 also inhibited tumor cell growth *in vivo*. Together, miR-205 inhibits proto-oncogenic Src family of kinases indicating its therapeutic potential in the treatment of renal cancer [26].

The oncogenic miR-185 is another miRNA with potentially important implications in RCC development. It was found to be significantly up-regulated in RCC and anti-correlated with tumor suppressor gene PTEN which is mutated or down-regulated in many advanced cancers [27]. Subfamily of potassium channel membrane proteins, which is another target of miR-185, KCNJ16, member of, is also suggested in anticancer therapies due to its important role in cell growth [28]. Such membrane proteins are known to be down-regulated in RCC [11].

Despite growing number of miRNAs as potential cancer therapeutic targets there are still some limitations which need to be addressed. Up-to-date literature provides only a tight insight into the construct of „miRNA - chemotherapeutic agent" interactions which might be extremely complex and complicated, and detailed mechanisms and intracellular pathways involved in the miRNA-mediated effects are not fully understood. Furthermore, exosomal-derived miRNA profiling has not yet been analysed regarding its potential to predict response to an anticancer treatment. For above mentioned reasons and also because there is no evidence of a tolerance of such a treatment in humans, additional studies have to be undertaken to validate the safety and efficiency of miRNA-based treatment in clinical settings.

## Acknowledgment

This work was supported by grants NS 10361-3/2009, NR/9814-4/2008, NS 10352-3/2009, NT/11214-4/2010 of Czech Ministry of Health, Project No. MZ0MOU2005 of the Czech Ministry of Health and by the project "CEITEC – Central European Institute of Technology" (CZ.1.05/1.1.00/02.0068).

## References

[1] Gottardo F, Liu CG, Ferracin M, Calin GA, Fassan M, Bassi P, Sevignani C, Byrne D, Negrini M, Pagano F, Gomella L, Croce CM, Baffa R: Micro-RNA profiling in kidney and bladder cancers. *Urol. Oncol.* 2007 25:387-92.
[2] White NMA, Yousef GM: MicroRNAs: exploring a new dimension in the pathogenesis of kidney cancer. *BMC Med* 2010 8:65.
[3] Lin J, Horikawa Y, Tamboli P, Clague J, Wood CG, Wu X: Genetic variations in microRNA-related genes are associated with survival and recurrence in patients with renal cell carcinoma. *Carcinogenesis* 2010 31:1805-12.
[4] Van Spronsen DJ, Mulders PF, De Mulder PH: Novel treatments for metastatic renal cell carcinoma. *Crit Rev Oncol Hematol* 2005 55:177-91.
[5] Campbell SC, Novick AC, Bukowski RM: Renal tumors. In Campbell-Wals Urology, 9th edn, Wein AJ, Kavoussi LR, Novick AC, Partin AW, Peters CA (eds). Saunders: Philadelphia, PA, 2007 1567-637.
[6] Yi Z, Fu Y, Zhao S, Zhang X, Ma C: Differential expression of miRNA patterns in renal cell carcinoma and nontumorous tissues. *J. Cancer Res. Clin. Oncol.* 2010 136:855-62.
[7] Chow TF, Youssef YM, Lianidou E, Romaschin AD, Honey RJ, Stewart R, Pace KT, Yousef GM: Differential expression profiling of microRNAs and their potential involvement in renal cell carcinoma pathogenesis. *Clin. Biochem.* 2010 43:150-8.

[8] Huang Y, Dai Y, Yang J, Chen T, Yin Y, Tang M, Hu C, Zhang L: Microarray analysis of microRNA expression in renal clear cell carcinoma. *Eur. J. Surg. Oncol.* 2009 35:1119-23.

[9] Calzada MJ, del Peso L: Hypoxia-inducible factors and cancer. *Clin. Transl. Oncol.* 2007 9:278-89.

[10] Redova M, Svoboda M, Slaby O: MicroRNAs and their target gene networks in renal cell carcinoma. *Biochem. Biophys. Res. Commun.* 2011 405:153-6.

[11] Liu H, Brannon AR, Reddy AR, Alexe G, Seiler MW, Arreola A, Oza JH, Yao M, Juan D, Liou LS, Ganesan S, Levine AJ, Rathmell WK, Bhanot GV: Identifying mRNA targets of microRNA dysregulated in cancer: with application to clear cell Renal Cell Carcinoma. *BMC Syst. Biol.* 2010 4:51.

[12] Janzen NK, Kim HL, Figlin RA, Belldegrun AS: Surveillance after radical or partial nephrectomy for localized renal cell carcinoma and management of recurrent disease. *Urol. Clin. North Am.* 2003 30:843-52.

[13] Escudier B: Advanced renal cell carcinoma: current and emerging management strategies. *Drugs* 2007 67:1257-64.

[14] Horikawa Y, Wood CG, Yang H, Zhao H, Ye Y, Gu J, Lin J, Habuchi T, Wu X: Single nucleotide polymorphisms of microRNA machinery genes modify the risk of renal cell carcinoma. *Clin. Cancer Res.* 2008 14:7956-62.

[15] Petillo D, Kort EJ, Anema J, Furge KA, Yang XJ, The BT: MicroRNA profiling of human kidney cancer subtypes. *Int. J. Oncol.* 2009 35:109-14.

[16] Nakada C, Matsuura K, Tsukamoto Y, Tanigawa M, Yoshimoto T, Narimatsu T, Nguyen LT, Hijiya N, Uchida T, Sato F, Mimata H, Seto M, Moriyama M: Genome-wide microRNA expression profiling in renal cell carcinoma: significant down-regulation of miR-141 and miR-200c. *J. Pathol.* 2008 216:418-27.

[17] Slaby O, Jancovicova J, Lakomy R, Svoboda M, Poprach A, Fabian P, Kren L, Michalek J, Vyzula R: Expression of miRNA-106b in conventional renal cell carcinoma is a potential marker for prediction of early metastasis after nephrectomy. *J. Exp. Clin. Cancer Res.* 2010 29:90.

[18] Neal CS, Michael MZ, Rawlings LH, Van der Hoek MB, Gleadle JM: The VHL-dependent regulation of microRNAs in renal cancer. *BMC Med.* 2010 8:64.

[19] Camps C, Buffa FM, Colella S, Moore J, Sheldon H, Harris AL, Gleadle JM, Ragoussis J: hsa-miR-210 is induced by hypoxia and is an independent prognostic factor in breast cancer. *Clin. Cancer Res.* 2008 14:1-8.

[20] Gee HE, Camps C, Buffa FM, Colella S, Sheldon H, Gleadle JM, Ragoussis J, Harris AL: MicroRNA-10b and breast cancer metastasis. *Nature* 2008 455:E8-E9.

[21] Gee HE, Camps C, Buffa FM, Patiar S, Winter SC, Betts G, Homer J, Corbridge R, Cox G, L.West CM, Ragoussis J, Harris AL: hsa-mir-210 is a marker of tumor hypoxia and a prognostic factor in head and neck cancer. *Cancer* 2010 116:2148-58.

[22] Hummel R, Hussey DJ, Haier J: MicroRNAs: Predictors and modifiers of chemo- and radiotherapy in different tumour types. *Eur. J. Cancer* 2010 46:298-311.

[23] Juan D, Alexe G, Antes T, Liu H, Madabhushi A, Delisi C, Ganesan S, Bhanot G, Liou LS: Identification of a microRNA panel for clear-cell kidney cancer. *Urology* 2010 75:835-41.

[24] Park SM, Gaur AB, Lengyel E, Peter ME: The miR-200 family determines the epithelial phenotype of cancer cells by targeting the E-cadherin repressors ZEB1 and ZEB2. *Genes Dev.* 2008 22:894-907.

[25] Jung M, Mollenkopf HJ, Grimm C, Wagner I, Albrecht M, Waller T, Pilarsky C, Johannsen M, Stephan C, Lehrach H, Nietfeld W, Rudel T, Jung K, Kristiansen G: MicroRNA profiling of clear cell renal cell cancer identifies a robust signature to define renal malignancy. *J. Cell Mol. Med.* 2009 13:3918-28.

[26] Majid S, Saini S, Dar AA, Hirata H, Shahryari V, Tanaka Y, Yamamura S, Ueno K, Zaman MS, Singh K, Chang I, Deng G, Dahiya R: MicroRNA-205 inhibits Src-mediated oncogenic pathways in renal cancer. *Cancer Res.* 2011 DOI: 10.1158/0008-5472.CAN-10-3666.

[27] Hara S, Oya M, Mizuno R, Horiguchi A, Marumo K, Murai M: Akt activation in renal cell carcinoma: contribution of a decreased PTEN expression and the induction of apoptosis by an Akt inhibitor. *Ann. Oncol.* 2005 16:928-33.

[28] Felipe A, Vicente R, Villalonga N, Roura-Ferrer M, Martínez-Mármol R, Solé L, Ferreres JC, Condom E: Potassium channels: new targets in cancer therapy. *Cancer Detect Prev.* 2006 30:375-85.

In: MicroRNAs in Solid Cancer
Editor: Ondrej Slaby

ISBN: 978-61324-514-9
©2012 Nova Science Publishers, Inc.

*Chapter X*

# MicroRNAs and Hepatocellular Carcinoma

*Martina Redova*
Masaryk Memorial Cancer Institute, Brno, Czech Republic

## Abstract

Hepatocellular carcinoma (HCC) is the fifth most prevalent cancer in the world and is the third leading cause of cancer-related death. Because of its high fatality rates, the incidence and mortality rates are almost equal. From these reasons, it is necessary to identify powerful biological markers that can be used to screen high-risk patients in order to allow better HCC detection, earlier intervention, and to increase the likelihood of successful treatment. Accumulating evidence has linked the dysregulated miRNA levels to a variety of malignancies, including HCC. Several investigations have also described the ability of specific miRNA expression profiles to predict prognosis, and potential of selected miRNAs as novel therapeutic targets in HCC patients.

## 10.1. Introduction

Hepatocellular carcinoma accounts for 80% to 90% of primary liver cancers and shows a wide geographical variation with high incidence areas in Africa and Asia. In endemic areas, HCC is strongly associated with chronic viral infections of hepatitis types B and C and liver cirrhosis [1]. Major features of HCC include chronic inflammation and the effects of cytokines on the development of fibrosis and liver cell proliferation. In addition, some viral genes can cause malignant transformation [2]. The high mortality associated with this disease is mainly caused by partial failure to diagnose HCC patients at an early stage and a lack of effective therapies for patients with advanced stage HCC [3]. Nowadays, the curative treatments for HCC detected at an early stage include surgical resection, liver transplantation, and percutaneous ablation, but although surgery remains the most effective treatment for

HCC, the majority of patients are inoperable at presentation because of late diagnosis [4]. Furthermore, despite surgical or locoregional therapies, prognosis remains poor because of high tumor recurrence or progression, and currently there are no well-established effective adjuvant therapies [5]. Hepatocarcinogenesis is a multistep process going from chronic hepatitis through cirrhosis and/or dysplastic nodule (DN) to HCC [6]. Like many other tumors, HCC seems to develop via a multistage process with an accumulation of genetic and epigenetic alterations in regulatory genes or mechanisms. Several important intracellular signaling pathways such as the Ras/Raf/MAPK pathway and PI3K/Akt/mTOR pathway have been recognized, and the roles of several growth factors and angiogenic factors such as EGF and VEGF have been confirmed [5,7]. TP53, RB, IGF2R, oncogenes, c-myc, CCND1, CTNNB1, and c-Met have been reported in hepatocarcinogenesis [4-10]. Activation of the matrix metalloproteinase family, angiopoietin, VEGF, and inactivation of E-cadherin have been reported to play important roles in invasion and metastasis of hepatocellular carcinoma [2]. Understanding the relationships between biological behavior and molecular changes in HCC is of main importance to set accurate and early diagnosis, to develop efficient treatment of HCC, and improve the prognosis of patients. Aberrant expression of several miRNAs was found to be involved in human hepatocarcinogenesis. MiRNA expression signatures were correlated with histopathological and clinical features of HCC. In some cases, aberrantly expressed miRNAs could be linked to cancer-associated pathways, indicating a direct role in liver tumorigenesis. The demonstration of *in vivo* efficacy and safety of anti-miRNA compounds has opened the way to their potential use as novel therapeutic targets.

## 10.2. Polymorphisms within Mature miRNA Sequence and miRNA Binding Regions and Risk of Cancer

Single nucleotide polymorphisms (SNPs) or mutations in mature miRNA sequence may alter miRNAs expression and influence variety of target genes. It has been well demonstrated that SNPs in protein-coding genes can affect the functions of proteins and in turn influence the individual susceptibility to cancers. To date, little is known about the impact of various SNPs in the miRNA genes.

Xu et al. (2008) dealt with the G>C polymorphism in miR-146a precursor and found out that it may result in important phenotypic traits with biomedical implications. Using multivariate unconditional logistic regression, with adjustment for sex, age and hepatitis B virus (HBV) status, they analyzed the association between genotype and risk of HCC. Their results revealed that male individuals with GG genotype were two-fold more susceptible to HCC (OR 2.016, 95% CI 1.056-3.848, $p = 0.034$) compared with those with CC genotype [8].

Furthermore, it was reported that SNPs in the promoters of genes may affect the binding efficiency or disrupt the binding of GATA, which subsequently caused changed transcription activities of the promoter. For example, to confirm the hypothesis that a potentially functional common SNP rs4938723, which was found in the promoter region of pri-miR-34b/c, and TP53 Arg72-Pro are independently or jointly associated with the risk of HCC, later on, Xu et al. (2011) genotyped the 2 SNPs in a case-control study of 501 HCC patients and 548 cancer-free controls in a Chinese population. They found out that the SNP rs4938723 located within the CpG island of pri-miR-34b/c might create a predicted GATA-binding site, and therefore, it may affect miR-34b/c expression by both genetic and epigenetic mechanisms. Furthermore, they revealed association between this SNP and a significantly increased risk of HCC. Moreover, from their results it is evident that miR-34b/c plays a less role in HBV- or HCV-positive HCC, which may have the inactivated p53-miR-34 pathway [9].

Additionally, Gao et al. (2009) identified a variant allele in the 3′ UTR of IL1A that alters miR-122 and miR-378 mediated regulation of IL1A expression and is associated with HCC risks in Chinese population. In other words, the risk variant alleles of rs3783553 (OR 0,62; 95% CI 0,49-0,78, for the variant homozygote) strengthens the binding of miR-122 and miR-378 with 3′ UTR of IL1A which in turn inhibit the expression of IL-1α, then attenuate the antitumor immunity of this cytokine and confer risk for HCC development. MiR-122 has been shown to play an important role in the process of metastasis of HCC, and a loss of miR-122 expression in liver cancer correlates with suppression of the hepatic phenotype and gain of metastatic properties [10,11]. Since IL-1α affects not only various phases of the malignant process, but also patterns of interactions between malignant cells and the host's immune system, IL-1α could serve as a promising target for immunotherapy, early diagnosis and intervention of HCC [5,12].

## 10.3. Serum and Plasma miRNAs: Early Detection of Disease Onset and Progression

Numerous studies have shown that aberrant miRNA expression is associated with the development and progression of various types of human cancer, including HCC, and interestingly, circulating miRNAs are emerging as promising biomarkers for several pathological conditions. This access further offers a sensitive and convenient means as earlier detection and a monitoring tool of the process to assess hepatocarcinogenesis and presumably many other neoplastic diseases in both experimental and clinical settings.

For example, Sukata et al. (2011) have successfully identified changes of circulating miRNAs in the sera of rats with preneoplastic or neoplastic lesions in the liver, concretely, let-7a, let-7f, and miR-98, known as the miRNAs related to carcinogenesis, showed statistically significant gradual increase in the serum from the rat with hepatocellular preneoplastic and neoplastic lesions [13].

From a clinical point of view, it is necessary to found biomarkers that would improve the diagnosis and management of patients with liver pathologies, particularly insidious liver impairment and early HCC. Facing such a challenge, Gui et al. (2011) chose five miRNAs (i.e. miR-885-5p, miR-574-3p, miR-224, miR-215, and miR-146a) that were up-regulated in the HCC and liver cirrhosis (LC) serum pools and further quantified them using qRT-PCR in patients with HCC, LC, CHB (chronic hepatitis B) or GC (gastric cancer) and in normal controls. Their study revealed that the levels of miR-885-5p were consistently and significantly up-regulated in sera from patients with HCC, LC and CHB than in healthy controls or GC patients. MiR-885-5p yielded an AUC of 0,904 (95% CI 0.837-0.951, $p < 0,0001$) with 90,53% sensitivity and 79,17% specificity in discriminating liver pathologies from healthy controls, suggesting that serum miR-885-5p could potentially serve as an independent and complementary liver pathology associated biomarker [14].

Additionally, study of Xu et al. (2011) demonstrated that three miRNAs commonly deregulated in primary HCC, miR-21, miR-122, and miR-223, are presented at higher levels in serum of patients with HCC compared with healthy individuals, suggesting that these serum miRNAs, especially miR-122 known to be liver specific, might serve as potential markers of cancer. Unfortunately, according to the fact that these miRNAs are also presented at significantly higher levels in serum of patients with chronic hepatitis, they are more likely to reflect liver injury caused by inflammation [15].

## 10.4. Tissue miRNA Signatures: Implications for Diagnostic Oncology

Considering that HCC subtypes has been shown to have distinct miRNA profiles which allow to distinguish between HCC and their adjacent non-tumorous liver tissues, among different HCC histological subtypes, and furthermore, whether it is cancer stem cell (CSC)-like or mature hepatocyte-like, malignant or benign, metastatic or non-metastatic, viral or non-viral in origin, and whether it is caused by hepatitis B or hepatitis C, miRNAs seem to be utilized as HCC biomarkers. Set of studies have identified a unique miRNA profile, unfortunately lacking any miRNAs in common - this might be caused by different ethnicities and/or different techniques used.

Beside liver-specific miR-122 which is significantly down-regulated in HCC tissues and which functions as a potential tumor suppressor, other miRNAs with altered expression, such as up-regulated miR-21, miR-224, miR-23a~27a~24, miR-17-29, miR-221, miR-146a, and miR-18a, and down-regulated miR-125, miR-223, and miR-101, are involved in promoting loss of cell cycle control in HCC [16-24]. Results of Yamashita et al. (2009) support the possible biomarker role of miR-181 family members to identify HCC cases with a cancer stem cell feature, which is an activity contributing metastatic dissemination and resistance to chemotherapy [25]. In term of distinguishing between HCC from adjacent non-tumor liver tissue, Wong et al. (2008) revealed that deregulation of miR-222 and miR-223 could serve as an unequivocally discriminator [23].

Furthermore, it has been described that HCCs have increased levels of miR-21, miR-10b, miR-222, which can be used for differentiating HCC from benign tumors, which in contrast show decreased expression of miR-200c and miR-203 [26]. In addition, the combination of miR-200c and miR-141, miRNAs that promote epithelial phenotypes and are described to have significantly higher levels in non-hepatic epithelial tumors, and endothelial-associated and highly conserved miR-126 which shows higher expression levels in hepatocellular carcinomas, might accurately identified primary hepatocellular carcinoma from metastatic adenocarcinoma in the liver [27].

Study of Ladeiro et al. (2008) also characterized and validated that low levels of miR-126* are seen in HCC associated with alcohol consumption subgroups and high levels of miR-96 in HCC associated with hepatitis B virus infection [26]. Interestingly, miR-18a was found to be much higher expressed in female HCC than male HCC.

**Table 10.1. List of representative miRNAs differentially expressed in HCC mentioned in at least two microRNA profiling studies (* SAM, significance analysis of microarrays)**

| Up-regulated miRNAs in HCC | | Down-regulated miRNAs in HCC | |
|---|---|---|---|
| miRNA | Reference, Fold Change (FC), p-value | miRNA | Reference, Fold Change (FC), p-value |
| miR-25 | [18] FC = 3.396 [19] FC = 3.230; p = 0.045 [29] FC = 2.0; p □0.01 [41] 2.65*; p = 0.021 | miR-29c | [18] FC = 0.269 [19] FC = 0.174; p = 0.007 |
| miR-93 | [18] FC = 4.111; p = 0.024 [29] FC = 3.0; p □0.01 [41] 2.77*; p = 0.049 | miR-101 | [18] FC = 0.212 [19] FC = 0.214; p = 0.009 |
| miR-222 | [16] FC = 4.993 [18] FC = 5.238 [19] FC = 4.964; p = 0.011 | miR-199a | [19] FC = 0.149; p = 0.014 [41] -5.163*; p = 0.0004 |
| miR-18a | [19] FC = 3.223; p = 0.039 [29] FC = 3.1; p □0.01 | miR-424 | [18] FC = 0.284 [19] FC = 0.092; p = 0.001 |
| miR-210 | [19] FC = 3.785; p = 0.04 [41] 3.22*; p = 0.002 | | |
| miR-221 | [16] FC = 2.97 [18] FC = 6.516 | | |
| miR-224 | [16] FC = 11.314 [19] FC = 27.231; p □0.001 | | |

Through targeting the estrogen receptor, the high expression levels of miR-18a in HCC are believed to contribute to HCC cell proliferation [28]. Increased expression of miR-18a was also described by Li et al. [29].

Because it is well known that HCC develops in a multistep process, from chronic hepatitis, cirrhosis through dysplastic nodules (DN) to small and large HCCs, investigations on the precancerous lesions and early-staged HCC have significant clinical values and help to gain insight on the molecular mechanisms of hepatocarcinogenesis. The results of Gao et al. (2010) suggests that down-regulation of miR-145 frequently observed in human DNs and HCC samples may play a role in immortalization of non-tumorigenic cells and its further loss may facilitate cellular transformation [31]. Most recently, miR-145 has also been implicated in controlling the stemness of embryonic cells [30]. They have also confirmed that underexpression of miR-199b, and overexpression of miR-224 in particular, is common in pre-malignant lesions and may accumulate throughout the multistep hepatocarcinogenesis [31]. Other dysregulated microRNAs are listed in Table 10.1.

## 10.5. MiRNAs Expression in Prognosis and Response Prediction

Although surgery remains the most effective treatment modality for HCC, the indispensable majority of patients are inoperable at presentation because of late diagnosis [3]. The consequent improvement in long-term survival of postsurgery patients is only modest because of a high recurrence rate of intrahepatic metastases [1]. Summarizing these reasons, understanding the relationships between phenotypic and molecular changes in HCC is of paramount importance to improve the prognosis of diagnosed patients.

Regarding such a request, Budhu et al. (2008), using a large and clinically well-defined cohort, identified a unique 20-miRNA signature that can predict primary HCC tissues with venous metastases and disease-free and overall survival in an independent cohort of HCC cases including early stage HCC. These miRNAs are: in metastatic HCC up-regulated miR-338, miR-219-1, miR-207, miR-185, and down-regulated miR-30c-1, -1-2, -34a, -19a, -148a, -124a-2, -9-2, -148b, -122a, -125b-2, -194, -30a, -126, -15a, -30e, and let-7g. The procedure of defining this metastasis signature may provide a simple and useful profiling method to assist in identifying HCC patients who are likely to develop metastases or suffer recurrence. This miRNA set also highlights particular biomarkers that may be useful to identify HCC patients who would benefit from adjuvant therapy to reduce the chance of metastasis and recurrence [32].

MiR-122 has been previously described as a liver specific miRNA. Burchard et al. (2010) observed a miR-122 decrease in HBV-associated HCC. They also confirmed the correlation between miR-122 loss and the decrease of mitochondrion-related metabolic pathway gene expression in HCC and in non-tumor liver tissues. Therefore, beside inhibition of HCC cell growth through induction of apoptosis, miR-122 also regulates mitochondrial metabolism and its loss may be detrimental to sustaining critical liver function and contribute to morbidity and mortality of liver cancer patients [1,33].

Another miRNA known to be frequently down-regulated in HCC, is miR-125b which is conversely correlated with Ki-67 and which might inhibit HCC cell growth *in vitro* and *in vivo* by induction of cell cycle arrest in G1/S transition. Altogether, the suppressive effects of miR-125b on HCC cell growth and metastasis might contribute to the poor prognosis of HCC patients with low expression of miR-125b [34,35].

The list of miRNAs which could potentially serve as a prognostic tool may be supplemented by miR-152, whose expression is frequently down-regulated in HBV-related HCC tissues in comparison with adjacent non-cancerous hepatic tissues and is described to be inversely correlated to DNA methyltransferase 1 (DNMT1) mRNA expression in HBV-related HCCs [36], whereas increased protein expression of DNMT1 has been significantly correlated with the malignant potential and poor prognosis of human HCC [37]. Moreover, miR-101 which plays a fundamental role in the adaptation of cancer cells to low nutrition, and whose reduced expression is frequently observed in both hepatoma cell lines and human HCC tissues, is associated with worse survival of HCC patients [19]. Another potential predictor of poor prognosis in HCC patients is miR-29, which is also frequently down-regulated in HCC tissues and which play an important role in the regulation of apoptosis and generally in the molecular etiology of HCC [38]. Study of Lan et al. (2011) demonstrates a strong correlation between the inhibitory effect of let-7g on the proliferation of HepG2 cells and the oncogene c-Myc. According to the fact that the over-expression of c-Myc is involved in a wide spectrum of human cancers and is associated with high aggressiveness and poor prognosis, let-7g might fulfill the pool of prognostic markers in HCC [39].

According to the alarming reality, that patients who undergo curative resection of HCC tumors frequently have tumor recurrence, and the postoperative 5-year survival is only 30-40% [40], clarification of the molecular mechanisms underlying HCC recurrence might help to identify therapeutic targets for the prevention of HCC recurrence. Results of Chung et al.

(2010) indicate that miR-15b expression in HCC tissues may predict a low risk of tumor recurrence following curative resection, suggesting its prognostic significance. In addition, the modulation of miR-15b expression may be useful as an apoptosis-sensitizing strategy for HCC treatment [41]. Also TGFβ mediated up-regulation of hepatic miR-181b is promoting hepatocarcinogenesis by targeting TIMP3. Promotion of HCC cell invasion by miR-181b and up-regulation of miR-181b in highly invasive HCCs suggests that miR-181b could serve as a prognostic marker for HCC [42,43].

## 10.6. MiRNAs as Potential Therapeutic Targets

The high mortality associated with HCC is mainly attributed to the failure to diagnose HCC patients at an early stage and a lack of effective therapies for patients with advanced stage. Although surgery remains the most effective treatment for HCC, the majority of patients are inoperable because of late diagnosis. Small molecule intervention of miRNA misregulation has the potential to provide new therapeutic approaches to such diseases. Furthermore, the discovery of the aberrantly expressed miRNAs and their corresponding targets has opened a novel avenue to investigate the molecular basis of HCC carcinogenesis and to develop potential therapeutics against HCC.

MiR-122 is a liver specific miRNA with described decreasing expression during the carcinogenesis. Restoration of miR-122 in liver cancer cells selectively induced apoptosis through caspase activation, thus having implications in cancer chemotherapy [44]. It is also known that miR-122 sensitizes cells to doxorubicin-induced apoptosis either through a p53-dependent and p53-independent mechanism [4]. These findings make miR-122 a suitable target for miRNA-based therapy.

Among other therapeutically relevant miRNAs should be mentioned miR-143 whose up-regulated expression transcribed by NFκB in HBV-HCC promotes cancer cell invasion/migration and tumor metastasis by repression of fibronectin type III domain containing 3B (FNDC3B) [45]; miR-191 whose inhibition decreased cell proliferation and induced apoptosis *in vitro* and significantly reduced tumor masses *in vivo* in an orthotopic xenograft mouse model of HCC [46]; miR-22, which in a down-regulated status, has an anti-proliferative effect on HCC cells both *in vitro* and *in vivo* [47]; miR-199a-3p which is down-regulated in several human malignancies including HCC and whose restored attenuated levels may leed to G(1)-phase cell cycle arrest, reduced invasive capability, enhanced susceptibility to hypoxia, and increased sensitivity to doxorubicin-induced apoptosis [48]; miR-152 whose enhanced expression by gene transfer could reverse the malignant phenotype of HCC cells [36]; miR-26a whose systemic administration in a mouse model results in inhibition of HCC cell proliferation, induction of tumor-specific apoptosis, and dramatic protection from disease progression without toxicity [49]; miR-15b whose modulation may be therapeutically useful as an apoptosis sensitizing strategy [41]; miR-196 whose up-regulation may be an additional new therapeutic approach to prevent or ameliorate hepatitis C infection [50]; and miR-34a [51], miR-101 [19], miR-125b [34], miR-181 [43], miR-193b [52], miR-195 [53], miR-199a-3p [48], miR-375 [54], miR-29 [38], miR-21 [55], and miR-17-5p [56].

## Acknowledgment

This work was supported by grants NS 10361-3/2009, NR/9814-4/2008, NS 10352-3/2009, NT/11214-4/2010 of Czech Ministry of Health, Project No. MZ0MOU2005 of the Czech Ministry of Health.

## References

[1] Burchard J, Zhang C, Liu AM, Poon RT, Lee NP, Wong KF, Sham PC, Lam BY, Ferguson MD, Tokiwa G, Smith R, Leeson B, Beard R, Lamb JR, Lim L, Mao M, Dai H, Luk JM: microRNA-122 as a regulator of mitochondrial metabolic gene network in hepatocellular carcinoma. *Mol. Syst. Biol.* 2010 6:402.
[2] Huang YS, Dai Y, Yu XF, Bao SY, Yin YB, Tang M, Hu CX: Microarray analysis of microRNA expression in hepatocellular carcinoma and non-tumorous tissues without viral hepatitis. *J. Gastroenterol. Hepatol.* 2008 23:87-94.
[3] Lee NP, Cheung ST, Poon RT, Fan ST, Luk JM: Genomic and proteomic biomarkers for diagnosis and prognosis of hepatocellular carcinoma. *Biomarkers Med.* 2007 1:273-84.
[4] Fornari F, Gramantieri L, Giovannini C, Veronese A, Ferracin M, Sabbioni S, Calin GA, Grazi GL, Croce CM, Tavolari S, Chieco P, Negrini M, Bolondi L: MiR-122/cyclin G1 interaction modulates p53 activity and affects doxorubicin sensitivity of human hepatocarcinoma cells. *Cancer Res.* 2009 69:5761-7.
[5] Gao Y, He Y, Ding J, Wu K, Hu B, Liu Y, Wu Y, Guo B, Shen Y, Landi D, Landi S, Zhou Y, Liu H: An insertion/deletion polymorphism at miRNA-122-binding site in the interleukin-1α´ untranslated region confers risk for hepatocellular carcinoma. *Carcinogenesis* 2009 30:2064-9.
[6] Kudo M: Multistep human hepatocarcinogenesis: correlation of imaging with pathology. *J. Gastroenterol.* 2009 44 Suppl 19:112-8.
[7] Pang RW, Poon RT: From molecular biology to targeted therapies for hepatocellular carcinoma: the future is now. *Oncology* 2007 72 Suppl 1:30-44.
[8] Xu T, Zhu Y, Wei QK, Yuan Y, Zhou F, Ge YY, Yang JR, Su H, Zhuang SM: A functional polymorphism in the miR-146a gene is associated with the risk for hepatocellular carcinoma. *Carcinogenesis* 2008 29:2126-31.
[9] Xu Y, Liu L, Liu J, Zhang Y, Zhu J, Chen J, Liu S, Liu Z, Shi H, Shen H, Hu Z: A potentially functional polymorphism in the promoter region of miR-34b/c is associated with an increased risk for primary hepatocellular carcinoma. *Int. J. Cancer* 2011 128:412-7.
[10] Tsai WC, Hsu PW, Lai TC, Chau GY, Lin CW, Chen CM, Lin CD, Liao YL, Wang JL, Chau YP, Hsu MT, Hsiao M, Huang HD, Tsou AP: MicroRNA-122, a tumor suppressor microRNA that regulates intrahepatic metastasis of hepatocellular carcinoma. *Hepatology* 2009 49:1571-82.
[11] Coulouarn C, Factor VM, Andersen JB, Durkin ME, Thorgeirsson SS: Loss of miR-122 expression in liver cancer correlates with suppression of the hepatic phenotype and gain of metastatic properties. *Oncogene* 2009 28:3526-36.

[12] Apte RN, Voronov E: Is interleukin-1 a good or bad 'guy' in tumor immunobiology and immunotherapy? *Immunol. Rev.* 2008 222:222-41.

[13] Sukata T, Sumida K, Kushida M, Ogata K, Miyata K, Yabushita S, Uwagawa S: Circulating microRNAs, possible indicators of progress of rat hepatocarcinogenesis from early stages. *Toxicol. Lett.* 2011 200:46-52.

[14] Gui J, Tian Y, Wen X, Zhang W, Zhang P, Gao J, Run W, Tian L, Jia X, Gao Y: Serum microRNA characterization identifies miR-885-5p as a potential marker for detecting liver pathologies. *Clin. Sci. (Lond)* 2011 120:183-93.

[15] Xu J, Wu C, Che X, Wang L, Yu D, Zhang T, Huang L, Li H, Tan W, Wang C, Lin D: Circulating MicroRNAs, miR-21, miR-122, and miR-223, in patients with hepatocellular carcinoma or chronic hepatitis. *Mol. Carcinog.* 2011 50:136-42.

[16] Wang Y, Lee AT, Ma JZ, Wang J, Ren J, Yang Y, Tantoso E, Li KB, Ooi LL, Tan P, Lee CG: Profiling microRNA expression in hepatocellular carcinoma reveals microRNA-224 up-regulation and apoptosis inhibitor-5 as a microRNA-224-specific target. *J. Biol. Chem.* 2008 283:13205-15.

[17] Meng F, Henson R, Wehbe-Janek H, Ghoshal K, Jacob ST, Patel T: MicroRNA-21 regulates expression of the PTEN tumor suppressor gene in human hepatocellular cancer. *Gastroenterology* 2007 133:647-58.

[18] Li W, Xie L, He X, Li J, Tu K, Wei L, Wu J, Guo Y, Ma X, Zhang P, Pan Z, Hu X, Zhao Y, Xie H, Jiang G, Chen T, Wang J, Zheng S, Cheng J, Wan D, Yang S, Li Y, Gu J: Diagnostic and prognostic implications of microRNAs in human hepatocellular carcinoma. *Int. J. Cancer* 2008 123:1616-22.

[19] Su H, Yang JR, Xu T, Huang J, Xu L, Yuan Y, Zhuang SM: MicroRNA-101, down-regulated in hepatocellular carcinoma, promotes apoptosis and suppresses tumorigenicity. *Cancer Res.* 2009 69:1135-42.

[20] Huang S, He X, Ding J, Liang L, Zhao Y, Zhang Z, Yao X, Pan Z, Zhang P, Li J, Wan D, Gu J: Upregulation of miR-23a approximately 27a approximately 24 decreases transforming growth factor-beta-induced tumor-suppressive activities in human hepatocellular carcinoma cells. *Int. J. Cancer* 2008 123:972-8.

[21] Connolly E, Melegari M, Landgraf P, Tchaikovskaya T, Tennant BC, Slagle BL, Rogler LE, Zavolan M, Tuschl T, Rogler CE: Elevated expression of the miR-17-92 polycistron and miR-21 in hepadnavirus-associated hepatocellular carcinoma contributes to the malignant phenotype. *Am. J. Pathol.* 2008 173:856-64.

[22] Fornari F, Gramantieri L, Ferracin M, Veronese A, Sabbioni S, Calin GA, Grazi GL, Giovannini C, Croce CM, Bolondi L, Negrini M: MiR-221 controls CDKN1C/p57 and CDKN1B/p27 expression in human hepatocellular carcinoma. *Oncogene* 2008 27:5651-61.

[23] Wong QW, Lung RW, Law PT, Lai PB, Chan KY, To KF, Wong N: MicroRNA-223 is commonly repressed in hepatocellular carcinoma and potentiates expression of Stathmin1. *Gastroenterology* 2008 135:257-69.

[24] Ji J, Wang XW: New kids on the block: diagnostic and prognostic microRNAs in hepatocellular carcinoma. *Cancer Biol. Ther.* 2009 8:1686-93.

[25] Yamashita T, Ji J, Budhu A, Forgues M, Yang W, Wang HY, Jia H, Ye Q, Qin LX, Wauthier E, Reid LM, Minato H, Honda M, Kaneko S, Tang ZY, Wang XW: EpCAM-positive hepatocellular carcinoma cells are tumor-initiating cells with stem/progenitor cell features. *Gastroenterology* 2009 136:1012-24.

[26] Ladeiro Y, Couchy G, Balabaud C, Bioulac-Sage P, Pelletier L, Rebouissou S, Zucman-Rossi J: MicroRNA profiling in hepatocellular tumors is associated with clinical features and oncogene/tumor suppressor gene mutations. *Hepatology* 2008 47:1955-63.

[27] Barshack I, Meiri E, Rosenwald S, Lebanony D, Bronfeld M, Aviel-Ronen S, Rosenblatt K, Polak-Charcon S, Leizerman I, Ezagouri M, Zepeniuk M, Shabes N, Cohen L, Tabak S, Cohen D, Bentwich Z, Rosenfeld N: Differential diagnosis of hepatocellular carcinoma from metastatic tumors in the liver using microRNA expression. *Int. J. Biochem. Cell Biol.* 2010 42:1355-62.

[28] Liu WH, Yeh SH, Lu CC, Yu SL, Chen HY, Lin CY, Chen DS, Chen PJ: MicroRNA-18a prevents estrogen receptor-alpha expression, promoting proliferation of hepatocellular carcinoma cells. *Gastroenterology* 2009 136:683-93.

[29] Li Y, Tan W, Neo TW, Aung MO, Wasser S, Lim SG, Tan TM: Role of the miR-106b-25 microRNA cluster in hepatocellular carcinoma. *Cancer Sci.* 2009 100:1234-42.

[30] Xu N, Papagiannakopoulos T, Pan G, Thomson JA, Kosik KS: MicroRNA-145 regulates OCT4, SOX2, and KLF4 and represses pluripotency in human embryonic stem cells. *Cell* 2009 137:647-58.

[31] Gao P, Chak-Lui Wong C, Kwok-Kwan Tung E, Man-Fong Lee J, Wong C-M, Oi-Lin Ng I: Deregulation of microRNA expression occurs early and accumulates in early stages of HBV-associated multistep hepatocarcinogenesis. *Journal of Hepatology* 2010 doi: 10.1016/j.jhep.2010.09.023.

[32] Budhu A, Jia HL, Forgues M, Liu CG, Goldstein D, Lam A, Zanetti KA, Ye QH, Qin LX, Croce CM, Tang ZY, Wang XW: Identification of metastasis-related microRNAs in hepatocellular carcinoma. *Hepatology* 2008 47:897-907.

[33] Diao S, Zhang JF, Wang H, He ML, Lin MC, Chen Y, Kung HF: Proteomic identification of microRNA-122a target proteins in hepatocellular carcinoma. *Proteomics* 2010 10:3723-31.

[34] Liang L, Wong CM, Ying Q, Fan DN, Huang S, Ding J, Yao J, Yan M, Li J, Yao M, Ng IO, He X: MicroRNA-125b suppressesed human liver cancer cell proliferation and metastasis by directly targeting oncogene LIN28B2. *Hepatology* 2010 52:1731-40.

[35] Li W, Xie L, He X, Li J, Tu K, Wei L, Wu J, Guo Y, Ma X, Zhang P, Pan Z, Hu X, Zhao Y, Xie H, Jiang G, Chen T, Wang J, Zheng S, Cheng J, Wan D, Yang S, Li Y, Gu J: Diagnostic and prognostic implications of microRNAs in human hepatocellular carcinoma. *Int. J. Cancer* 2008 123:1616-22.

[36] Huang J, Wang Y, Guo Y, Sun S: Down-regulated microRNA-152 induces aberrant DNA methylation in hepatitis B virus-related hepatocellular carcinoma by targeting DNA methyltransferase 1. *Hepatology* 2010 52:60-70.

[37] Saito Y, Kanai Y, Nakagawa T, Sakamoto M, Saito H, Ishii H, Hirohashi S: Increased protein expression of DNA methyltransferase (DNMT) 1 is significantly correlated with the malignant potential and poor prognosis of human hepatocellular carcinomas. *Int. J. Cancer* 2003 105:527-32.

[38] Xiong Y, Fang JH, Yun JP, Yang J, Zhang Y, Jia WH, Zhuang SM: Effects of microRNA-29 on apoptosis, tumorigenicity, and prognosis of hepatocellular carcinoma. *Hepatology* 2010 51:836-45.

[39] Lan FF, Wang H, Chen YC, Chan CY, Ng SS, Li K, Xie D, He ML, Lin MC, Kung HF: Hsa-let-7g inhibits proliferation of hepatocellular carcinoma cells by downregulation of c-Myc and upregulation of p16(INK4A). *Int. J. Cancer* 2011 128:319-31.

[40] Blum HE: Hepatocellular carcinoma: therapy and prevention. *World J Gastroenterol* 2005 11:7391-400.

[41] Chung GE, Yoon JH, Myung SJ, Lee JH, Lee SH, Lee SM, Kim SJ, Hwang SY, Lee HS, Kim CY: High expression of microRNA-15b predicts a low risk of tumor recurrence following curative resection of hepatocellular carcinoma. *Oncol. Rep.* 2010 23:113-9.

[42] Ji J, Yamashita T, Budhu A, Forgues M, Jia HL, Li C, Deng C, Wauthier E, Reid LM, Ye QH, Qin LX, Yang W, Wang HY, Tang ZY, Croce CM, Wang XW: Identification of microRNA-181 by genome-wide screening as a critical player in EpCAM-positive hepatic cancer stem cells. *Hepatology* 2009 50:472-80.

[43] Wang B, Hsu SH, Majumder S, Kutay H, Huang W, Jacob ST, Ghoshal K: TGFbeta-mediated upregulation of hepatic miR-181b promotes hepatocarcinogenesis by targeting TIMP3. *Oncogene* 2010 29:1787-97.

[44] Young DD, Connelly CM, Grohmann C, Deiters A: Small molecule modifiers of microRNA miR-122 function for the treatment of hepatitis C virus infection and hepatocellular carcinoma. *J. Am .Chem. Soc.* 2010 132:7976-81.

[45] Zhang X, Liu S, Hu T, Liu S, He Y, Sun S: Up-regulated microRNA-143 transcribed by nuclear factor kappa B enhances hepatocarcinoma metastasis by repressing fibronectin expression. *Hepatology* 2009 50:490-9.

[46] Elyakim E, Sitbon E, Faerman A, Tabak S, Montia E, Belanis L, Dov A, Marcusson EG, Bennett CF, Chajut A, Cohen D, Yerushalmi N: hsa-miR-191 is a candidate oncogene target for hepatocellular carcinoma therapy. *Cancer Res.* 2010 70:8077-87.

[47] Zhang J, Yang Y, Yang T, Liu Y, Li A, Fu S, Wu M, Pan Z, Zhou W: microRNA-22, downregulated in hepatocellular carcinoma and correlated with prognosis, suppresses cell proliferation and tumourigenicity. *Br. J. Cancer* 2010 103:1215-20.

[48] Fornari F, Milazzo M, Chieco P, Negrini M, Calin GA, Grazi GL, Pollutri D, Croce CM, Bolondi L, Gramantieri L: MiR-199a-3p regulates mTOR and c-Met to influence the doxorubicin sensitivity of human hepatocarcinoma cells. *Cancer Res.* 2010 70:5184-93.

[49] Kota J, Chivukula RR, O'Donnell KA, Wentzel EA, Montgomery CL, Hwang HW, Chang TC, Vivekanandan P, Torbenson M, Clark KR, Mendell JR, Mendell JT: Therapeutic microRNA delivery suppresses tumorigenesis in a murine liver cancer model. *Cell* 2009 137:1005-17.

[50] Hou W, Tian Q, Zheng J, Bonkovsky HL: MicroRNA-196 represses Bach1 protein and hepatitis C virus gene expression in human hepatoma cells expressing hepatitis C viral proteins. *Hepatology* 2010 51:1494-504.

[51] Li N, Fu H, Tie Y, Hu Z, Kong W, Wu Y, Zheng X: miR-34a inhibits migration and invasion by down-regulation of c-Met expression in human hepatocellular carcinoma cells. *Cancer Lett.* 2009 275:44-53.

[52] Xu C, Liu S, Fu H, Li S, Tie Y, Zhu J, Xing R, Jin Y, Sun Z, Zheng X: MicroRNA-193b regulates proliferation, migration and invasion in human hepatocellular carcinoma cells. *Eur. J. Cancer* 2010 46:2828-36.

[53] Xu T, Zhu Y, Xiong Y, Ge YY, Yun JP, Zhuang SM: MicroRNA-195 suppresses tumorigenicity and regulates G1/S transition of human hepatocellular carcinoma cells. *Hepatology* 2009 50:113-21.

[54] Liu AM, Poon RT, Luk JM: MicroRNA-375 targets Hippo-signaling effector YAP in liver cancer and inhibits tumor properties. *Biochem. Biophys. Res. Commun.* 2010 394:623-7.

[55] Liu C, Yu J, Yu S, Lavker RM, Cai L, Liu W, Yang K, He X, Chen S: MicroRNA-21 acts as an oncomir through multiple targets in human hepatocellular carcinoma. *J. Hepatol.* 2010 53:98-107.

[56] Yang F, Yin Y, Wang F, Wang Y, Zhang L, Tang Y, Sun S: miR-17-5p Promotes migration of human hepatocellular carcinoma cells through the p38 mitogen-activated protein kinase-heat shock protein 27 pathway. *Hepatology* 2010 51:1614-23.

*Chapter XI*

# MicroRNAs and Pancreatic Cancer

*Martina Redova*
Masaryk Memorial Cancer Institute, Brno, Czech Republic

## Abstract

Pancreatic cancer (i.e. pancreatic adenocarcinoma, PDAC) remains one of the most lethal malignancies, with most cases diagnosed during the late stages after metastatic spread, rendering the carcinoma surgically inoperable. The major biological characteristic of pancreatic adenocarcinomas are early and aggressive local invasion, metastasis and resistance to chemotherapy and radiotherapy. From this point of view, the discovery of miRNA alterations in this malignancy helps not only to improve the understanding of the PDAC biology, but more importantly, provides new diagnostic, prognostic and even therapeutic strategies.

## 11.1. Introduction

Pancreatic cancer is one of the most devastating and rapidly fatal cancer. It is the fourth leading cause of cancer related death in Western countries and has one of the lowest 5-year survival rates (4 %) among solid cancers [1,2]. Median survival in patients with locally advanced/metastatic disease is less than 12 months despite aggressive multimodality treatment. Furthermore, due to non-specific symptoms, aggressive growth and early dissemination, PDAC patients are often diagnosed during the late stages. As pancreatic cancer is notoriously known to be resistant to chemotherapy and radiotherapy, surgical resection offers the ideal treatment selection with prolonged survival for patients with resectable disease. Unfortunately, surgery is feasible only in 15-20% of patients and, even after complete resection, prognosis remains dismal [3]. Moreover, pancreatic adenocarcinomas have a predisposition for early vascular dissemination and metastasis to distant organs. Not only new therapeutic targets but also reliable and non-invasive tumor biomarkers which may facilitate early diagnosis and have the potential for use in monitoring response to cancer therapies are urgently needed. This might be a potential field for recently discovered miRNAs in the sense of fulfilling a task of suitable biomarkers or even therapeutic modalities. Although the association between miRNAs and their roles in PDAC progression remains unclear, the miRNAs dysregulation suggests that they might be involved in pancreatic tumorigenesis by acting as tumor suppressors or oncogenes.

## 11.2. Serum and Plasma miRNAs: Early Detection of Disease Onset and Progression

According to the fact that tissue-based diagnosis remains invasive and time-consuming, serum and plasma have been extensively researched, and in 2008 Lawrie et al. established the existence of miRNA in circulation. It has highlighted the potential of miRNAs as non-invasive diagnostic biomarkers and their promising applications in therapy and prognostication of various malignancies [4]. Although the enigmatic mechanism of miRNAs existence in serum/plasma remains to be elucidated, their stability has been already established and due to the stability, abundance and relatively easy accessibility from serum or plasma, such circulating blood-based biomarkers remain one of the most promising means of diagnosis, potential prediction of clinical behavior of individual cancers and monitoring therapeutic response.

Based on the fact that PDAC exhibit extremely hypoxic signatures which are considered to be associated with poorer prognosis and marked resistance to chemotherapy and radiation, Ho et al. (2010) hypothesized that miR-210 may serve as a diagnostic marker for screening or surveillance in pancreatic cancer. They have finally proved that plasma miR-210 expression from patients with newly diagnosed locally advanced PDACs was significantly elevated in comparison to age-matched controls (4× over-expression, $p < 0.00004$), and thus miR-210 may serve as a reliable blood-based biomarker, using a minimum amount of sample (100 μl) [5]. In other words, elevated levels of miR-210 which is believed to suppress normoxic genes that are no longer necessary for adaptation [6] and survival in a hypoxic environment and which has been also found to promote cell cycle progression by activating c-Myc through inhibition of a c-Myc antagonist [7], could also facilitate earlier diagnosis and treatment of this malignancy.

Kong et al. (2010) investigated a set of PDAC-associated miRNAs (miR-21, miR-155, miR-196a, miR-181a, miR-181b, miR-221, and miR-222) in serum of PDAC patients and found out that serum miRNA signature is not fully consistent with that of PDAC tissues. They have also revealed that serum miR-196a expression level in the unresectable group of patients (stage III and IV) was significantly higher than that in the resectable group of patients (stage I and II, $p = 0.001$). MiR-196a serum expression levels were observed to be associated with the TNM staging of PDAC and thus miR-196a may provide objective clues for the selection of patients for laparotomy. They have found no significant correlation between expression levels of the other six miRNAs (miR-21, miR-155, miR-181a, miR-181b, miR-221, miR-222) and resectable status. On the basis of different expression levels of miR-21 in serum, they were able to differentiate PDAC patients from those with benign pancreas (chronic pancreatitis/normal; $p = 0.033$ and $0.001$), whereas miR-155 and miR-196a could differentiate sick pancreas (PDAC/chronic pancreatitis; $p = 0.0002$ and $0.010$) from normal pancreas [8]. Results of these studies imply that a cluster of dysregulated miRNAs combined with protein-based biomarkers might notably improve the diagnosis of pancreatic adenocarcinomas.

## 11.3. Tissue miRNA Signatures: Implications for Diagnostic Oncology

According to the hypothesis that reliable tumor markers may facilitate earlier diagnosis and have the potential for development of new diagnostic tools and therapeutic strategies and use in monitoring response to cancer therapies, it is important to discover a unique miRNA profiling pattern for pancreatic cancer and identify considerable molecular targets. From the diagnostic point of view, it is very important to have a powerfull tool enabling differentiation between PDAC and healthy pancreatic tissue. Furthermore, because it is generally known that PDAC often occurs in a background of chronic pancreatitis (CP), it is also worth seeking for a possibility to distinguish among healthy parenchyma, CP and PDAC. Dysregulated miRNAs expression is considered a common and relevant feature in human malignancies, facilitating proliferation, differentiation, apoptosis, invasion, metastatic potential and resistance to chemotherapeutic agents.

In a profiling study of 95 miRNAs in PDAC Zhang et al. (2009) identified a set of 8 up-regulated miRNAs (miR-196, miR-190, miR-186, miR-221, miR-222, miR-200b, miR-15b, and miR-95) to be significantly increased (3.3-fold, $p = 0.05$) in PDAC in comparison with normal pancreatic tissue [10]. Their observations indicate that these miRNAs may share common pathways in the pancreatic cancer pathogenesis [9]. Other studies have confirmed the potential of miR-196a to distinguish between PDAC and healthy tissue and even to differentiate between long and short-term survivors, whereas increased expression level of miR-196a was associated with poor survival [8,10].

A combination of oncogenic miR-21 whose inhibition could suppress cell cycle and induce apoptosis, miR-210 which tends to be increased under hypoxia conditions, miR-155 which in the state of over-expression enhances the tumorigenicity by repressing the function of pro-apoptotic p53-induced nuclear protein 1 (TP53INP1), and miR-196a known to promote cell invasion and metastasis, to differentiate PDAC and healthy tissue, has been established [2,5,8]. While deregulation of miR-21 expression levels occurs later during the process of carcinogenesis, either at the stage of carcinoma-in-situ or in invasive adenocarcinomas, deregulation of miR-155 is considered to be an early event in the multistep process of pancreatic cancer development [2,9]. Furthermore, in the study of Zhao et al., miR-217 which serves as a potential tumor suppressing miRNA in PDAC development was found to be frequently down-regulated ($p < 0.01$) [13].

Employing hierarchical clustering Lee et al. (2007) were able to distinguish tumor from normal pancreas, pancreatitis and cell lines. They found one hundred miRNA precursors aberrantly expressed in pancreatic cancer or desmoplasia ($p < 0.01$), including miRNAs previously reported as differentially expressed in other human cancers (miR-155, miR-21, miR-221, and miR-222).

**Table 11.1. List of representative miRNAs differentially expressed in PDAC mentioned in at least two microRNA profiling studies**

| Up-regulated miRNAs in PDAC | |
|---|---|
| miRNA | Reference, Fold Change (FC), p-value |
| miR-221 | [11] FC = 3.42* [12] FC = 26.2; p = 5.66E-05 [9] FC = 6.6; p = 0.01 [10] FC = 32; p □ 0.01 |
| miR-100 | [11] FC = 32.49* [12] FC = 36.90; p = 4.40E-06 [9] FC = 3.8; p = 0.01 |
| miR-21 | [11] FC = 3.08* [12] FC = 15.70; p = 2.00E-04 [9] FC = 12.1; p = 0.0004 |
| miR-181a | [11] FC = 3.01* [12] FC = 18.6; p = 8.31E-04 [9] FC = 7.7; p = 0.01 |
| miR-181c | [11] FC = 2.36* [12] FC = 18.6; p = 8.31E-04 [9] FC = 9.5; p = 0.005 |
| miR-155 | [11] FC = 2.1* [12] FC = 14.0; p = 1.51E-03 [9] FC = 11.6; p = 0.005 |
| miR-107 | [11] FC = 2.28* [12] FC = 8.2; p = 3.86E-05 [9] FC = 10.8; p = 0.01 |
| miR-210 | [11] FC = 2.97* [9] FC = 5.7; p = 0.005 |
| miR-222 | [11] FC = 2.7* [10] FC = 32.0; p □ 0.01 |
| miR-15b | [12] FC = 8.55; p = 4.00E-04 [10] FC = 20.18; p □ 0.01 |

Used method: [11] - miRNA microarray + quantitative qRT-PCR; * Significance Analysis of Microarrays (SAM) version 3.0 application with a threshold difference in expression set to 2, s0 percentile centile set to 0.05 (default),and the number of permutations set to 100 (default); [12] qRT-PCR profiling of microRNA precursors; [9] quantitative RT-PCR; [10] real time RT-PCR.

They also confirm that aberrant miRNA expression may offer new clues to pancreatic tumorigenesis and may provide diagnostic biomarkers for pancreatic adenocarcinoma [12]. For detailed information about other dysregulated miRNA see Table 11.1.

## 11.4. MiRNAs Expression in Prognosis and Response Prediction

Beside diagnostic impact, the discovery of miRNA alterations in PDAC improve not only understanding of the pathogenesis and biology of this disease, but more importantly provides also new prognostic strategies. Additionally, specific miRNAs dysregulation appear to be correlated with clinically malignancy or metastatic phenotypes, and may predict the clinical outcome even better than the mRNA expression data [10,14].

In addition to previously mentioned prognostic value of plasma miR-196a, Bloomstom et al. (2007) have confirmed also the power of tissue miR-196a-2 to predict poor survival in PDAC patients [11]. In PDAC which is characterized by a dismal prognosis, the high risk of recurrence following surgical resection provides the rationale for adjuvant therapy. Unfortunately, only a subset of PDAC patients benefit from this therapy. From this point of view, miR-21 whose expression is associated with increased proliferation, invasiveness and gemcitabine chemoresistance seems to be a very interesting target. MiR-21 has been observed as over-expressed in PDAC tissue and could be a potential predictor of overall survival (OS) and disease free survival (DFS) [15,17].

Furthermore, when PDAC patients were stratified according to the adjuvant therapy response, the group of adjuvant treated patients with low miR-21 expression were shown to have a favorable outcome compared to patients with high miR-21 expression. These results indicate that miR-21 may allow stratification for adjuvant therapy, thus offering a potential new biomarker for treatment selection and more individualized therapy. Additionally, high miR-21 expression was observed to be associated with an increased distant recurrence rate, suggesting a role in the metastatic behavior of pancreatic adenocarcinoma. Accordingly, high miR-21 expression levels correlated with increased proliferation and occurrence of liver metastasis in studies in PDAC cells and in pancreatic endocrine tumors [16,17,18].

Also miR-34a expression was associated with decreased DFS at the multivariate analysis in the not adjuvantly treated patients. Furthermore, Hwang et al. (2010) found a significant correlation between high miR-34a expression and high VEGF and p-c-Met levels, which have been correlated with increased microvessel density, tumor metastatic potential, local disease progression and chemoresistance in a variety of malignancies, including PDAC [16,19,20].

Results of Greither et al. study (2010) provide an evidence for an oncogenic activity of miR-155, miR-203, miR-210, and miR-222 in the development of pancreatic cancer since the elevated expression of these miRNAs in PDAC is associated with poorer survival [21].

## 11.5. MiRNAs as Potential Therapeutic Targets

According to the ascertainment that miRNA may regulate multiple oncogenic pathways and may serve as potential targets for cancer therapy, it is worth finding detailed miRNA profile pattern in PDAC. As PDACs are known to be chemo- and radioresistant and according to the deleterious side effects of oncologic treatment that augment mortality and morbidity, it is a major challenge to develop safe and clinically efficacious therapeutic agents. For example, antagomirs and chemically modified antisense nucleotides for miRNAs can be used to silence specific endogenous miRNA in vivo [10,22]. This may provide a novel strategy to treat pancreatic cancer.

Hwang et al. (2010) have transfected the PANC-1 cells with miR-21 precursors and observed reduced gemcitabine sensitivity [16]. On the contrary, antisense inhibition of miR-21 in HS766T cells led to cell cycle arrest, induced apoptosis and sensitized these cells to the effects of gemcitabine [23]. Although miR-21 expression was correlated with resistance to several anticancer agents in different models, these results suggest a key role of miR-21 in modulating the response to this specific drug in PDAC cells [16,24].

Also results of Ma et al. (2010) show that oncogenic miR-27a possess a potential to serve as a tool in the treatment of pancreatic adenocarcinoma by modulating the malignant behavior of pancreatic cancer cells, and by targeting Sprouty2 (Spry2), an important regulator of KRAS, which showed low expression level in the pancreatic cancer samples. They show that transfection of the miR-27a inhibitor suppressed cell proliferation, colony formation and migration of both PANC-1 and MIA PaCa-2 cell lines, indicating the oncogenic role of miR-27a in pancreatic cancer cells. They also found that inhibition of miR-27a up-regulated the Spry2 expression and suppressed the phospho-Erk1/2 levels, indicating that miR-27a may participate in the modulation of malignant biological behavior. Spry2 down-regulation by miR-27a provides anti-apoptotic action for tumor cells by permitting unchecked activation of the Ras/MAPK pathway [1].

In study of Zhao et al. (2010), they found that over-expression of miR-217 significantly reduced PDAC cell growth and anchorage-independent colony formation. Furthermore, in vivo xenograft tumor growth curves revealed a significant decrease in tumor growth rates following treatment with the miR-217 expression vector. These results indicate that miR-217 can reverse the malignant behavior of PDAC cells and may have a promising future for the treatment of PDAC [13].

## Acknowledgment

This work was supported by grants NS 10361-3/2009, NR/9814-4/2008, NS 10352-3/2009, NT/11214-4/2010 of Czech Ministry of Health, Project No. MZ0MOU2005 of the Czech Ministry of Health.

## References

[1] Ma Y, Yu S, Zhao W, Lu Z, Chen J: miR-27a regulates the growth, colony formation and migration of pancreatic cancer cells by targeting Sprouty2. *Cancer Lett.* 2010 298:150-8.

[2] Ryu JK, Hong SM, Karikari CA, Hruban RH, Goggins MG, Maitra A: Aberrant MicroRNA-155 expression is an early event in the multistep progression of pancreatic adenocarcinoma. *Pancreatology* 2010 10:66-73.

[3] Zuckerman DS, Ryan DP: Adjuvant therapy for pancreatic cancer: a review. *Cancer* 2008 112:243-9.

[4] Lawrie CH, Gal S, Dunlop HM, Pushkaran B, Liggins AP, Pulford K, Banham AH, Pezzella F, Boultwood J, Wainscoat JS, Hatton CS, Harris AL: Detection of elevated levels of tumour-associated microRNAs in serum of patients with diffuse large B-cell lymphoma. *Br. J. Haematol.* 2008 141:672-5.

[5] Ho AS, Huang X, Cao H, Christman-Skieller C, Bennewith K, Le QT, Koong AC: Circulating miR-210 as a Novel Hypoxia Marker in Pancreatic Cancer. *Transl. Oncol.* 2010 3:109-13.

[6] Huang X, Ding L, Bennewith KL, Tong RT, Welford SM, Ang KK, Story M, Le QT, Giaccia AJ: Hypoxia-inducible mir-210 regulates normoxic gene expression involved in tumor initiation. *Mol. Cell* 2009 35:856-67.

[7] Zhang AY, Obagi S: Diagnosis and management of skin resurfacing-related complications. *Oral. Maxillofac. Surg. Clin. North Am.* 2009 21:1-12, v.

[8] Kong X, Du Y, Wang G, Gao J, Gong Y, Li L, Zhang Z, Zhu J, Jing Q, Qin Y, Li Z: Detection of differentially expressed microRNAs in serum of pancreatic ductal adenocarcinomapPatients: miR-196a could be a potential marker for poor prognosis. *Dig Dis Sci* 2010 [Epub ahead of print].

[9] Habbe N, Koorstra JB, Mendell JT, Offerhaus GJ, Ryu JK, Feldmann G, Mullendore ME, Goggins MG, Hong SM, Maitra A: MicroRNA miR-155 is a biomarker of early pancreatic neoplasia. *Cancer Biol. Ther.* 2009 8:340-6.

[10] Zhang Y, Li M, Wang H, Fisher WE, Lin PH, Yao Q, Chen C: Profiling of 95 microRNAs in pancreatic cancer cell lines and surgical specimens by real-time PCR analysis. *World J. Surg.* 2009 33:698-709.

[11] Bloomston M, Frankel WL, Petrocca F, Volinia S, Alder H, Hagan JP, Liu CG, Bhatt D, Taccioli C, Croce CM: MicroRNA expression patterns to differentiate pancreatic adenocarcinoma from normal pancreas and chronic pancreatitis. *JAMA* 2007 297:1901-8.

[12] Lee EJ, Gusev Y, Jiang J, Nuovo GJ, Lerner MR, Frankel WL, Morgan DL, Postier RG, Brackett DJ, Schmittgen TD: Expression profiling identifies microRNA signature in pancreatic cancer. *Int. J. Cancer* 2007 120:1046-54.

[13] Zhao WG, Yu SN, Lu ZH, Ma YH, Gu YM, Jie Chen J: The miR-217 microRNA functions as a potential tumor suppressor in pancreatic ductal adenocarcinoma by targeting KRAS. *Carcinogenesis* 2010 31:1726-33.

[14] Jeffrey SS: Cancer biomarker profiling with microRNAs. *Nat. Biotechnol.* 2008 26:400-1.

[15] Dillhoff M, Liu J, Frankel W, Croce C, Bloomston M: MicroRNA-21 is overexpressed in pancreatic cancer and a potential predictor of survival. *J. Gastrointest. Surg.* 2008 12:2171-6.

[16] Hwang JH, Voortman J, Giovannetti E, Steinberg SM, Leon LG, Kim YT, Funel N, Park JK, Kim MA, Kang GH, Kim SW, Del Chiaro M, Peters GJ, Giacconel G: Identification of microRNA-21 as a biomarker for chemoresistance and clinical outcome following adjuvant therapy in resectable pancreatic cancer. *PloS One* 2010 5:e10630.

[17] Gironella M, Seux M, Xie MJ, Cano C, Tomasini R, Gommeaux J, Garcia S, Nowak J, Yeung ML, Jeang KT, Chaix A, Fazli L, Motoo Y, Wang Q, Rocchi P, Russo A, Gleave M, Dagorn JC, Iovanna JL, Carrier A, Pébusque MJ, Dusetti NJ: Tumor protein 53-induced nuclear protein 1 expression is repressed by miR-155, and its restoration inhibits pancreatic tumor development. *Proc. Natl. Acad. Sci. USA* 2007 104:16170-5.

[18] Roldo C, Missiaglia E, Hagan JP, Falconi M, Capelli P, Bersani S, Calin GA, Volinia S, Liu CG, Scarpa A, Croce CM: MicroRNA expression abnormalities in pancreatic endocrine and acinar tumors are associated with distinctive pathologic features and clinical behavior. *J. Clin. Oncol.* 2006 24:4677-84.

[19] Shah AN, Summy JM, Zhang J, Park SI, Parikh NU, Gallick GE: Development and characterization of gemcitabine-resistant pancreatic tumor cells. *Ann. Surg. Oncol.* 2007 14:3629-37.

[20] Itakura J, Ishiwata T, Friess H, Fujii H, Matsumoto Y, Büchler MW, Korc M: Enhanced expression of vascular endothelial growth factor in human pancreatic cancer correlates with local disease progression. *Clin. Cancer Res.* 1997 3:1309-16.

[21] Greither T, Grochola LF, Udelnow A, Lautenschläger C, Würl P, Taubert H: Elevated expression of microRNAs 155, 203, 210 and 222 in pancreatic tumors is associated with poorer survival. *Int. J. Cancer* 2010 126:73-80.

[22] Krützfeldt J, Rajewsky N, Braich R, Rajeev KG, Tuschl T, Manoharan M, Stoffel M: Silencing of microRNAs in vivo with 'antagomirs'. *Nature* 2005 438:685-9.

[23] Park JK, Lee EJ, Esau C, Schmittgen TD: Antisense inhibition of microRNA-21 or -221 arrests cell cycle, induces apoptosis, and sensitizes the effects of gemcitabine in pancreatic adenocarcinoma. *Pancreas* 2009 38:e190-9.

[24] Meng F, Henson R, Lang M, Wehbe H, Maheshwari S, Mendell JT, Jiang J, Schmittgen TD, Patel T: Involvement of human micro-RNA in growth and response to chemotherapy in human cholangiocarcinoma cell lines. *Gastroenterology* 2006 130:2113-29.

In: MicroRNAs in Solid Cancer
Editor: Ondrej Slaby

ISBN: 978-61324-514-9
©2012 Nova Science Publishers, Inc.

*Chapter XII*

# MicroRNAs and Gastric Cancer

*Ondrej Slaby*
*Masaryk Memorial Cancer Institute, Brno, Czech Republic*
*Central European Institute of Technology, Masaryk University, Brno, Czech Republic*

## Abstract

Gastric cancer is the fourth most common cancer in the world. Polymorphisms within miRNA genes have been described as new risk factors for atrophic gastritis and gastric cancer. A substantial number of miRNAs show differential expression in gastric cancer tissues. Genes coding for these miRNAs have been characterized as novel protooncogenes and tumor-suppressor genes based on findings that these miRNAs control malignant phenotypes of gastric cancer cells and the carcinogenic effect of *Helicobacter pylori* infection. Several investigations have also described the ability of specific miRNA expression profiles to predict prognosis, and potential of selected miRNAs as therapeutic targets in gastric cancer patients.

## 12.1. Introduction

Gastric cancer (GC) is one of the most common cancers in the world. It is considered as the second frequent cause of cancer-related death worldwide, with particularly high frequencies in East Asia. Even after a curative resection alone or after adjuvant therapy, nearly 60% of those patients affected die from GC [1,2]. Approximately two thirds of patients have locally advanced or metastatic disease at diagnosis, and up to one half of patients have recurrent disease after curative surgery. The median survival time for these patients is only 6-9 months [3].

GC is thought to result from a combination of environmental factors and the accumulation of generalized and specific genetic alterations, and consequently affects mainly older patients often after a long period of atrophic gastritis. The commonest cause of gastritis is infection by *H. pylori*, which is the single most common cause of gastric cancer [4] and has been classified by the World Health Organization (WHO) as a class I carcinogen since 1994 [5] and the causal role has been extensively studied in animal models [6]. The response to *H. pylori* infection and the subsequent pattern of gastritis depends on the genotype of the patients and in particular a polymorphism in interleukin 1 beta, an inflammatory mediator triggered by *H. pylori* infection [7,8].

The most commonly used classifications of GC are the WHO two main histological types, diffuse and intestinal [9], which have different clinicopathological characteristics. Diffuse cancer occurs more commonly in young patients, can be multifocal, is not often accompanied by intestinal metaplasia and can be hereditary [10-12]. Intestinal type is more frequently observed in older patients and follows multifocal atrophic gastritis [8].

For the diagnosis of GC, few highly sensitive or highly specific tumor markers are available, and current diagnostic tools for GC, including the serological markers carbohydrate antigen 19-9 (CA19-9) and carcinoembryonic antigen (CEA), have low specificity and sensitivity. Several groups have undertaken high-throughput analyses of GC expression profiles by DNA microarrays and microdissection. Good markers for diagnosis and progression of GC, however, have not yet been identified [13,14].

Molecular studies have provided evidence that GC arises not only from the combined effects of environmental factors and susceptible genetic variants but also from the accumulation of genetic and epigenetic alterations that play crucial roles in the process of cellular immortalization and tumorigenesis. Recent studies have confirmed the altered expression profile of miRNAs in gastric cancer (for review [15,16]). This chapter will focus on research related to the miRNAs involved in the pathogenesis of gastric cancer and discuss their possible use as markers for diagnosis and prognosis, and eventually as new targets for a specific therapy.

## 12.2. Polymorphisms within Mature miRNA Sequence and miRNA Binding Regions and Risk of Cancer

Sun et al. (2010) designed the study to determine whether A/G polymorphism (rs895819) within mir-27a is associated with a risk of gastric cancer. Authors also investigated miR-27a and its target gene Zinc finger and BTB domain containing 10 (ZBTB1) expression in consideration of the genotype [17]. In the case-control study based on 304 gastric cancer cases and 304 cancer-free controls, they found that subjects with the variant genotypes (AG + GG) showed a significantly increased risk of gastric cancer relative to AA carriers (adjusted OR 1.48; 95% CI 1.06-2.05; $p = 0.019$). A significant association of hsa-mir-27a variant genotypes with lymph node metastasis was also observed. Further functional analyses indicated that variant genotypes might be responsible also for elevated miR-27a levels and reduced ZBTB10 mRNA [17].

The most frequently studied miRNA SNP, rs11614913 in miR-196a-2, was studied also in the gastric cancer. Peng et al. (2010) conducted hospital-based case-control study from 213 gastric cancer patients and 213 age- and sex-matched controls in Chinese population. They found significantly increased risk of gastric cancer in subjects with the variant homozygote

CC of miR-196a-2 compared with wild-type homozygote TT and heterozygote CT carriers (adjusted OR 1.57; 95% CI 1.03-2.39; *p = 0.038*).

Stratified analyses indicated that the variant homozygote CC genotype had a strong association with lymph node metastasis of gastric cancer (adjusted OR 2.25, 95% CI 1.21-4.18, *p = 0.011*). These findings suggest that both, genetic variant within miR-196a-2 and miR-27a could play an important role in the development and progression of gastric cancer [18].

## 12.3. Serum and Plasma miRNAs: Early Detection of Disease Onset and Progression

Growing number of studies have shown that tumor-derived miRNAs are present in circulation in stable form and the levels of circulating miRNAs are detectable and could be quantified with current available and standardized methods [19]. A recent study examined the concentration of tumor-derived miRNAs in patients with gastric cancer to assess their clinical application for diagnosing and monitoring diseases and showed that levels of four miRNAs (miR-17-5p, miR-21, miR-106a, miR-106b) were significantly elevated and let-7a was lower in plasma of gastric cancer patients than controls and the elevated miRNAs were significantly reduced in postoperative samples.

The value of the area under the receiver-operating characteristic curve can be achieved as high as 0.879 for the miR-106a/let-7a ratio assay [20]. High levels of miR-17 and miR-106a in peripheral blood of gastric cancer patients have also been confirmed in another study in which the value of the area under the receiver-operating characteristic curve for combined miR-17/miR-106a assay was 0.741 [21].

Also the study of Liu et al. (2010) aimed a serum miRNAs expression profile that can serve as a novel diagnostic biomarker for GC detection and to assess its clinical applications in monitoring disease progression. Serum samples were taken from 164 GC patients and 127 age- and gender-matched tumor-free controls. An initial screening of miRNA expression by Solexa sequencing was performed using serum samples pooled from 20 patients and 20 controls, respectively. Differential expression was validated using qRT-PCR in individual samples.

The Solexa sequencing results demonstrated that 19 serum miRNAs were markedly upregulated in the GC patients compared to the controls. The qRT-PCR analysis further identified a profile of five serum miRNAs (miR-1, miR-20a, miR-27a, miR-34, and miR-423-5p) as a biomarker for GC detection. The analysis results showed that the expression level of five serum miRNAs was correlated to tumor stage. The areas under ROC curve of this five-serum miRNA signature were 0.879 (95% CI 0.822-0.936) and 0.831 (95% CI 0.767-0.898) for the two sets of serum samples, respectively, markedly higher than those of the biomarkers carcinoembryonic antigen (CEA) (0.503) and carbohydrate antigen 19-9 (CA19-9) (0.600). These findings together suggest that miRNAs may be useful biomarkers for diagnosis of gastric cancer [22].

## 12.4. Tissue miRNA Signatures: Implications for Diagnostic Oncology

Katada et al. (2009) comprehensively investigated miRNA expression profile in 42 undifferentiated gastric cancer tissues and paired normal gastric tissue. QRT-PCR was performed for a set of 72 miRNAs. The expression levels of 3 miRNAs (mir-34b, mir-34c, and mir-128a) were significantly up-regulated and 3 miRNAs (mir-128b, mir-129, and mir-148) were down-regulated in undifferentiated gastric cancer tissue when compared with those of the paired normal tissues [23].

The purpose of the study of Guo et al. (2009) was to determine the miRNA expression profile of gastric cancer by use of hybridization microarray technology. The most highly expressed miRNAs in non-tumorous tissues were miR-768-3p, miR-139-5p, miR-378, miR-31, miR-195, miR-497, and miR-133b. Three of them, miR-139-5p, miR-497, and miR-768-3p, were first found in non-tumorous tissues. The most highly expressed miRNAs in gastric cancer tissues were miR-20b, -20a, -17, -106a, -18a, -21, -106b, -18b, -421, -340*, -19a, and -658. Among them, miR-340*, miR-421, and miR-658 were found highly expressed in cancer cells for the first time. Also the expression of some target genes (such as Rb and PTEN) in cancer tissues was found to be decreased [24].

In the study of Ueda et al. (2010), a large group of 353 gastric samples from two independent subsets of patients from Japan were analysed by miRNA microarray. MiRNA expression patterns were compared between non-tumor mucosa and cancer samples, graded by diffuse and intestinal histological types and by progression-related factors (e.g. depth of invasion, metastasis, and stage). In 160 paired samples of non-tumor mucosa and cancer, 22 microRNAs were up-regulated and 13 were down-regulated in gastric cancer; 292 (83%) samples were distinguished correctly by this signature. The two histological subtypes of gastric cancer showed different miRNA signatures: eight miRNAs were up-regulated in diffuse-type and four in intestinal-type cancer [25].

To identify the specific miRNAs in gastric carcinoma, expression level of miRNAs in 24 gastric carcinoma and 3 normal gastric samples were detected by miRNA gene chip in the study of Luo et al. (2009). They found 19 miRNAs and 7 miRNAs were down-regulated and up-regulated, respectively. Compared with normal gastric tissue samples, miR-9 and miR-433 were down-regulated in gastric carcinoma [26].

Tsukamoto et al. (2010) investigated miRNA expression profiles in gastric carcinomas by use of a miRNA microarray platform covering a total of 470 human miRNAs. They identified 39 differentially expressed miRNAs in gastric carcinoma, of which six were significantly down-regulated and the other 33 were up-regulated. MiR-375 was the most down-regulated and its ectopic expression in gastric carcinoma cells markedly reduced cell viability via the caspase-mediated apoptosis pathway [27].

With high-throughput profiling method, Matsushima et al. (2010) found that 31 miRNAs were significantly deregulated in *H. pylori*-positive gastric mucosa versus *H. pylori*-negative mucosa. Severity of active and chronic inflammation in mucosa correlated significantly with the expression levels of several miRNAs, suggesting the involvement of miRNAs in host immune response to *H. pylori* infection. Although the exact relationship between miRNAs and *H. pylori*-induced inflammation remains unclear, some of the deregulated miRNAs (e.g. miR-155) is believed to play a role in regulation of inflammation and not just a consequence

**Table 12.1. List of representative miRNAs differentially expressed in GC mentioned in at least two miRNA profiling studies**

| Up-regulated miRNAs in GC | | Down-regulated miRNAs in GC | |
|---|---|---|---|
| miRNA | Reference, Fold Change (p-value) | miRNA | Reference, Fold Change (p-value) |
| miR-17-5p | [24] (0.018) [25] 1.7 (<0.00001) [27] 9.0 (0.01) | miR-148a | [23] <0.5 [25] 0.2 (<0.00001) [27] 0.2 (0.03) |
| miR-18a | [24] (0.03) [25] 1.7 (<0.00001) [27] 10.7 (0.01) | miR-29c | [25] 0.7 (<0.00001) [27] 0.2 (0.01) |
| miR-19a | [24] (0.05) [25] 1.5 (<0.0008) [27] 7.8 (0.01) | miR-375 | [25] 0.3 (<0.00001) [27] 0.2 (0.02) |
| miR-20a | [24] (0.02) [25] 1.8 (<0.00001) [27] 7.6 (0.01) | | |
| miR-20b | [24] (0.006) [25] 1.9 (<0.00001) [27] 6.8 (0.01) | | |
| miR-21 | [24] (0.03) [25] 2.0 (<0.00001) [27] 4.1 (0.01) | | |
| miR-25 | [25] 1.7 (<0.00001) [27] 5.6 (0.01) | | |
| miR-92 | [25] 1.7 (<0.00001) [27] 5.2 (0.01) | | |
| miR-106a | [24] (0.02) [25] 1.7 (<0.00001) [27] 9.0 (0.01) | | |
| miR-106b | [24] (0.04) [25] 1.6 (<0.00001) [27] 4.3 (0.01) | | |
| miR-320 | [26] (0.02) [27] 4.2 (0.01) | | |
| miR-425-5p | [25] 2.2 (<0.00001) [27] 5.3 (0.01) | | |

of immune response [28]. MiR-155 is the most studied miRNA regulator of immune response [29]. Continuous *H. pylori* infection could probably induce gastric carcinogenesis through altering the expression of some cancer associated miRNAs. Expression of some miRNAs including oncogenic (miR-106b, miR-21) and tumor suppressor miRNAs (let-7) could be significantly decreased following *H. pylori* infection, indicating a dysregulation of cancer-related miRNAs caused by *H. pylori* [28]. Ando et al. (2009) found that the methylation levels of the three tumor suppressor miRNAs (miR-124a-1, miR-124a-2, and miR-124a-3) were significantly higher in *H. pylori*-infected mucosa, suggesting a mechanism of *H. pylori's* modulation of miRNAs expression [15,30].

## 12.5. MiRNAs Expression in Prognosis and Response Prediction

Development of sensitive and specific biomarkers for gastric cancer will improve current management of the malignant disease including cancer early detection, differentiation, progression and recurrence monitoring and treatment response evaluation. Accumulating studies have investigated the diagnostic and prognostic values of miRNAs in gastric cancer.

Low expression of let-7g (HR 2.6; 95% CI 1.3-4.9) and miR-433 (HR 2.1; 95% CI 1.1-3.9) and high expression of miR-214 (HR 2.4; 95% CI 1.2-4.5) were associated with unfavourable outcome in overall survival independent of clinical covariates, including depth of invasion, lymph-node metastasis, and stage in the study performed by Ueda et al. (2009) described in detail above [25].

MiRNA expression profile was analysed by qRT-PCR in 100 gastric cancer patients, who were randomly assigned to either the training set or the testing set and stratified according to their prognosis. [31] Cox proportional hazard regression and risk-score analysis were used to identify a stage-independent set of seven-miRNA signature (miR-10b, miR-21, miR-223, miR-338, let-7a, miR-30a-5p, miR-126) in the training set that could classify patients with significantly different prognosis: according to overall survival ($p = 0.0009$) and relapse-free survival ($p = 0.0005$). Multivariate analysis showed that the risk signature was an independent predictor of overall survival (HR 3.046; 95% CI 1.246-7.445, $p = 0.015$) and relapse-free survival (HR 3.337; 95% CI 1.298-8.580, $p = 0.012$). Furthermore, the predictive value of this seven-miRNA signature was validated in the testing set of 50 patients and an independent set of 60 GC patients [31].

Prognosis of patients with undifferentiated gastric cancer is generally poor. In the study of Katada et al. (2009), the probability of survival was significantly lower in patients with high expression levels of mir-20b or miR-150. Also a correlation between mir-27a and lymph node metastasis was observed [23].

More recently, the expression of Dicer and Drosha was studied by immunohistochemistry in 332 gastric cancers and correlated with clinico-pathological patient characteristics. Differential expression of miRNAs was analyzed through miRNA Microarray Probe Set NCode (Invitrogen) containing 857 mammalian probes in a test set of six primary gastric cancers (three with and three without lymph node metastases). Differential expression was validated by qRT-PCR on an independent validation set of 20 patients with gastric cancer. Dicer and Drosha were differentially expressed in non-neoplastic and neoplastic gastric tissue. The expression of Drosha correlated with local tumor growth and was a significant independent prognosticator ($p = 0.026$) of patient survival. Twenty miRNAs were up- and two down-regulated in gastric carcinoma compared with non-neoplastic tissue. Six of these miRNAs separated node-positive from node-negative gastric cancers: miR-103, miR-21, miR-145, miR-106b, miR-146a, and miR-148a. These changes correlate independently with patient prognosis and probably influence local tumor growth and nodal spread [32].

## 12.6. MiRNAs as Potential Therapeutic Targets

The association of miRNA deregulation with pathogenesis and progression of malignant disease illustrates great potential of utilizing miRNAs as targets for therapeutic intervention. The basic strategy of current miRNA-based treatment studies is either to antagonize the expression of target miRNAs with antisense technology or to restore or strengthen the function of given miRNAs in order to inhibit the expression of certain protein-coding genes

[15]. There is a number of experimentally, *in vitro* or/and *in vivo*, proved miRNAs presenting potential therapeutic targets in gastric cancer. Here, only selected examples are discussed.

Ji et al. (2008) demonstrated that in p53-deficient human gastric cancer cells, restoration of functional miR-34 inhibits cell growth and induces chemosensitization and apoptosis, indicating that miR-34 may restore p53 function. Restoration of miR-34 inhibits tumorsphere formation and growth, which is reported to be correlated to the self-renewal of cancer stem cells. The mechanism of miR-34-mediated suppression of self-renewal appears to be related to the direct modulation of downstream targets Bcl-2, Notch, and HMGA2, indicating that miR-34 may be involved in gastric cancer stem cell self-renewal/differentiation decision-making. These data suggests that restoration of the tumor suppressor miR-34 may provide a novel molecular therapy for p53-mutant gastric cancer [33]. Inhibition of miR-372 using antisense miR-372 oligonucleotide (AS-miR-372) suppressed proliferation, arrested the cell cycle at G2/M phase, and increased apoptosis of AGS gastric cancer cells. Furthermore, AS-miR-372 treatment increased expression of LATS2. Over-expression of LATS2 induced changes in AGS cells similar to those in AGS cells treated with AS-miR-372, indicating an oncogenic role for miR-372 in controlling cell growth, cell cycle, and apoptosis through down-regulation of a tumor suppressor gene, LATS2 [34]. Results of Chun-Zhi et al. (2010) demonstrate that miR-221 and miR-222 regulate radiosensitivity, and cell growth and invasion of SGC7901 gastric cancer cells, possibly via direct modulation of PTEN expression [35]. After knockdown of miR-27a in gastric cancer cells, mRNA level and protein level of prohibitin are both elevated. Down-regulation of prohibitin by miR-27a may explain why suppression of miR-27a can inhibit gastric cancer cell growth, further supporting that miR-27a acts as an oncogene [36]. MiR-21 may be important in the initiation and progression of gastric cancers as an oncomiR, likely through regulating RECK. Observations of Zhang et al. (2008) suggest a potential regulatory pathway in which *H. pylori* infection up-regulates expression of miR-21, which in turn down-regulates RECK, and then leads to the development of gastric cancer [37]. Wang et al. (2010) reported that the expression of miR-101 is down-regulated in gastric cancer tissues and cells, and ectopic expression of miR-101 significantly inhibits cellular proliferation, migration and invasion of gastric cancer cells by targeting EZH2, Cox-2, Mcl-1 and Fos. Animal study also indicated that miR-101 could potentially suppress tumor growth *in vivo* [38]. Another potential therapeutic target presents miR-126 frequently down-regulated in gastric cancer tissue. Ectopic expression of miR-126 in SGC-7901 gastric cancer cells potently inhibited cell growth by inducing cell cycle arrest in G0/G1 phase, migration and invasion *in vitro* as well as tumorigenicity and metastasis *in vivo* [39]. Li et al. (2010) characterized Dicer1 as a direct target of miR-107. Their results suggested that miR-107 is an oncogenic miRNA promoting gastric cancer metastasis through downregulation of Dicer1 *in vitro* and *in vivo*. Inhibition of miR-107 or restoration of Dicer1 may represent a new potential therapeutic target for gastric cancer treatment [40]. Over-expression of miR-130b increased cell viability, reduced cell death and decreased expression of Bim in TGF-beta mediated apoptosis, subsequently to the down-regulation of RUNX3 protein expression in gastric cell lines. In 15 gastric tumors, miR-130b expression was significantly higher compared to matched normal tissue, and was inversely associated with RUNX3 hypermethylation [41].

Chemotherapy resistance remains one of the major obstacles to improvement overall survival and quality of life for gastric cancer patients. MiRNAs-based therapy could be used as a tool to modulate the response of cancer cells to chemotherapy. For instance, Xia et al.

(2008) found that miR-15b and miR-16 were down-regulated in a multi-drug resistant gastric cancer cell line SGC7901/VCR compared with its parental cell line SGC7901. Enforced overexpression of miR-15b or miR-16 could sensitize SGC7901/VCR cells to vincristine induced apoptosis. The chemotherapy sensitizing effect of the miRNAs was partly mediated by modulation of apoptosis via targeting Bcl2 [42]. Zhu et al. (2011) investigated the possible role of miRNAs in the development of multidrug resistance (MDR) in human gastric cancer cell line. They found that miR-497 was down-regulated in multidrug-resistant human gastric cancer cell line SGC7901/vincristine (VCR) and the down-regulation of miR-497 was concurrent with the up-regulation of Bcl2 protein, compared with the parental SGC7901 and A549 cell lines, respectively. *In vitro* drug sensitivity assay demonstrated that overexpression of miR-497 sensitized SGC7901/ cells to anticancer drugs [43].

Except the above mentioned research areas, the role of miRNAs in counteracting metastasis, angiogenesis, and radiotherapy resistance is yet to be investigated. There are several major challenges to overcome before the application of miRNA-based treatment. Firstly, the multitargeting nature of miRNAs gives the risk of unintended off-target effects that need to be carefully evaluated. Secondly, the expression of target gene may be controlled by several different miRNAs, which may compromise the effect of miRNA-based treatment. Finally, there is still lack of miRNA delivery system with enough specificity and efficacy [15].

## Acknowledgment

This work was supported by grants NS 10361-3/2009, NR/9814-4/2008, NS 10352-3/2009, NT/11214-4/2010 of Czech Ministry of Health, Project No. MZ0MOU2005 of the Czech Ministry of Health and by the project "CEITEC – Central European Institute of Technology" (CZ.1.05/1.1.00/02.0068).

## References

[1] Macdonald JS, Smalley SR, Benedetti J, Hundahl SA, Estes NC, Stemmermann GN, Haller DG, Ajani JA, Gunderson LL, Jessup JM, Martenson JA: Chemoradiotherapy after surgery compared with surgery alone for adenocarcinoma of the stomach or gastroesophageal junction. *N. Engl. J. Med.* 2001 345:725-30.

[2] Bonenkamp JJ, Hermans J, Sasako M, van de Velde CJ, Welvaart K, Songun I, Meyer S, Plukker JT, Van Elk P, Obertop H, Gouma DJ, van Lanschot JJ, Taat CW, de Graaf PW, von Meyenfeldt MF, Tilanus H; Dutch Gastric Cancer Group: Extended lymph-node dissection for gastric cancer. *N. Engl. J. Med.* 1999 340:908-14.

[3] Kaneko S, Yoshimura T: Time trend analysis of gastric cancer incidence in Japan by histological types, 1975-1989. *Br. J. Cancer* 2001 84:400-5.

[4] Forman D, Newell DG, Fullerton F, Yarnell JW, Stacey AR, Wald N, Sitas F: Association between infection with Helicobacter pylori and risk of gastric cancer: evidence from a prospective investigation. *BMJ* 1991 302:1302-5.

[5] Suerbaum S, Michetti P: Helicobacter pylori infection. *N. Engl. J. Med.* 2002 347:1175-86.

[6] Watanabe T, Tada M, Nagai H, Sasaki S, Nakao M: Helicobacter pylori infection induces gastric cancer in mongolian gerbils. *Gastroenterology* 1998 115:642-8.

[7] El-Omar EM, Carrington M, Chow WH, McColl KE, Bream JH, Young HA, Herrera J, Lissowska J, Yuan CC, Rothman N, Lanyon G, Martin M, Fraumeni JF Jr, Rabkin CS: Interleukin-1 polymorphisms associated with increased risk of gastric cancer. *Nature* 2000 404:398-402.

[8] Milne AN, Carneiro F, O'Morain C, Offerhaus GJ: Nature meets nurture: molecular genetics of gastric cancer. *Hum. Genet.* 2009 126:615-28.

[9] Lauren P: The Two Histological Main Types of Gastric Carcinoma: Diffuse and So-Called Intestinal-Type Carcinoma. An Attempt at a Histo-Clinical Classification. *Acta Pathol. Microbiol. Scand.* 1965 64:31-49.

[10] Matley PJ, Dent DM, Madden MV, Price SK: Gastric carcinoma in young adults. *Ann. Surg.* 1988 208:593-6.

[11] Kokkola A, Sipponen P: Gastric carcinoma in young adults. *Hepatogastroenterology* 2001 48:1552-5.

[12] Carneiro F, Huntsman DG, Smyrk TC, Owen DA, Seruca R, Pharoah P, Caldas C, Sobrinho-Simoes M: Model of the early development of diffuse gastric cancer in E-cadherin mutation carriers and its implications for patient screening. *J. Pathol.* 2004 203:681-7.

[13] Kochi M, Fujii M, Kanamori N, Kaiga T, Kawakami T, Aizaki K, Kasahara M, Mochizuki F, Kasakura Y, Yamagata M: Evaluation of serum CEA and CA19-9 levels as prognostic factors in patients with gastric cancer. *Gastric. Cancer* 2000 3:177-86.

[14] Takahashi Y, Takeuchi T, Sakamoto J, Touge T, Mai M, Ohkura H, Kodaira S, Okajima K, Nakazato H: The usefulness of CEA and/or CA19-9 in monitoring for recurrence in gastric cancer patients: a prospective clinical study. *Gastric. Cancer* 2003 6:142-5.

[15] Wang J, Wang Q, Liu H, Hu B, Zhou W, Cheng Y: MicroRNA expression and its implication for the diagnosis and therapeutic strategies of gastric cancer. *Cancer Lett.* 2010 297:137-43.

[16] Wu WK, Lee CW, Cho CH, Fan D, Wu K, Yu J, Sung JJ: MicroRNA dysregulation in gastric cancer: a new player enters the game. *Oncogene* 2010 29:5761-71.

[17] Sun Q, Gu H, Zeng Y, Xia Y, Wang Y, Jing Y, Yang L, Wang B: Hsa-mir-27a genetic variant contributes to gastric cancer susceptibility through affecting miR-27a and target gene expression. *Cancer Sci.* 2010 101:2241-7.

[18] Peng S, Kuang Z, Sheng C, Zhang Y, Xu H, Cheng Q: Association of microRNA-196a-2 gene polymorphism with gastric cancer risk in a Chinese population. *Dig. Dis. Sci.* 2010 55:2288-93.

[19] Cortez MA, Calin GA: MicroRNA identification in plasma and serum: a new tool to diagnose and monitor diseases. *Expert Opin. Biol. Ther.* 2009 9:703-11.

[20] Tsujiura M, Ichikawa D, Komatsu S, Shiozaki A, Takeshita H, Kosuga T, Konishi H, Morimura R, Deguchi K, Fujiwara H, Okamoto K, Otsuji E: Circulating microRNAs in plasma of patients with gastric cancers. *Br. J. Cancer* 2010 102:1174-9.

[21] Zhou H, Guo JM, Lou YR, Zhang XJ, Zhong FD, Jiang Z, Cheng J, Xiao BX: Detection of circulating tumor cells in peripheral blood from patients with gastric cancer using microRNA as a marker. *J. Mol. Med.* 2010 88:709-17.

[22] Liu R, Zhang C, Hu Z, Li G, Wang C, Yang C, Huang D, Chen X, Zhang H, Zhuang R, Deng T, Liu H, Yin J, Wang S, Zen K, Ba Y, Zhang CY: A five-microRNA signature identified from genome-wide serum microRNA expression profiling serves as a fingerprint for gastric cancer diagnosis. *Eur. J. Cancer* 2010 [Eub ahead of print].

[23] Katada T, Ishiguro H, Kuwabara Y, Kimura M, Mitui A, Mori Y, Ogawa R, Harata K, Fujii Y: microRNA expression profile in undifferentiated gastric cancer. *Int. J. Oncol.* 2009 34:537-42.

[24] Guo J, Miao Y, Xiao B, Huan R, Jiang Z, Meng D, Wang Y: Differential expression of microRNA species in human gastric cancer versus non-tumorous tissues. *J. Gastroenterol. Hepatol.* 2009 24:652-7.

[25] Ueda T, Volinia S, Okumura H, Shimizu M, Taccioli C, Rossi S, Alder H, Liu CG, Oue N, Yasui W, Yoshida K, Sasaki H, Nomura S, Seto Y, Kaminishi M, Calin GA, Croce CM: Relation between microRNA expression and progression and prognosis of gastric cancer: a microRNA expression analysis. *Lancet Oncol.* 2010 11:136-46.

[26] Luo H, Zhang H, Zhang Z, Zhang X, Ning B, Guo J, Nie N, Liu B, Wu X: Down-regulated miR-9 and miR-433 in human gastric carcinoma. *J. Exp. Clin. Cancer Res.* 2009 28:82.

[27] Tsukamoto Y, Nakada C, Noguchi T, Tanigawa M, Nguyen LT, Uchida T, Hijiya N, Matsuura K, Fujioka T, Seto M, Moriyama M: MicroRNA-375 is downregulated in gastric carcinomas and regulates cell survival by targeting PDK1 and 14-3-3zeta. *Cancer Res* 70:2339-49.

[28] Matsushima K, Isomoto H, Inoue N, Nakayama T, Hayashi T, Nakayama M, Nakao K, Hirayama T, Kohno S: MicroRNA signatures in Helicobacter pylori-infected gastric mucosa. *Int. J. Cancer* 2011 128:361-70.

[29] Tsitsiou E, Lindsay MA: microRNAs and the immune response. *Curr. Opin. Pharmacol.* 2009 9:514-20.

[30] Ando T, Yoshida T, Enomoto S, Asada K, Tatematsu M, Ichinose M, Sugiyama T, Ushijima T: DNA methylation of microRNA genes in gastric mucosae of gastric cancer patients: its possible involvement in the formation of epigenetic field defect. *Int. J. Cancer* 2009 124:2367-74.

[31] Li X, Zhang Y, Ding J, Wu K, Fan D: Survival prediction of gastric cancer by a seven-microRNA signature. *Gut* 2010 59:579-85.

[32] Tchernitsa O, Kasajima A, Schafer R, Kuban RJ, Ungethum U, Gyorffy B, Neumann U, Simon E, Weichert W, Ebert MP, Rocken C: Systematic evaluation of the miRNA-ome and its downstream effects on mRNA expression identifies gastric cancer progression. *J. Pathol.* 2010 222:310-9.

[33] Ji Q, Hao X, Meng Y, Zhang M, Desano J, Fan D, Xu L: Restoration of tumor suppressor miR-34 inhibits human p53-mutant gastric cancer tumorspheres. *BMC Cancer* 2008 8:266.

[34] Cho WJ, Shin JM, Kim JS, Lee MR, Hong KS, Lee JH, Koo KH, Park JW, Kim KS: miR-372 regulates cell cycle and apoptosis of ags human gastric cancer cell line through direct regulation of LATS2. *Mol. Cells* 2009 28:521-7.

[35] Chun-Zhi Z, Lei H, An-Ling Z, Yan-Chao F, Xiao Y, Guang-Xiu W, Zhi-Fan J, Pei-Yu P, Qing-Yu Z, Chun-Sheng K: MicroRNA-221 and microRNA-222 regulate gastric carcinoma cell proliferation and radioresistance by targeting PTEN. *BMC Cancer* 2010 10:367.

[36] Liu T, Tang H, Lang Y, Liu M, Li X: MicroRNA-27a functions as an oncogene in gastric adenocarcinoma by targeting prohibitin. *Cancer Lett.* 2009 273:233-42.

[37] Zhang Z, Li Z, Gao C, Chen P, Chen J, Liu W, Xiao S, Lu H: miR-21 plays a pivotal role in gastric cancer pathogenesis and progression. *Lab. Invest.* 2008 88:1358-66.

[38] Wang HJ, Ruan HJ, He XJ, Ma YY, Jiang XT, Xia YJ, Ye ZY, Tao HQ: MicroRNA-101 is down-regulated in gastric cancer and involved in cell migration and invasion. *Eur. J. Cancer* 2010 46:2295-303.

[39] Feng R, Chen X, Yu Y, Su L, Yu B, Li J, Cai Q, Yan M, Liu B, Zhu Z: miR-126 functions as a tumour suppressor in human gastric cancer. *Cancer Lett.* 2010 298:50-63.

[40] Li X, Zhang Y, Shi Y, Dong G, Liang J, Han Y, Wang X, Zhao Q, Ding J, Wu K, Fan D: MicroRNA-107, an Oncogene MicroRNA that Regulates Tumor Invasion and Metastasis By Targeting DICER1 in Gastric Cancer: MiR-107 promotes gastric cancer invasion and metastasis. *J. Cell Mol. Med.* 2010 [Epub ahead of print].

[41] Lai KW, Koh KX, Loh M, Tada K, Subramaniam MM, Lim XY, Vaithilingam A, Salto-Tellez M, Iacopetta B, Ito Y, Soong R: MicroRNA-130b regulates the tumour suppressor RUNX3 in gastric cancer. *Eur. J. Cancer* 2010 46:1456-63.

[42] Wang HJ, Ruan HJ, He XJ, Ma YY, Jiang XT, Xia YJ, Ye ZY, Tao HQ: MicroRNA-101 is down-regulated in gastric cancer and involved in cell migration and invasion. *Eur. J. Cancer* 2010 46:2295-303.

[43] Zhu W, Zhu D, Lu S, Wang T, Wang J, Jiang B, Shu Y, Liu P: miR-497 modulates multidrug resistance of human cancer cell lines by targeting BCL2. *Med. Oncol.* 2011 [Epub ahead of print].

In: MicroRNAs in Solid Cancer
Editor: Ondrej Slaby

ISBN: 978-61324-514-9
©2012 Nova Science Publishers, Inc.

*Chapter XIII*

# MicroRNAs and Thyroid Cancer

*Martina Redova*
Masaryk Memorial Cancer Institute, Brno, Czech Republic

## Abstract

Thyroid cancer is the most common endocrine malignancy with incidence significantly increasing over last few decades. MiRNAs have tremendous potential for use in the diagnosis and prognosis of thyroid tumors carcinogenesis, and their deregulated expression together with their biological roles suggest a correlation with diagnosis, prognosis, and even therapeutic approaches.

## 13.1. Introduction

Thyroid cancer is a relatively rare disease, accounting for approximately 1% of all new cases per year, but it represents the most common endocrine malignancy. The incidence in female is higher, with ratio 3:1 [1].

The thyroid gland is composed of two distinct hormone-producing cell types: follicular cells, which are present in the monolayer epithelium, are responsible for iodine uptake and thyroid hormone synthesis, and parafollicular C-cells, which are responsible for the production of the calcium-regulating hormone calcitonin and from which the medullary carcinoma (MC) accounting for less than 5% of thyroid tumors originates. The majority of the thyroid tumors (more than 95%) are derived from the follicular cells and are commonly divided into (i) well-differentiated thyroid carcinoma (WDTC), comprehensive of papillary thyroid carcinoma (PTC) and follicular thyroid carcinoma (FTC) types, (ii) poorly differentiated thyroid carcinoma (PDTC), and (iii) undifferentiated types depending on various histological and clinical factors [2,3]. PTCs, which account for approximately 80% of all cases and are responsible for the overall increase in incidence of thyroid cancer, are often multifocal and tend to metastasize to the regional lymph nodes, and are characterized by classical papillary architecture and cells with typical nuclear alterations [4]. FTC accounts for about 10% of all thyroid carcinomas and may be of conventional or oncocytic (Hurthle cell) type. FTC is well differentiated, usually unifocal, encapsulated, with a tendency to metastasize via the vascular system to the bones and lungs [3]. Both PTCs and FTCs may progress to poorly differentiated carcinoma (PDTC) or may completely loose differentiation and transform to anaplastic carcinoma (ATC), which accounts for very rare tumors estimated to comprise about 2-5% of thyroid malignancies and which are extremely aggressive and insensitive to conventional radiotherapy and chemotherapy [5].

Radiation exposure is the major risk factor for PTCs. The incidence of FTCs is higher in areas of iodine deficiency. Moreover, several oncogenes have been involved in thyroid carcinoma development - in PTCs, non-overlapping mutations of genes involved in the activation pathway of mitogen-activated protein kinase (MAPK), such as RET, TRK, RAS, and BRAF, have been found in about 70% of the cases [6]. Indeed, a fraction of about 30% of PTCs present a typical gene alteration consisting in the rearrangement of RET proto-oncogene [7].

The current standard of care for patients with papillary thyroid cancer includes total thyroidectomy and a therapeutic lymph node dissection for patients presenting with clinically evident nodal disease [8]. Regarding the preoperative diagnosis, fine-needle aspiration (FNA) of thyroid nodules is a safe and accurate tool. The major challenge is to differentiate between the follicular-patterned thyroid cancers and hyperplastic nodules, which are common in general population. Therefore, a diagnostically useful assay has to distinguish thyroid cancer not only from normal thyroid tissue but also from hyperplastic nodules. The diagnostic benefits of miRNA detection in freshly collected FNA samples obtained for pre-operative evaluation of thyroid nodules have been explored [9].

## 13.2. Polymorphisms within Mature miRNA Sequence and miRNA Binding Regions and Risk of Cancer

Although papillary thyroid carcinoma displays strong heritability, no predisposing germ-line mutations have been found. It has been reported that miR-146, which represents one of the most up-regulated miRNAs in PTCs and which identifies two different miRNAs differing only for two nucleotides (miR-146a on chromosome 5q33 and miR-146b on chromosome 10q24), can interact with a domain in the exon 18 region of the c-KIT mRNA. KIT, whose transcript levels are known to be extremely low in PTC tumor cells, is an important tyrosine kinase receptor in cell differentiation and growth. Intriguingly, there is a single-nucleotide polymorphism (SNP; 2607G>C) located in the crucial region of the c-KIT mRNA pairing with miR-146. This event could lead to changes in the duplex conformation between miRNA and mRNA and result in hybridization with a different region, modulating the expression of the target gene in a different manner [3,10].

In an effort to elucidate the putative role of miR-146 in PTC, Jazdzewski et al. (2008) sequenced the pri-miR-146a and pri-miR-146b in the genomic DNA and in the pre-miR-146a they noted a common G/C polymorphism designated rs2910164. The rarer C allele causes mispairing within the hairpin and taken together, the SNP might reduce the stability of the pri-miRNA, the efficiency of processing of pri-miRNA into pre-miRNA, or the efficiency of processing the pre-miRNA into the mature miRNA. This polymorphism shows marked difference in genotype distribution and possibly affect the predisposition to PTCs, i.e. an increased risk to develop PTCs is associated with the GC heterozygous status. This is a rare phenomenon (overdominance) in which heterozygosity is a genetic risk rather than homozygosity [11].

In a sequent work, they showed that in the case of miR-146a the presence of the SNP potentially generates two isoforms (marked *): miR-146a*G from the allele carrying G, and miR-146a*C from the C allele. Thus, GG and CC homozygotes each produce two mature molecules (miR-146a from the leading strand, and miR-146a*G or *C, respectively, from the passenger strand) whereas GC heterozygotes differ from both homozygotes by producing three mature miRNAs (miR-146a and both miR-146a*G and miR-146a*C). Because each mature miRNA binds to a distinct set of target genes, different target genes are affected by the miRNAs produced by GG or CC homozygotes. Finally, they propose that the production of distinct miRs and regulation of different target genes by heterozygotes compared with homozygotes may explain the predisposition to PTC displayed by individuals who are heterozygous [12].

Also miR-221 and miR-222, described as being among the most dramatically over-expressed miRNAs in PTCs, could be affected by SNPs. By sequencing the regions harboring two binding domains, one for miR-221 and miR-222, He et al. (2005) identified a polymorphism in each recognition site - the 3169G3A SNP (rs17084733) located within the crucial region of the miR-221 and miR-222 domain in the KIT 3` UTR region. It is likely that variants within the binding regions can acquire new miRNAs as regulating factors due to sequence changes such as SNPs, and moreover, that not only changes in miRNAs but also in their target genes profoundly influence PTC carcinogenesis [10].

## 13.3. Tissue miRNA Signatures: Implications for Diagnostic Oncology

As palpable thyroid nodules are common, the fine-needle aspiration is considered a safe and accurate tool in the diagnosis of thyroid cancer. Although diagnostics might be improved by supplementary testing of FNA material for somatic mutations known to occur in thyroid tumors, such testing could be limited because a significant proportion of PTCs and FTCs do not harbor any known mutations. These cases may benefit from additional diagnostic modalities, such as miRNA profiling. Regarding the preoperative diagnostics, the major challenge is to clearly differentiate between the follicular patterned thyroid cancers and hyperplastic nodules [13].

Recent studies have confirmed the set of seven miRNAs including miR-221, miR-222, miR-146, miR-21, miR-155, miR-181a, and miR-181b, up-regulated in PTCs compared with the normal thyroid tissue and hyperplastic nodules, respectively [10,14,15]. Surprisingly, miRNA profiling studies reveled no global down-regulation of miRNA expression in less differentiated carcinomas as compared to well-differentiated thyroid carcinomas (PTCs, FTCs, MCs), which is in contrast with reported study that found overall decrease in miRNA expression in poorly differentiated tumors as compared with their well-differentiated counterparts in various cancers [16]. Regarding diagnosis, miR-181b was found up-regulated in both thyroid tumors and hyperplastic nodules [9].

During examination of a correlation between miRNA expression and known somatic mutations, it was observed that papillary carcinomas positive for BRAF, RET/PTC, and RAS mutations, and those with no known mutations demonstrated significant differences in the expression of certain miRNAs. For example, miR-187 was expressed at high levels in PTCs harboring RET/PTC rearrangements, whereas miR-221 and miR-222 were found at the highest levels in BRAF- and RAS-positive PTCs and tumors with no known mutations, and the highest expression level of miR-146b were found in PTCs carrying RAS mutations [9].

As for other thyroid tumors, the most highly up-regulated miRNAs in conventional FTCs were miR-187, miR-224, miR-155, miR-222, and miR-221, and those in oncocytic variants were miR-187, miR-221, miR-339, miR-183, miR-222, and miR-197, whereas the most highly up-regulated miRNAs in conventional FTAs were miR-339, miR-224, miR-205, miR-210, miR-190, miR-328, and miR-342, and those in oncocytic variants were miR-31, miR-339, miR-183, miR-221, miR-224, and miR-203 [9]. In addition, Weber et al. (2006) identified four miRNAs differentially expressed between FTCs and FTAs (miR-192, miR-197, miR-328, and miR-346) [17]. Regarding anaplastic thyroid carcinomas, miR-302c, miR-205, and miR-137 were found to be up-regulated in ATCs as compared to hyperplastic nodules. On the contrary, a significant decrease in expression of miR-30d, miR-125b, miR-26a, and miR-30a-5p was detected [18]. Furthermore, the miR-17-92 cluster (miR-17-5p, miR-17-3p, miR-18a, miR-19a, miR-19b, miR-20a, miR-92-1) as well as miR-106a and miR-106b were reported as being over-expressed in ATC cell lines [19].

Other dysregulated miRNAs are listed in Table 13.1.

**Table 13.1. List of representative miRNAs differentially expressed in PTC mentioned in at least two microRNA profiling studies (* SAM, significance analysis of microarrays)**

| Up-regulated miRNAs in PTC | |
|---|---|
| miRNA | Reference, Fold Change (FC) / SAM*, p-value |
| miR-221 | [9] FC = 19.1 [10] 12.3* [14] FC = 12.64; p = 0.014 [15] 7.26* |
| miR-222 | [9] FC = 17.2 [10] 10.9* [14] FC = 24.76; p = 0.0026 [15] 7.04* |
| miR-181a | [10] 2.6* [14] FC = 3.66; p = 0.0002 [15] 3.1* |
| miR-181b | [9] FC = 14.4 [14] FC = 7.83; p = 3.68E-05 [15] 3.63* |
| miR-224 | [9] FC = 6.2 [14] FC = 3.46; p = 0.042 [15] 2.51* |
| miR-34a | [10] 1.8* [14] FC = 2.41; p = 0.014 [15] 3.97* |
| miR-146 | [9] FC = 10.5 [10] 19.3* |
| miR-155 | [9] FC = 9.5 [10] 2.2* |
| miR-31 | [9] FC = 7.5 [15] 4.27* |
| miR-21 | [10] 4.3* [15] 4.06* |
| miR-220 | [10] 4.0* [14] FC = 5.1; p = 0.004 |
| miR-181c | [10] 2.4* [14] FC = 3.34; p = 7.88E-05 |
| miR-213 | [10] 1.9* [14] FC = 4.38; p = 0.0006 |
| Down-regulated miRNA in PTC | |
| miR-345 | [10] 0.6* [15] -2.77* |

## 13.4. MiRNAs Expression in Prognosis and Response Prediction

Thyroid neoplasms serve as a good model systems to study changes in molecular events because they comprise a wide variety of different grades of malignancy with differentiated carcinomas (e.g. follicular carcinoma and papillary carcinoma) which have a good prognosis to poorly differentiated and anaplastic carcinomas which are aggressive and have poor prognosis. MicroRNAs have tremendous potential for use in the diagnosis and prognosis of thyroid tumors carcinogenesis, and their deregulated expression together with their biological role suggest a correlation with diagnosis, prognosis, and even therapeutic approaches. For example, results of He et al. (2005) from the prediction analysis of microarrays analysis indicated that five over-expressed miRNAs (miR-221, miR-222, miR-146, miR-21, and miR-181a) were sufficient to successfully predict cancer status [10]. Additionally, discovery of specific miRNAs which could portend progression of thyroid tumors to poorly differentiated or anaplastic carcinoma would be highly useful and could potentially identify tumors with no anaplastic features or poorly differentiated areas which might still need aggressive treatment [20].

## 13.5. MiRNAs as Potential Therapeutic Targets

As various preclinical studies have identified numerous over- or under-expressed proteins that affect critical cellular processes, including transcription, signaling, mitosis, proliferation, cell cycle, apoptosis and adhesion, newer therapeutic modalities are worth finding, and more effective combinations are needed to improve patient outcomes.

Also, identification of miRNAs and their putative target genes lays the groundwork for therapeutic advances in terms of small molecular inhibitors, kinase inhibitors, gene therapy, etc. [20].

From this point of view, inhibition of mostly up-regulated miRNAs such as miR-221, miR-222, and miR-146, with „antagomirs" or „locked nucleic acid-modified anti-miRs", is an attractive direction for individualised targeted therapy [3].

Moreover, the inhibition of miR-17-3p, miR-17-5p, and miR -19a, resulted in a reduced cell growth. On the basis of these findings and the fact that retinoblastoma protein (RB1) and PTEN have been previously confirmed as direct targets of these miRNAs, an oncogenic potential could be suggested [19]. On the contrary, restoration of down-regulated miRNAs as well would be a tool to improve the thyroid cancer patients management and response to applied treatment. \

The recent results of Kota et al. (2009) reporting the restoration of miR-26a expression levels in hepatocellular carcinoma suggest a possible use of miR-26a restoration also in ATC that is well known to be refractory to any conventional radiotherapy and chemotherapy [3,21].

## Acknowledgment

This work was supported by grants NS 10361-3/2009, NR/9814-4/2008, NS 10352-3/2009, NT/11214-4/2010 of Czech Ministry of Health, Project No. MZ0MOU2005 of the Czech Ministry of Health and by the project "CEITEC – Central European Institute of Technology" (CZ.1.05/1.1.00/02.0068).

## References

[1] Greco A, Borrello MG, Miranda C, Degl'Innocenti D, Pierotti MA: Molecular pathology of differentiated thyroid cancer. *Q. J. Nucl. Med. Mol. Imaging* 2009 53:440-53.

[2] Kondo T, Ezzat S, Asa SL: Pathogenetic mechanisms in thyroid follicular-cell neoplasia. *Nat. Rev. Cancer* 2006 6:292-306.

[3] Pallante P, Visone R, Croce CM, Fusco A: Deregulation of microRNA expression in follicular-cell-derived human thyroid carcinomas. *Endocr. Relat. Cancer* 2010 17:F91-104.

[4] Davies L, Welch HG: Increasing incidence of thyroid cancer in the United States, 1973-2002. *JAMA* 2006 295:2164-7.

[5] Yau T, Lo CY, Epstein RJ, Lam AK, Wan KY, Lang BH: Treatment outcomes in anaplastic thyroid carcinoma: survival improvement in young patients with localized disease treated by combination of surgery and radiotherapy. *Ann. Surg. Oncol.* 2008 15:2500-5.

[6] Frattini M, Ferrario C, Bressan P, Balestra D, De Cecco L, Mondellini P, Bongarzone I, Collini P, Gariboldi M, Pilotti S, Pierotti MA, Greco A: Alternative mutations of BRAF, RET and NTRK1 are associated with similar but distinct gene expression patterns in papillary thyroid cancer. *Oncogene* 2004 23:7436-40.

[7] Santoro M, Carlomagno F, Melillo RM, Fusco A: Dysfunction of the RET receptor in human cancer. *Cell Mol. Life Sci.* 2004 61:2954-64.

[8] Moo TA, Fahey TJ, 3rd: Lymph node dissection in papillary thyroid carcinoma. *Semin. Nucl. Med.* 2011 41:84-8.

[9] Nikiforova MN, Tseng GC, Steward D, Diorio D, Nikiforov YE: MicroRNA expression profiling of thyroid tumors: biological significance and diagnostic utility. *J. Clin. Endocrinol. Metab.* 2008 93:1600-8.

[10] He H, Jazdzewski K, Li W, Liyanarachchi S, Nagy R, Volinia S, Calin GA, Liu CG, Franssila K, Suster S, Kloos RT, Croce CM, de la Chapelle A: The role of microRNA genes in papillary thyroid carcinoma. *Proc. Natl. Acad. Sci. USA* 2005 102:19075-80.

[11] Jazdzewski K, Murray EL, Franssila K, Jarzab B, Schoenberg DR, de la Chapelle A: Common SNP in pre-miR-146a decreases mature miR expression and predisposes to papillary thyroid carcinoma. *Proc. Natl. Acad. Sci. USA* 2008 105:7269-74.

[12] Jazdzewski K, Liyanarachchi S, Swierniak M, Pachucki J, Ringel MD, Jarzab B, de la Chapelle A: Polymorphic mature microRNAs from passenger strand of pre-miR-146a contribute to thyroid cancer. *Proc. Natl. Acad. Sci. USA* 2009 106:1502-5.

[13] Nikiforova MN, Chiosea SI, Nikiforov YE: MicroRNA expression profiles in thyroid tumors. *Endocr. Pathol.* 2009 20:85-91.

[14] Pallante P, Visone R, Ferracin M, Ferraro A, Berlingieri MT, Troncone G, Chiappetta G, Liu CG, Santoro M, Negrini M, Croce CM, Fusco A: MicroRNA deregulation in human thyroid papillary carcinomas. *Endocr. Relat. Cancer* 2006 13:497-508.

[15] Tetzlaff MT, Liu A, Xu X, Master SR, Baldwin DA, Tobias JW, Livolsi VA, Baloch ZW: Differential expression of miRNAs in papillary thyroid carcinoma compared to multinodular goiter using formalin fixed paraffin embedded tissues. *Endocr. Pathol.* 2007 18:163-73.

[16] Lu J, Getz G, Miska EA, Alvarez-Saavedra E, Lamb J, Peck D, Sweet-Cordero A, Ebert BL, Mak RH, Ferrando AA, Downing JR, Jacks T, Horvitz HR, Golub TR: MicroRNA expression profiles classify human cancers. *Nature* 2005 435:834-8.

[17] Weber F, Teresi RE, Broelsch CE, Frilling A, Eng C: A limited set of human MicroRNA is deregulated in follicular thyroid carcinoma. *J. Clin. Endocrinol. Metab.* 2006 91:3584-91.

[18] Visone R, Pallante P, Vecchione A, Cirombella R, Ferracin M, Ferraro A, Volinia S, Coluzzi S, Leone V, Borbone E, Liu CG, Petrocca F, Troncone G, Calin GA, Scarpa A, Colato C, Tallini G, Santoro M, Croce CM, Fusco A: Specific microRNAs are downregulated in human thyroid anaplastic carcinomas. *Oncogene* 2007 26:7590-5.

[19] Takakura S, Mitsutake N, Nakashima M, Namba H, Saenko VA, Rogounovitch TI, Nakazawa Y, Hayashi T, Ohtsuru A, Yamashita S: Oncogenic role of miR-17-92 cluster in anaplastic thyroid cancer cells. *Cancer Sci.* 2008 99:1147-54.

[20] Menon MP, Khan A: Micro-RNAs in thyroid neoplasms: molecular, diagnostic and therapeutic implications. *J. Clin. Pathol.* 2009 62:978-85.

[21] Kota J, Chivukula RR, O'Donnell KA, Wentzel EA, Montgomery CL, Hwang HW, Chang TC, Vivekanandan P, Torbenson M, Clark KR, Mendell JR, Mendell JT: Therapeutic microRNA delivery suppresses tumorigenesis in a murine liver cancer model. *Cell* 2009 137:1005-17.

In: MicroRNAs in Solid Cancer
Editor: Ondrej Slaby

ISBN: 978-61324-514-9
©2012 Nova Science Publishers, Inc.

*Chapter XIV*

# MicroRNAs and Glioblastoma

*Jiri Sana, Radek Lakomy, Marian Hajduch and Ondrej Slaby*

Masaryk Memorial Cancer Institute, Brno, Czech Republic
Laboratory of Experimental Medicine,
Institute of Molecular and Translational Medicine,
Faculty of Medicine and Dentistry, Palacky University and University,
Hospital in Olomouc, Czech Republic

## Abstract

Glioblastoma is the highly malignant brain tumor with very poor prognosis. Despite great progress, current therapeutic approaches are insufficient for total cure of patients afflicted with this malignancy. MiRNAs represent promising therapeutic targets in glioblastoma. In this chapter we summarize the current knowledge about miRNAs significance in glioblastoma, with special focus on their involvement in core signaling pathways, their roles in drug resistance and potential clinical implications.

## 14.1. Introduction

Glioblastoma (GBM), a WHO grade IV malignant glioma, is the most frequent and lethal primary brain tumor, with an incidence 3.55 new cases per 100,000 Caucasians per year. Despite modern therapeutic approaches in oncology, GBM remains associated with very poor prognosis and a median survival rates range from 12 to 15 months [1,2,3]. This tumor is characterized by rapid diffusely infiltrative growth and high level of cellular heterogeneity associated with therapeutic resistance. Furthermore, GBM is also characterized by multiple genetic alternations. Epidermal growth factor receptor (EGFR) amplification and PTEN mutations are typical for primary GBM arising *de novo*, whereas TP53 mutations are typical for secondary glioblastoma developing from lower grade astrocytomas. Nevertheless, this distinction is not absolute and both glioblastoma types may harbour other gene and chromosome changes, e.g. the loss of heterozygosity (LOH) 10q is the most frequent aberration in both primary and secondary glioblastomas [1,4,5].

MiRNAs in GBM have been extensively studied in recent years. Here, we summarize these studies, with emphasis on their alterations and roles in GBM pathogenesis and their potential usage as disease biomarkers or novel therapeutic targets.

## 14.2. Polymorphisms within Mature microRNA Sequence and miRNA Binding Regions and Risk of Cancer

In gliomas, only one polymorphism within mature miRNA sequence, specifically rs11614913 gene variant of miR-196a, was studied till now [6]. Reached data suggest that the CC genotype of miR-196a SNP is associated with decreased risk of glioma in the Chinese population (OR 0.74; 95% CI, 0.56-0.98).

Significant association was observed also between these genotype and risk of particular glioma subgroups: patients over 18 years (OR 0.73; 95% CI, 0.55-0.98), male glioma patients (OR 0.69; 95% CI, 0.48-0.99) and patients with high grade glioma-glioblastoma (OR 0.58; 95% CI, 0.37-0.91). In contrast to other solid cancers, such as lung and breast cancer, data in glioblastoma showed opposite association between miR-196a genotype and cancer risk. This may be related to the diversity on the tissues origin, and characteristic molecular alterations in different cancers [6].

## 14.3. Tissue miRNA Signatures: Implications for Diagnostic Oncology

Two independent research groups performed analyses of the miRNA expression profiles of glioblastoma tissues. Both studies have described significant up-regulation of miR-21. This finding fully corresponds to the expression level of miR-21 observed in other cancers [7,8,9]. Furthermore, miR-125b was over-expressed, and miR-128a and miRNA-181 family were significantly down-regulated in both studies.

Interestingly, Ciafré et al. (2005) described miR-221 as up-regulated, whereas, Slaby et al. (2010) observed approximately four-fold lower levels of the same miRNA in glioblastomas in comparison to the adult brain tissue [10,11]. Authors discussed this phenomenon and conclude that it is likely that the brain tissue (used as control in their study), though excised from the margin of resection material, contained traces of micro-capillaries from around the arteriovenous malformation.

It is largely known that miR-221/222 is found in the highest levels in endothelial cells [11]. For a summary of miRNAs with changed expression in the glioblastoma tissues in both studies see Table 14.1.

Table 14.1. List of representative miRNAs differentially expressed in GBM mentioned in both miRNA profiling studies, C/P ratios from [10] represents the range of ratio between tumor samples values (C, center of the tumor) and the control samples values (P, peripheral brain area from the same patient)

| Up-regulated miRNAs in GBM | | Down-regulated miRNAs in GBM | |
|---|---|---|---|
| miRNA | Reference + C/P ratio or fold change | miRNA | Reference + C/P ratio or fold change |
| miR-21 | [10] 1.81-9.3 [11] 8.35 | miR-128a | [10] 0.34 - 0.56 [11] 0.03 |
| miR-125b | [11] 1.45 | miR-181a | [10] 0.082 - 0.56 [11] 0.4 |
| miR-125b-1 | [10] 2.19-2.73 | miR-181b | [10] 0.098 - 0.56 [11] 0.28 |
| miR-125b-2 | [10] 1.95-2.88 | miR-181c | [10] 0.096 - 0.56 [11] 0.29 |

Table 14.2. Differential expression of miRNAs in glioblastoma versus anaplastic astrocytoma (according to [12])

| Up-regulated miRNAs in GBM | | Down-regulated miRNAs in GBM | |
|---|---|---|---|
| miRNA | fold change (p-value) | miRNA | fold change (p-value) |
| miR-196a | 105.6 (0.00384) | miR-105 | 0.029 (0.0177) |
| miR-15b | 3.3 (0.00734) | miR-367 | 0.036 (0.021) |
| miR-196b | 11.8 (0.0371) | miR-184 | 0.101 (0.0361) |
| miR-363 | 27 (0.0371) | miR-504 | 0.072 (0.0374) |
| miR-21 | 3.6 (0.0421) | miR-302b | 0.061 (0.0415) |
| miR-135b | 5 (0.0487) | miR-128b | 0.15 (0.0421) |
| | | miR-601 | 0.289 (0.0421) |
| | | miR-517c | 0.081 (0.0462) |
| | | miR-302d | 0.136 (0.0487) |
| | | miR-383 | 0.156 (0.0487) |

## 14.4. MiRNAs Expression in Prognosis and Response Prediction

The clinical significance of miRNA expression profiles in malignant gliomas is not yet much explored. Nevertheless, a set of 16 candidate miRNAs associated with the malignant progression from anaplastic astrocytomas to glioblastomas was published (see Table 14.2). Among these miRNAs, the members of miR-196 family, indicated the highest level of significance. MiR-196 expression levels significantly correlated with poor survival by Kaplan-Meier method (p = 0.0073) and, moreover, multivariate analysis showed that its expression levels were an independent predictor of overall survival in glioblastoma patients (p = 0.021; HR 2.81) [12]. Another research group investigated miRNA expression profiles in patients who developed progression to secondary glioblastomas. They identified 12 miRNAs (miR-9, -15a, -16, -17, -19a, -20a, -21, -25, -28, -130b, -140, and -210) showing increased expression, and two miRNAs (miR-184 and miR-328) with reduced expression upon progression [13].

MiRNA expression could be potentially used also in therapy response prediction. Expression levels of miR-181b and miR-181c in glioblastoma tissued was successfully associated with response to concomitant chemoradiotherapy with temozolomide (RT/TMZ). MiR-181b and miR-181c were significantly down-regulated in patients who responded to RT/TMZ (p = 0.016; p = 0.047, respectively) in comparison to patients with progredient disease [11]. In other study, miR-195, miR-455-3p, and miR-10a* were the three most up-regulated miRNAs in the TMZ-resistant cell lines. Moreover, knockdown of miRNA-195 in the TMZ-resistant cell line led to overcome of TMZ resistance and increase the cell killing effect of TMZ [14].

## 14.5. MiRNAs as Potential Therapeutic Targets

The involvement of miRNAs in regulation of many important cell processes and dysregulation of miRNAs in glioblastoma, led to the suggestion that miRNAs could serve as a potential therapeutic targets.

The most frequently explored miRNA is the miR-21, which has been found to act as an oncogene. It is evident that miR-21 influences multiple important components of oncogenic signaling pathways including p53 and TGF-β. Direct targets of miR-21 are p63, p53 activators JMY, TOPORS, TP53BP2, TGFBR2/3, DAXX, and HNRNPK that can stabilize p53 protein levels by interfering with MDM2 and/or act as p53 transcriptional cofactors. Furthermore, an increase of endogenous levels of tumor suppressor PDCD4 in dependence on miR-21 inhibition was described [15]. The protein PDCD4 inhibits translation by its interaction with a factor that initiates translation of eIF4A and eIF4G. PDCD4 also inhibits proliferation via activation of p21 [4,16]. Corsten et al. (2007) show that the combined supression of miR-21 and neural precursor cells expressing S-TRAIL (a secretable variant of the cytotoxic agent tumor necrosis factor-related apoptosis inducing ligand) leads to synergistic increase in caspase activity and significantly decreased cell viability in human glioma cells *in vitro*. This phenomenon persists *in vivo*, as they observed complete eradication of LNA-antimiR-21 treated gliomas in the murine brain [17]. Thus, these findings suggest that the therapeutic influencing of miR-21 levels in the glioblastoma cells leads to decreasing of their tumorigenicity *in vitro* and could repress tumor growth *in vivo*.

MiR-21 also contributes to the drug resistance. Recently, Shi et al. (2010) observed that TMZ resistance in U87MG cells was associated with over-expression of miR-21, and as cosequence with decreased Bax/Bcl-2 ratio, caspase-3 activity, and reduction of TMZ-induced apoptosis [18]. Moreover, the miR-21 inhibitor enhanced the chemosensitivity of human glioblastoma cells to taxol by inhibiting STAT3 expression and phosphorylation [19]. In accordance these observations, the suppression of miR-21 by specific antisense oligonucleotides led to enhanced cytotoxicity of VM-26 (Teniposide) against U373MG glioblastoma cells [20].

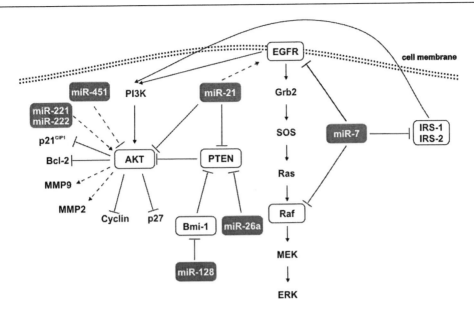

Figure 14.1. miRNAs involved in EGFR and PI3K/AKT signaling pathways.

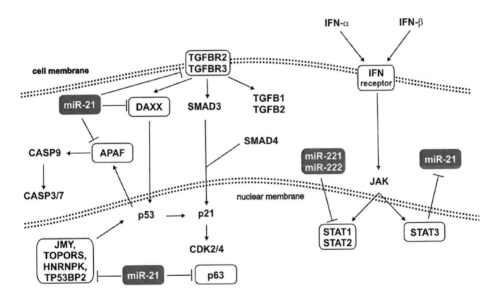

Figure 14.2. miRNAs involved in TGF-β and IFN-alfa/IFN-beta signaling pathways.

Furthermore, miR-21 contributes to invasiveness of glioma cells by regulating the activity of matrix metalloproteinases (MMPs) inhibitors RECK and TIMP3. The direct target of miR-21 seems to be only RECK, however, the expression level of TIMP3 also decreases as the level of miR-21 increases [4,21]. Therefore, miR-21 plays a key role in the glioblastoma pathology and its targeted down-regulation in tumor tissue could offer a new therapeutic approach.

Other two studies also documented a link between miR-328, and miR-451, respectively, and chemotherapeutic agents efficiency. ABCG2, the target gene for miR-328, is associated with multi-drug resistance and its high expression was previously confirmed in glioblastomas. Li et al. (2010) hypothesize that modulating ABCG2 expression by targeting miR-328, which is under-expressed in GBM, could contribute to increased sensitivity to the chemotherapeutic agents [22]. Another research group described enhancing effect of miR-451 transfection on treatment with Imatinib mesylate. Moreover, up-regulation of miR-451 led to GBM stem cells differentiation [23]. An important role of miR-451 in glioblastoma was confirmed by further studies. Akt1, CyclinD1, MMP-2, MMP-9, and Bcl-2 protein expression decreased, and p27 expression increased in a dose-dependent manner by use of miR-451 mimic oligonucleotides. Hence, the authors have proposed that this miRNA influences cell proliferation, invasion and apoptosis, perhaps via regulation of the PI3K/AKT pathway [24]. Additionally, miR-451 is also a regulator of the LKB1/AMPK signaling pathway, and may contribute to cellular adaptation in response to metabolic stress acting on glioma cells [25]. Involvement of particular miRNAs in core signaling pathways in GBM pathogenesis is illustrated in detail in Figures 14.1 and 14.2.

## Acknowledgment

This work was supported by grants NS 10361-3/2009, NR/9814-4/2008, NS 10352-3/2009, NT/11214-4/2010 of Czech Ministry of Health, Project No. MZ0MOU2005 of the Czech Ministry of Health and by the project "CEITEC – Central European Institute of Technology" (CZ.1.05/1.1.00/02.0068) and project "Institute of Molecular and Translational Medicine" was supported from the Operational Programme Research and Development for Innovations (project CZ.1.05/2.1.00/01.0030).

## References

[1] Ohgaki H, Dessen P, Jourde B, Horstmann S, Nishikawa T, Di Patre PL, Burkhard C, Schüler D, Probst-Hensch NM, Maiorka PC, Baeza N, Pisani P, Yonekawa Y, Yasargil MG, Lütolf UM, Kleihues P: Genetic pathways to glioblastoma: a population-based study. *Cancer Res.* 2004 64:6892-9.

[2] Ohgaki H: Genetic pathways to glioblastomas. *Neuropathology* 2005 25:1-7.

[3] Sana J, Hajduch M, Michalek J, Vyzula R, Slaby O. microRNAs and glioblastoma: roles in core signalling pathways and potential clinical implications. *J. Cell Mol. Med.* 2011, doi: 10.1111/j.1582-4934.2011.01317.x..

[4] Novakova J, Slaby O, Vyzula R, Michalek J: MicroRNA involvement in glioblastoma pathogenesis. *Biochem. Biophys. Res. Commun.* 2009 386:1-5.

[5] Schwartzbaum JA, Fisher JL, Aldape KD, Wrensch M: Epidemiology and molecular pathology of glioma. *Nat. Clin. Pract. Neurol.* 2006 2:494-503.

[6] Dou T, Wu Q, Chen X, Ribas J, Ni X, Tang C, Huang F, Zhou L, Lu D: A polymorphism of microRNA196a genome region was associated with decreased risk of glioma in Chinese population. *J. Cancer Res. Clin. Oncol.* 2010 136:1853-9.

[7] Zhang B, Farwell MA: microRNAs: a new emerging class of players for disease diagnostics and gene therapy. *J. Cell Mol. Med.* 2008 12:3-21.

[8]  Chan JA, Krichevsky AM, Kosik KS: MicroRNA-21 is an antiapoptotic factor in human glioblastoma cells. *Cancer Res.* 2005 65:6029-33.

[9]  Esquela-Kerscher A, Slack FJ: Oncomirs - microRNAs with a role in cancer. *Nat. Rev. Cancer* 2006 6:259-69.

[10] Ciafrè SA, Galardi S, Mangiola A, Ferracin M, Liu CG, Sabatino G, Negrini M, Maira G, Croce CM, Farace MG: Extensive modulation of a set of microRNAs in primary glioblastoma. *Biochem. Biophys. Res. Commun.* 2005 334:1351-8.

[11] Slaby O, Lakomy R, Fadrus P, Hrstka R, Kren L, Lzicarova E, Smrcka M, Svoboda M, Dolezalova H, Novakova J, Valik D, Vyzula R, Michalek J: MicroRNA-181 family predicts response to concomitant chemoradiotherapy with temozolomide in glioblastoma patients. *Neoplasma* 2010 57:264-9.

[12] Guan Y, Mizoguchi M, Yoshimoto K, Hata N, Shono T, Suzuki SO, Araki Y, Kuga D, Nakamizo A, Amano T, Ma X, Hayashi K, Sasaki T: MiRNA-196 is upregulated in glioblastoma but not in anaplastic astrocytoma and has prognostic significance. *Clin. Cancer Res.* 2010 16:4289-97.

[13] Malzkorn B, Wolter M, Liesenberg F, Grzendowski M, Stühler K, Meyer HE, Reifenberger G: Identification and functional characterization of microRNAs involved in the malignant progression of gliomas. *Brain Pathol.* 2010 20:539-50.

[14] Ujifuku K, Mitsutake N, Takakura S, Matsuse M, Saenko V, Suzuki K, Hayashi K, Matsuo T, Kamada K, Nagata I, Yamashita S: miR-195, miR-455-3p and miR-10a(*) are implicated in acquired temozolomide resistance in glioblastoma multiforme cells. *Cancer Lett.* 2010 296:241-8.

[15] Chen Y, Liu W, Chao T, Zhang Y, Yan X, Gong Y, Qiang B, Yuan J, Sun M, Peng X: MicroRNA-21 down-regulates the expression of tumor suppressor PDCD4 in human glioblastoma cell T98G. *Cancer Lett.* 2008 272:197-205.

[16] Papagiannakopoulos T, Shapiro A, Kosik KS: MicroRNA-21 targets a network of key tumor-suppressive pathways in glioblastoma cells. *Cancer Res.* 2008 68:8164-72.

[17] Corsten MF, Miranda R, Kasmieh R, Krichevsky AM, Weissleder R, Shah K: MicroRNA-21 knockdown disrupts glioma growth in vivo and displays synergistic cytotoxicity with neural precursor cell delivered S-TRAIL in human gliomas. *Cancer Res.* 2007 67:8994-9000.

[18] Shi L, Chen J, Yang J, Pan T, Zhang S, Wang Z: MiR-21 protected human glioblastoma U87MG cells from chemotherapeutic drug temozolomide induced apoptosis by decreasing Bax/Bcl-2 ratio and caspase-3 activity. *Brain Res.* 2010 1352:255-64.

[19] Ren Y, Zhou X, Mei M, Yuan XB, Han L, Wang GX, Jia ZF, Xu P, Pu PY, Kang CS: MicroRNA-21 inhibitor sensitizes human glioblastoma cells U251 (PTEN-mutant) and LN229 (PTEN-wild type) to taxol. *BMC Cancer* 2010 10:27.

[20] Li Y, Li W, Yang Y, Lu Y, He C, Hu G, Liu H, Chen J, He J, Yu H: MicroRNA-21 targets LRRFIP1 and contributes to VM-26 resistance in glioblastoma multiforme. *Brain Res.* 2009 1286:13-8.

[21] Gabriely G, Wurdinger T, Kesari S, Esau CC, Burchard J, Linsley PS, Krichevsky AM: MicroRNA 21 promotes glioma invasion by targeting matrix metalloproteinase regulators. *Mol. Cell Biol.* 2008 28:5369-80.

[22] Li WQ, Li YM, Tao BB, Lu YC, Hu GH, Liu HM, He J, Xu Y, Yu HY: Downregulation of ABCG2 expression in glioblastoma cancer stem cells with miRNA-328 may decrease their chemoresistance. *Med. Sci. Monit.* 2010 16:HY27-30.

[23] Gal H, Pandi G, Kanner AA, Ram Z, Lithwick-Yanai G, Amariglio N, Rechavi G, Givol D: MIR-451 and Imatinib mesylate inhibit tumor growth of Glioblastoma stem cells. *Biochem. Biophys. Res. Commun.* 2008 376:86-90.

[24] Nan Y, Han L, Zhang A, Wang G, Jia Z, Yang Y, Yue X, Pu P, Zhong Y, Kang C: MiRNA-451 plays a role as tumor suppressor in human glioma cells. *Brain Res.* 2010 1359:14-21.

[25] Godlewski J, Nowicki MO, Bronisz A, Williams S, Otsuki A, Nuovo G, Raychaudhury A, Newton HB, Chiocca EA, Lawler S: Targeting of the Bmi-1 oncogene/stem cell renewal factor by microRNA-128 inhibits glioma proliferation and self-renewal. *Cancer Res.* 2008 68:9125-30.

# Abbreviations

| | |
|---|---|
| 3-UTR | 3'untranslated region |
| 5-FU | 5-fluorouracil |
| ABCG2 | ATP-binding cassette, sub-family G, member 2 |
| AC | adenocarcinoma |
| ac-pre-miRNA | the Ago2-cleaved precursor miRNA |
| ADARs (1 and 2) | adenosine deaminases acting on RNA (1 and 2) |
| ADT | androgen-deprivation therapy |
| Ago | Argonaute |
| AIB1 | amplified in breast cancer 1 |
| AKT | serine/threonine protein kinase Akt |
| AMOs | anti-miRNA oligonucleotides |
| ANN | analysis artificial neural networks analysis |
| ATC | anaplastic carcinoma |
| ATM | Ataxia telangiectasia mutated |
| AUC | area under the ROC curve |
| Bak1 | BCL2-antagonist/killer 1 |
| BC | breast cancer |
| Bcl-2 | B-cell CLL/lymphoma 2 protein |
| BMP4 | bone morphogenetic protein 4 |
| BMPR1B | bone morphogenetic protein receptor, type IB |
| BPH | benign prostate hyperplasia |
| BRAF | v-raf murine sarcoma viral oncogene homologB1 |
| BRCA (1 and 2) | breast cancer type 1 and 2 susceptibility protein |
| CA19-9 | carbohydrate antigen 19-9 |
| CAIX | carbonic anhydrase IX |
| CAPZB | capping protein (actin filament) muscle Z-line, beta |
| CCND1 | cyclin D1 |
| CDK (4 and 6) | cyclin-dependent kinase (4 and 6) |
| CEA | carcinoembryonic antigen |
| CI | confidential interval |
| CKI | cyclin-dependent kinase inhibitor |
| c-Met | growth factor receptor c-met |

| | |
|---|---|
| c-myb | cellular v-myb myeloblastosis viral oncogene homolog |
| c-myc | cellular v-myc myelocytomatosis viral oncogene homolog |
| CNAs | circulating nucleic acids |
| CP | chronic pancreatitis |
| C-P4H(I) | type I collagen prolyl-4-hydroxylase |
| CPT-11 | irinotecan |
| CRC | colorectal carcinoma |
| CREB | cAMP response element-binding protein |
| CSC | cancer stem cell |
| CTNNB1 | catenin (cadherin-associated protein), beta 1 |
| CUP | cancer of unknown primary sites |
| DAXX | death-domain associated protein |
| dbSNP | SNP database |
| DFI | disease-free interval |
| DFS | disease-free survival |
| DGCR8 | DiGeorge critical region 8 |
| DN | dysplastic nodule |
| DNMT1 | DNA (cytosine-5-)-methyltransferase 1 |
| DNMT3b | DNA (cytosine-5-)-methyltransferase 3 beta |
| DOX | doxorubicin |
| dsRNA | double stranded RNA |
| DTL | denticleless protein homolog |
| E2F | E2F transcription factor |
| E2F1 | E2F transcription factor 1 |
| ECM | extracellular matrix |
| EGF | epidermal growth factor |
| eIF4 | eukaryotic translation initiation factor 4 |
| ELK1 | ELK1, member of ETS oncogene family |
| EMT | epithelial-mesenchymal transition |
| EPO | erythropoietin |
| ErbB | v-erb-b2 erythroblastic leukemia viral oncogene homolog |
| ERK1/2 | extracellular signal-regulated kinase 1/2 |
| ERK5 | mitogen-activated protein kinase |
| ERs (α and β) | estrogen receptors (α and β) |
| ES cells, eSCs | embryonic stem cells |
| ESR1 | estrogen receptor 1 |
| EZH2 | enhancer of zeste homolog 2 |
| Fas | Fas - TNF receptor superfamily, member 6 |
| FFPE | formalin-fixed and paraffin-embedded |
| FNA | fine-needle aspiration |
| FNDC3B | fibronectin type III domain containing 3B |
| Foxp3 | forkhead box P3 |
| FTA | follicular thyroid adenoma |
| FTC | follicular thyroid carcinoma |
| FXR1 | fragile X-related protein 1 |

# Abbreviations

| | |
|---|---|
| GBM | glioblastoma |
| GC | gastric cancer |
| GEMIN3 | gem (nuclear organelle) associated protein 3 |
| GEMIN4 | gem (nuclear organelle) associated protein 4 |
| Gfi1 | growth factor independent 1 |
| GSP | gene-specific primer |
| GWAS | genome-wide association study |
| HBV | hepatitis B virus |
| HCC | hepatocellular carcinoma/cancer |
| HCV | hepatitis C virus |
| HER2 | human epidermal growth factor receptor 2 |
| HGFR | hepatocyte growth factor receptor |
| HGS | hepatocyte growth factor-regulated tyrosine kinase substrate |
| HIF | hypoxia-induced factor |
| HIV | Human Immunodeficiency Virus |
| HMGA2 | high mobility group AT-hook 2 |
| HNF-1alfa | HNF1 homeobox A |
| HNPCC | non-polyposis colorectal cancer |
| hnRNP A1 | heterogeneous nuclear ribonucleoprotein A1 |
| HNRNPK | heterogeneous nuclear ribonucleoprotein K |
| HoxD10 | homeobox D10 |
| HPC1 | hereditary prostate cancer locus-1 |
| HRPC | hormone-refractory prostate cancer |
| HS | healthy subjects |
| HSP90 | chaperone heat shock protein 90 |
| hTERT | human telomere reverse transcriptase |
| CHB | chronic hepatitis B |
| CHEK2 | CHK2 checkpoint homolog |
| IDC-NOS | invasive ductal carcinomas not otherwise specified |
| IDC-NST | invasive ductal carcinomas no special type |
| IGF2R | insulin-like growth factor 2 receptor |
| IGF-IR | type 1 insulin-like growth factor receptor |
| ISH | in situ hybridization |
| IL1A | interleukin 1, alpha |
| INSR | insulin receptor |
| IRFs | interferon regulatory factors |
| IRS-1 | insulin receptor substrate-1 |
| ITGB4 | integrin, beta 4 |
| JMY | junction mediating and regulatory protein, p53 cofactor |
| KCNJ16 | potassium inwardly-rectifying channel, subfamily J, member 16 |
| KRAS | v-Ki-ras2 Kirsten rat sarcoma viral oncogene homolog |
| KRASwt | KRAS wild-type |
| LATS2 | large tumor suppressor 2 |
| LC | liver cirrhosis |
| LCC | large cell carcinoma |

| | |
|---|---|
| LCS | Let-7 complementary sites |
| LIN-28 | lin-28 homolog |
| LNA | locked nucleic acid |
| LNN | lymph node negative |
| LOH | loss of heterozygosity |
| L-OHP | oxaliplatin |
| MAPK | mitogen activated protein kinase |
| MARCKS | myristoylated alanine-rich protein kinase C substrate |
| mat-miRNA | mature miRNA |
| MC | medullary carcinoma |
| mCRC | metastatic colorectal cancer |
| MDM2 | Mdm2 p53 binding protein homolog |
| MDR | multidrug resistance |
| MDR1 | mulridrug resistance 1 gene |
| Mef2 | myocyte enhancer factor 2 |
| miRAGE | miRNA serial analysis of gene expression |
| miRBase | microRNA database |
| miRISC | miRNA-induced silencing complex |
| miRNA | microRNA |
| MRI | magnetic resonance imaging |
| mRLC | miRISC loading complex |
| mRNA | messenger RNA |
| MSI | microsatellite instability |
| MSI-H | high levels of microsatellite instability |
| MSR1 | macrophage scavenger receptor 1 |
| MSS | microsatellite stability |
| mTOR | mammalian target of rapamycin |
| MYC | v-myc myelocytomatosis viral oncogene homolog (avian) |
| MYCN | v-myc myelocytomatosis viral related oncogene, neuroblastoma derived (avian) |
| MyoD | myogenic differentiation 1 |
| NFATc3 | nuclear factor of activated T-cells, cytoplasmic, calcineurin dependent 3 |
| NFI-A | nuclear factor I/A |
| NF-kappaB | nuclear factor of kappa light polypeptide gene enhancer in B-cells |
| NGS | next generation sequencing, also called deep sequencing |
| Nkx2-5 | NK2 transcription factor related, locus 5 |
| NSCLC | non-small cell lung cancer |
| OR | odds ratio |
| ORR | objective response rate |
| OS | overall survival |
| PACT | protein activator of PKR |
| PC | prostate cancer |
| PDAC | pancreatic cancer, pancreatic adenocarcinoma |
| PDCD4 | programmed cell death-4 |

# Abbreviations

| | |
|---|---|
| PDGFR | platelet derived growth factor receptor |
| PDTC | poorly differentiated thyroid carcinoma |
| PE | primer-extension |
| PI-3-K | phosphatidylinositol-3-kinase |
| Pitx3 | paired-like homeodomain 3 |
| PON1 | paraoxonase 1 |
| PPP2R2A | protein phosphatase 2, regulatory subunit B, alpha |
| PR | progesterone |
| pre-miRNA | precursor-miRNA |
| PRIMA1 | prolin rich membrane anchor 1 |
| pri-miRNA | miRNA primary transcript |
| PSA | Prostate-specific antigen |
| PTC | comprehensive of papillary thyroid carcinoma |
| PTCs | papillary thyroid carcinomas |
| PTEN | phosphatase and tensin homolog |
| PTPN12 | protein tyrosine phosphatase |
| PU.1 | transcription factor protein |
| qRT-PCR | quantitative reverse transcriptase-polymerase chain reaction |
| RAN | GTP-binding nuclear protein Ran, member RAS oncogene family |
| Rb | retinoblastoma protein |
| RbL2 | retinoblastoma-like protein 2 |
| RCC | renal cell carcinoma |
| RCCC, ccRCC | clear cell renal cell carcinoma |
| RECK | reversion-inducing-cysteine-rich protein with kazal motifs |
| REST | RE1-silencing transcription factor |
| RET | ret proto-oncogene |
| RFS | relapse-free survival |
| RhoA | ras homolog gene family, member A |
| RhoC | ras homolog gene family, member C |
| RNA | ribo-nucleic acid |
| RNAi | RNA interference |
| RNASEL | ribonuclease L (2',5'-oligoisoadenylate synthetase-dependent) |
| ROC | receiver operating characteristic |
| ROCK1 | Rho-associated, coiled-coil containing protein kinase 1 |
| ROS | reactive oxygen species |
| RP | reverse primer |
| RT | reverse transcription |
| RT/TMZ | concomitant chemoradiotherapy with temozolomide |
| RTKs | receptor tyrosin-kinases |
| RUNX3 | runt-related transcription factor 3 |
| SAM | self-assembling monolayer |
| SCC | small cell carcinoma |
| SCLC | small cell lung cancer |
| SET8 | also known as PR-SET7 encodes a histone H4–Lys-20–specific methyltransferase |

| | |
|---|---|
| siRNA | small interfering RNA |
| SLITRK1 | SLIT and NTRK-like family, member 1 |
| SMAD | mothers against decapentaplegic homolog |
| SNIP1 | SMAD nuclear interacting protein 1 |
| SNPs | single nucleotide polymorphisms |
| SPRY2 | sprouty homolog 2 |
| SqCC | squamous cell carcinoma |
| SRF | serum response factor |
| STAT3 | signal transducer and activator of transcription 3 (acute-phase response factor) |
| S-TRAIL | secretable variant of the cytotoxic agent tumor necrosis factor-related apoptosis inducing ligand |
| TFs | transcription factors |
| TGFα | transforming growth factor alpha |
| TGFβ | transforming growth factor beta |
| TGIFB | TGFB-induced factor homeobox 2 |
| TIMP3 | tissue inhibitor of metalloproteinase 3 |
| TLDA | TaqMan low density arrays |
| TMAC | tetra-methyl ammonium chloride |
| TNFSF10 | tumor necrosis factor (ligand) superfamily, member 10 |
| TNFα | tumor necrosis factor |
| TNRC6A | trinucleotide repeat-containing gene 6A protein |
| TNRC6C | trinucleotide repeat-containing gene 6C protein |
| TOPORS | topoisomerase I binding, arginine/serine-rich, E3 ubiquitin protein ligase |
| TP53BP2 | tumor protein p53 binding protein, 2 |
| TP53INP1 | tumor protein p53 inducible nuclear protein 1 |
| TPM1 | tropomyosin 1 |
| TRAIL | tumor necrosis factor-related apoptosis inducing ligand |
| TRBP | the Tar RNA-binding protein |
| TRIM71 | tripartite motif containing 71 |
| TRK | tyrosin kinase |
| TSP1 | thrombospondin 1 |
| TTP | time to progression |
| TUT4 | terminal (U) transferase 4 |
| Twist-1 | twist homolog 1 |
| UICC | International Union Against Cancer |
| UP | universal primer |
| uPAR | Urokinase-Type Plasminogen Activator Receptor |
| VCR | vincristine |
| VEGF | vascular endothelial growth factor |
| VEGFR | vascular endothelial growth factor receptor |
| VHL | von Hippel-Lindau gene |
| VM-26 | Teniposide |
| WDTC | well-differentiated thyroid carcinoma |

| | |
|---|---|
| WHO | World Health Organization |
| XPO5 | exportin 5 |
| ZBTB1 | zinc finger and BTB domain containing 10 |
| ZEB1 | zinc finger E-box binding homeobox 1 |
| ZEB2 | zinc finger E-box binding homeobox 2 |

# Index

## #

5-fluorouracil, 83, 89, 197

## A

adaptor sequences, 34
adenocarcinoma, 81, 88, 89, 92, 108, 109, 111, 112, 113, 118, 120, 122, 128, 147, 164, 175, 178, 197
adenoma, 198
adhesion, 62, 64, 72, 96, 118, 186
adhesion molecule, 64, 72
age-matched control, 158
Agendia MammaPrint, 98
aggressiveness, 72, 83, 99, 104, 124, 128, 149
Ago2-cleaved precursor miRNA, 13, 197
Ago-catalyzed cleavage, 5, 14
amplification, 34, 36, 43, 47, 59, 74, 189
anaplastic carcinoma, 182, 186, 188, 197
anchorage-independent growth, 57, 101
androgen-deprivation therapy, 125, 197
angiogenesis, 53, 54, 61, 62, 64, 70, 85, 90, 134, 175
angiogenic switch, 61
angiopoietin, 144
animal model, 85, 168
anoikis, 57, 101
antagomirs, 85, 89, 101, 117, 162, 165, 186
anti-angiogenic factors, 61
antigrowth signals, 53
antisense, 2, 47, 48, 85, 99, 111, 162, 173, 174, 192
apoptosis, 2, 5, 19, 53, 57, 58, 59, 67, 68, 69, 92, 96, 100, 117, 118, 122, 128, 129, 131, 141, 149, 150, 152, 154, 159, 162, 165, 171, 173, 175, 178, 186, 192, 194, 195
apoptosis sensitizing strategy, 150
apoptosis-sensitizing strategy, 150
Argonaute family, 2
arteriovenous malformation, 190
astrocytoma, 191, 195
atrophic gastritis, 167
autocrine regulation, 55

## B

basal-like, 92, 95
Bcl2, 59, 69, 175
Bcl-2, 58
Bcl-2, 59
Bcl-2, 59
Bcl-2, 84
Bcl-2, 174
Bcl-2, 192
Bcl-2, 194
Bcl-2, 195
Bcl-2, 197
Bead Based Arrays, 47
benign stroma, 128
binding domain, 12, 183
biopsy, 94
blood vessels, 61, 62
blood-based biomarker, 158
bone morphogenetic protein, 9, 197
breast cancer, 6, 10, 18, 29, 30, 31, 32, 56, 59, 61, 64, 65, 66, 68, 70, 72, 91, 92, 93, 94, 95, 96, 97, 98, 99, 100, 101, 102, 103, 104, 105, 106, 137, 141, 190, 197
breast cancer subtype, 95

## C

calcitonin, 181
cancer risk, 26, 27, 29, 31, 76, 93, 108, 190
cancer stem cell, 146, 147, 154, 174, 195, 198
capecitabine, 83, 89
carbohydrate antigen 19-9, 168, 170, 197

carcinoembryonic antigen, 168, 170, 197
carcinoma in situ, 91
case-control association study, 29, 76
caspase, 59, 60, 69, 75, 84, 150, 171, 192, 195
castration-mediated growth arrest, 128
cDNA library, 34
cDNA-GSP chimera, 40
cell cycle, 5, 19, 57, 58, 60, 62, 67, 84, 95, 96, 99, 117, 118, 129, 135, 146, 149, 150, 158, 159, 162, 165, 174, 178, 186
cell cycle arrest, 5, 58, 62, 67, 95, 117, 149, 150, 162, 174
cell-cell interaction, 55
cell-matrix interaction, 58, 62
cetuximab, 32, 77, 87
chaperone heat shock protein 90, 14, 199
chemically modified, 85, 101, 162
chemosensitizing, 84
chemotaxis, 62
chemotherapeutic agent, 84, 100, 138, 139, 159, 193
chemotherapy, 73, 83, 85, 100, 107, 108, 116, 117, 121, 125, 130, 134, 137, 147, 150, 157, 158, 165, 175, 182, 186
chromosomal region, 74
chronic inflammation, 143, 171
chronic pancreatitis, 159, 164, 198
circulating nucleic acid, 198
classical forward genetics, 33
cleavage site, 2, 11
clinical outcome, 77, 84, 121, 134, 161, 164
cluster analysis, 81
c-Met, 55, 56, 144, 155, 162, 197
cohort, 83, 93, 94, 110, 112, 116, 128, 148
colony formation, 118, 139, 163
colorectal cancer, 18, 32, 66, 68, 75, 76, 81, 84, 86, 87, 88, 89, 199, 200
computational prediction, 33, 38
concomitant chemoradiotherapy, 192, 195, 201
covalent crosslinking, 46
Cox regression analysis, 82
CpG island, 5, 82, 145
cross-species conservation, 37
curative approach, 73
curcumin, 117
cyclin-dependent kinase inhibitor, 58, 197
cytokines, 55, 143
cytoskeleton, 64

## D

decay pathway, 134
desmoplasia, 160
detachment, 57, 62

DIANA-microT, 37, 50
differentiation, vii, 2, 6, 7, 9, 12, 20, 36, 51, 57, 59, 64, 92, 95, 108, 159, 172, 174, 182, 183, 194, 200
diffuse, 59, 163, 168, 170, 176
diffusely infiltrative growth, 189
dihydrotestosterone, 129
directional cloning, 34
disease-free survival, 198
DNA damage, 9, 58, 104, 117
DNA methyltransferase 1, 63, 149, 154
docetaxel, 117, 121, 125, 130
doubling time, 108
down-regulation, 59, 63, 84, 99, 100, 110, 111, 117, 126, 128, 138, 140, 148, 155, 163, 174, 175, 184, 193
doxorubicin, 100, 105, 117, 150, 151, 155, 198
Drosha, 2, 5, 7, 9, 10, 11, 20, 21, 26, 61, 70, 173
dysplastic nodule, 144, 148, 198
dysregulated miRNAs, 135, 159, 185

## E

E-cadherin, 64, 71, 138, 141, 144, 176
ectopic expression, 59, 100, 101, 171, 174
embryonic bodies, 36
endothelial cells, 61, 62, 70, 190
epigenetic mechanisms, 78, 145
epigenetic silencing, 74
epithelial cells, 10, 64
epithelial-mesenchymal transition, 20, 63, 64, 71, 74, 75, 96, 138, 198
ErbB2 receptor, 56
etiology, 123, 137, 149
etoposide, 117
exosomes-derived miRNAs, 111
exportin 5, 2, 203
expression profile, 52, 64, 73, 74, 78, 79, 80, 81, 82, 83, 84, 87, 88, 89, 95, 98, 109, 110, 111, 113, 116, 117, 121, 123, 126, 143, 167, 168, 169, 170, 171, 172, 177, 187, 188, 190, 191
expression vector, 163
extracellular matrix, 55, 74, 75, 198
extracellular signal-regulated kinase 1/2, 56, 198
extravasation, 62
extrinsic apoptotic pathway, 58

## F

fecal occult blood test, 77
FFPE, 116, 198
fibrosis, 143
fine-needle aspiration, 182, 184, 198
fingerprint, 81, 177

flow cytometry, 47
fluorescence, 41, 46
follicular cells, 181
follicular thyroid carcinoma, 181, 188, 198
frameshift mutation, 76

## G

G1 phase, 57, 58, 59, 174
gastric cancer, 19, 28, 31, 32, 67, 77, 146, 167, 168, 169, 170, 172, 173, 174, 175, 176, 177, 178, 199
GATA-binding site, 145
gemcitabine, 161, 162, 165
GEMIN3, 26, 27, 199
GEMIN4, 26, 27, 134, 135, 199
gene silencing, 12, 21, 22
gene-specific primer, 40, 199
genetic markers, 26
genitourinary malignancies, 133
genome-wide association study, 28, 199
genome-wide profiling, 73, 76
genomic cluster, 11, 57
genotype, 27, 76, 77, 84, 102, 109, 124, 145, 168, 169, 183, 190
germline mutation, 26, 124
Gibbs free energy, 29, 76
glandular epithelium, 128
Gleason score, 124, 125, 127
glioblastoma, 56, 68, 189, 190, 191, 192, 193, 194, 195, 199
glioma, 28, 31, 72, 189, 190, 192, 193, 194, 195, 196
growth factors, 11, 55, 65, 144
guide strand, 2, 22, 26

## H

hairpin, 4, 11, 13, 33, 36, 38, 44, 183
healthy subjects, 77, 103, 110, 199
hematuria, 134
hepatitis B, 31, 144, 146, 147, 154, 199
hepatitis C, 146, 151, 155, 199
hepatocarcinogenesis, 144, 145, 148, 150, 151, 152, 153, 154
hepatocellular carcinoma, 31, 56, 58, 67, 71, 144, 147, 151, 152, 153, 154, 155, 186, 199
hepatocyte growth factor receptor, 56, 199
HER2+, 95
hereditary prostate cancer locus-1, 123, 199
heterogeneous nuclear ribonucleoprotein A1, 11, 199
hierarchical clustering, 160
high-throughput profiling, 40, 171
high-troughput multiplexed detection, 33, 43
homeobox, 63, 64, 199, 202, 203

homeostasis, 57, 58, 61
homologous recombination, 60, 61
hormone-refractory prostate cancer, 125, 130, 199
hormone-related effect, 93
human embryonic stem cells, 20, 36, 49, 153
hyperplasia, 125, 126, 197
hyperplastic nodules, 182, 184
hypoxia, 19, 61, 62, 63, 64, 70, 98, 133, 135, 137, 141, 150, 160, 199
hypoxia inducible factor, 133
hypoxia-induced factor, 61, 199
hypoxic conditions, 133
hypoxic environment, 61, 158
hypoxic signature, 158

## I

illegitimate miRNA target sites, 28
Imatinib mesylate, 194, 196
immortalization, 148, 168
immune response, 19, 171, 172, 177
immunoblotting, 60
immunodeficient mice, 117
immunohistochemistry, 173
imperfect base-pairing, 37
*in silico* analysis, 93
*in situ* hybridization, 39, 51, 199
incidence, 29, 76, 91, 107, 108, 123, 143, 176, 181, 182, 187, 189
individualized therapy, 162
inflammatory bowel disease, 77
INSR genes, 29, 76
insulin receptor, 67, 134, 199
insulin receptor substrate-1, 67, 199
intergenic regions, 2, 27
interleukin 1 beta, 168
intestinal, 19, 168, 170
intrahepatic metastases, 148
intravasation, 56, 62
intrinsic apoptotic pathway, 58
invasion, 18, 53, 54, 62, 63, 64, 65, 66, 68, 69, 71, 72, 79, 85, 92, 95, 96, 99, 101, 104, 118, 122, 128, 131, 135, 139, 144, 150, 155, 157, 159, 160, 170, 172, 174, 178, 194, 195
invasive ductal carcinomas, 92, 199
invasiveness, 56, 65, 96, 117, 161, 193
iodine deficiency, 182
iodine uptake, 181

## K

Kaplan-Meier analysis, 82, 128

KRAS, 12, 29, 32, 56, 66, 74, 76, 83, 86, 109, 111, 116, 119, 162, 164, 199

## L

laparotomy, 159
large-cell carcinoma, 108
late diagnosis, 138, 144, 148, 150
lentiviral vector, 117
let-7, 5, 11, 14, 21, 22, 23, 32, 34, 44, 45, 48, 56, 57, 61, 66, 67, 76, 80, 83, 86, 89, 94, 95, 97, 98, 110, 111, 113, 114, 115, 116, 119, 121, 126, 127, 128, 145, 149, 154, 169, 172
let-7a, 56, 94, 97, 113, 114, 115, 116, 117, 121, 128, 145, 169, 172
let-7f, 97, 126, 145
let-7g, 80, 83, 89, 111, 116, 149, 154, 172
LIN-28, 11, 13, 200
LIN-28–let-7 regulatory system, 11, 13
linker, 46
liver cirrhosis, 143, 146, 199
lobules, 91
loss of heterozygosity, 95, 190, 200
luciferase, 138
luminal A, 95
luminal B, 95
lung cancer, 29, 31, 56, 62, 63, 65, 70, 77, 91, 107, 108, 109, 110, 111, 112, 113, 114, 115, 116, 118, 119, 120, 121, 122
lymph node, 63, 72, 82, 88, 96, 98, 99, 103, 104, 115, 168, 169, 173, 182, 200
lymph node metastasis, 82, 88, 98, 105, 115, 169, 173

## M

malignant potential, 53, 149, 154
matrix degradation, 64
matrix metalloproteinases, 64, 193
mature miRNA, 2, 8, 10, 13, 14, 25, 26, 27, 37, 38, 40, 41, 44, 74, 78, 80, 81, 83, 85, 99, 112, 144, 183, 190, 200
MDM2, 192, 200
medullary carcinoma, 181, 200
melting temperature, 40, 44, 46
metaplasia, 168
metastasis, 18, 19, 53, 54, 62, 63, 64, 65, 69, 71, 72, 82, 85, 88, 94, 96, 99, 101, 104, 105, 106, 115, 125, 127, 128, 131, 135, 138, 140, 141, 144, 145, 149, 150, 152, 153, 154, 155, 157, 158, 160, 162, 170, 172, 174, 175, 178
metastatic behaviour, 53
methotrexate, 84

methylation, 5, 6, 18, 63, 64, 70, 71, 82, 88, 105, 154, 172, 177
microarray, 35, 44, 46, 47, 49, 80, 97, 103, 110, 113, 137, 161, 170, 171
microfluidic card, 47
microprocessor, 2, 9, 10, 12, 26
microRNA (miRNA), 107
microsatellite instability, 76, 81, 88, 200
microvessel density, 162
miR-100, 84, 95, 125, 126, 127, 131, 160
miR-101, 146, 147, 149, 151, 174
miR-105, 191
miR-106a, 78, 79, 80, 82, 94, 110, 111, 113, 116, 125, 136, 138, 169, 172, 184
miR-106b, 6, 58, 67, 136, 138, 153, 169, 172, 173, 184
miR-107, 5, 62, 95, 160, 174
miR-122a, 98, 136
miR-125b, 32, 56, 66, 84, 96, 103, 125, 126, 127, 149, 151, 184, 190, 191
miR-125b-1, 191
miR-125b-2, 191
miR-128a, 99, 190, 191
miR-128b, 191
miR-135b, 77, 78, 79, 81, 97, 191
miR-141, 63, 116, 125, 135, 136, 138, 140, 147
miR-145, 5, 6, 9, 10, 19, 57, 68, 78, 79, 84, 85, 88, 98, 99, 100, 112, 113, 118, 126, 127, 129, 148, 173
miR-146, 6, 19, 28, 31, 77, 93, 95, 102, 108, 110, 111, 114, 125, 130, 144, 146, 151, 173, 182, 183, 184, 185, 186, 187
miR-146a, 6, 28, 31, 77, 93, 102, 108, 125, 130, 144, 146, 151, 173, 183, 187
miR-148a, 5, 63, 64, 82, 171, 173
miR-148b, 63, 64
miR-155, 6, 19, 65, 80, 81, 94, 95, 96, 97, 100, 110, 111, 112, 113, 114, 115, 116, 135, 136, 137, 138, 158, 160, 162, 164, 171, 184, 185
miR-15b, 80, 95, 116, 149, 150, 159, 161, 175, 191
miR-16, 9, 10, 26, 59, 69, 116, 127, 128, 175
miR-17-5p, 57, 80, 95, 126, 151, 155, 169, 171, 184, 186
miR-181a, 158, 160, 184, 185, 186, 191
miR-181b, 79, 82, 83, 89, 150, 154, 158, 184, 185, 191, 192
miR-181c, 81, 97, 160, 185, 191, 192
miR-182, 81, 84, 110, 112, 115, 127, 136
miR-183, 78, 80, 81, 184
miR-184, 126, 191, 192
miR-185, 136, 139, 149
miR-18a, 11, 21, 57, 80, 95, 146, 147, 148, 171, 184
miR-191, 79, 84, 110, 111, 115, 150, 155

# Index

miR-196a, 81, 93, 102, 108, 158, 159, 160, 161, 164, 169, 190, 191
miR-196-a2, 28, 108
miR-196b, 6, 20, 191
miR-199a, 6, 10, 20, 57, 94, 136, 147, 150
miR-19a, 57, 125, 171, 184
miR-200 family, 63, 64, 71, 96, 141
miR-200b, 63, 83, 112, 116, 117, 136, 159
miR-200c, 63, 79, 82, 135, 136, 138, 140, 147
miR-203, 80, 82, 110, 111, 113, 147, 162, 184
miR-205, 71, 98, 100, 101, 106, 110, 111, 112, 115, 120, 125, 127, 138, 184
miR-20a, 57, 67, 79, 80, 82, 111, 113, 128, 131, 170, 171, 184
miR-20b, 125, 170, 171
miR-21, 5, 6, 9, 19, 20, 56, 59, 62, 63, 64, 66, 68, 69, 78, 79, 80, 82, 83, 84, 85, 88, 89, 94, 96, 97, 98, 99, 100, 104, 105, 110, 111, 112, 113, 115, 116, 117, 118, 122, 125, 127, 128, 131, 135, 136, 137, 141, 146, 147, 149, 151, 152, 153, 158, 159, 160, 161, 162, 163, 164, 171, 172, 173, 174, 178, 184, 185, 186, 190, 191, 192, 193
miR-210, 62, 63, 64, 97, 99, 110, 111, 112, 113, 115, 135, 136, 137, 141, 147, 158, 159, 160, 162, 163, 184
miR-213, 62, 185
miR-220, 185
miR-221, 60, 62, 77, 80, 98, 115, 117, 126, 127, 128, 129, 131, 132, 135, 146, 148, 158, 159, 160, 174, 183, 184, 185, 186, 190
miR-222, 58, 60, 62, 67, 77, 84, 117, 127, 129, 131, 132, 135, 147, 158, 159, 160, 161, 162, 174, 183, 184, 185, 186
miR-223, 7, 71, 80, 81, 146, 152, 172
miR-224, 110, 136, 146, 148, 184, 185
miR-25, 58, 111, 115, 147, 171
miR-26a-1, 28
miR-27a, 5, 28, 31, 32, 62, 93, 102, 162, 163, 168, 169, 170, 174, 177
miR-29c, 147, 171
miR-302b, 191
miR-302d, 191
miR-31, 68, 78, 79, 81, 88, 96, 100, 101, 103, 118, 170, 184, 185
miR-320, 83, 97, 172
miR-345, 126, 185
miR-34a, 58, 59, 61, 67, 68, 94, 96, 100, 115, 116, 135, 151, 155, 162, 185
miR-363, 191
miR-367, 191
miR-370, 127
miR-375, 112, 127, 151, 171
miR-383, 191
miR-411, 136
miR-423, 28, 125, 170
miR-424, 7, 20, 117, 147
miR-425-5p, 172
miR-492, 28, 76
miR-504, 191
miR-514, 136
miR-517c, 191
miR-601, 191
miR-9 family, 63, 64
miR-92, 58, 77, 79, 80, 81, 84, 116, 171, 184
miR-93, 58, 84, 110, 113, 125, 147
miR-99a, 95, 126, 127
miRanda, 28, 37, 38, 76
miRank, 36
miRBase, 1, 17, 28, 38, 51, 76, 200
miRISC, 2, 12, 13, 14, 15, 16, 26, 135, 200
miRISC loading complex, 12, 200
miRNA biogenesis, 1, 2, 8, 9, 10, 14, 25, 26, 27, 84, 134
miRNA deregulation, 56, 123, 173
miRNA editing, 7
miRNA expression patterns, 82
miRNA function, 1, 27, 135
miRNA library, 47
miRNA metabolism, 1
miRNA mimics, 85
miRNA processing, 4, 7, 8, 9, 10, 12, 13, 14, 16, 22, 26, 27, 39, 61, 78, 135
miRNA profiling pattern, 159
miRNA quantification, 33
miRNA signature, 62, 63, 80, 95, 111, 115, 126, 148, 158, 170, 171, 172
miRNA turnover, 17
miRNA*, 2, 4
miRnalyzer, 36
miRNA-mRNA complementarity, 14
MiRscan, 36
miRseeker, 36
mirtrons, 2
mitochondria permeability, 58
mitogen-activated protein kinase, 56, 155, 182, 198
mitogenic signals, 55
monitoring response, 158, 159
monoclonal antibodies, 76
monolayer epithelium, 181
motility, 62, 64, 96, 101, 128
mRNA targets, 3, 12, 27, 74, 76, 140
mTOR pathway, 144
multidrug resistance, 100, 175, 178, 200
multifocal atrophic gastritis, 168
mutation, 25, 76, 82, 176
MYC-mediated tumorigenesis, 5

## N

negative feedback loop, 9, 14, 20, 71
neovascularization, 61
nephrectomy, 134, 138, 140
next generation sequencing, 33, 34, 49, 200
non-overlapping mutations, 182
non-small cell lung cancer, 32, 60, 69, 107, 115, 119, 120, 121, 122, 200
non-squamous carcinoma, 107
non-synonymous SNP, 27, 135
normal-like, 95
Northern blotting, 39
nuclear transport, 135
nucleosomal fragmentation, 59
nutrition, 149

## O

objective response rate, 200
oligonucleotide, 39, 40, 46, 51, 52, 101, 174
oncocytoma, 135
oncogene, 12, 18, 31, 54, 55, 56, 58, 60, 61, 67, 68, 95, 102, 149, 153, 154, 155, 174, 178, 182, 192, 196, 197, 198, 199, 200, 201
oncogenic polycistron miR-17-92, 11
OncoTypeDX, 98
organogenesis, 56
ovarian cancer, 31, 56, 66, 71, 93, 102
overall survival, 76, 107, 115, 148, 161, 172, 173, 174, 191, 200
overdominance, 183
over-expression, 59, 60, 82, 84, 96, 98, 109, 112, 115, 117, 118, 129, 139, 149, 158, 160, 163, 175, 192
oxaliplatin, 84, 89, 200
oxidative stress, 135

## P

p27 (Kip1), 129, 135
pancreatic adenocarcinoma, 157, 159, 161, 162, 163, 164, 165, 200
pancreatic cancer, 51, 63, 157, 158, 159, 160, 162, 163, 164, 165, 200
pancreatic endocrine tumors, 162
papillary renal cell carcinoma, 135
papillary thyroid carcinoma, 31, 58, 181, 182, 187, 188, 201
parafollicular C-cells, 181
parenchyma, 159
Pasha, 2, 26
passenger strand, 13, 183, 187
pathological conditions, 125, 145
paxillin, 118
P-bodies, 14, 22
PCR primers, 34
percutaneous ablation, 144
peripheral blood, 94, 169, 177
peripheral zone tissue, 126
phenotype, 25, 34, 53, 60, 63, 64, 65, 71, 72, 76, 99, 105, 108, 109, 118, 141, 145, 150, 152, 153
physiological conditions, 58
PI-3-K pathway, 56
PicTar, 28, 37, 38, 76
plasma, 77, 87, 94, 125, 158, 161, 169, 177
polyacrylamide gel electrophoresis, 34, 39
polyadenylation, 41
poly-ubiquitinylation, 133
polyuridylation, 11
poorly differentiated thyroid carcinoma, 181, 201
poorly differentiated tumors, 78, 81, 184
postmitotic state, 57
potassium channel membrane proteins, 139
preclinical studies, 186
predictive biomarkers, 98
pre-miRNAs, 2, 7, 9, 13, 26, 27, 125, 135
preoperative diagnosis, 182
primary tumor, 62, 63, 64, 81, 113, 124
primer-extension, 40, 42, 51, 201
pri-miRNAs, 2, 5, 9, 10, 26, 27
pro-angiogenic factors, 61
pro-apoptotic p53-induced nuclear protein 1, 160
probe, 35, 44, 47
prognosis, 25, 31, 64, 73, 74, 81, 82, 83, 86, 89, 92, 98, 99, 104, 105, 108, 113, 115, 120, 123, 127, 134, 137, 138, 143, 144, 148, 149, 151, 154, 155, 157, 158, 161, 164, 167, 168, 172, 173, 177, 181, 186, 189
programmed cell death-4, 56, 96, 200
progression, 55, 56, 57, 62, 64, 72, 76, 77, 83, 84, 85, 86, 92, 94, 96, 98, 99, 108, 116, 118, 123, 124, 125, 127, 132, 135, 144, 145, 150, 158, 162, 163, 165, 168, 169, 170, 172, 173, 174, 177, 178, 186, 191, 195, 202
progression-free survival, 76, 77, 83
prohibitin, 174, 178
proliferation, vii, 2, 55, 56, 57, 58, 64, 68, 81, 84, 85, 91, 92, 95, 98, 101, 103, 117, 118, 122, 128, 129, 131, 134, 135, 138, 143, 148, 149, 150, 153, 154, 155, 159, 161, 162, 163, 174, 178, 186, 192, 194, 196
promoters, 2, 5, 18, 145
prostate cancer, 19, 56, 60, 64, 66, 69, 123, 124, 125, 126, 127, 128, 129, 130, 131, 132, 200

prostate-specific antigen, 124
proteasomal degradation, 14
proteasome, 133
proteolysis, 59
proximal renal tubule, 133
PTEN, 56, 59, 64, 66, 75, 117, 122, 128, 139, 141, 152, 170, 174, 178, 186, 189, 195, 201
putative target, 186

## Q

qRT-PCR, 40, 41, 42, 43, 47, 77, 78, 82, 83, 110, 126, 130, 137, 146, 161, 169, 170, 172, 173, 201
quantification, 41, 43, 47, 51, 52, 94
quiescence, 57, 58

## R

radical prostatectomy, 123
radioactive tag, 39
radiotherapy, 85, 107, 116, 117, 121, 138, 141, 157, 175, 182, 186, 187
rearrangement, 14, 83, 182
RECK, 64, 75, 174, 193, 201
rectal tumor, 83
recurrence, 83, 85, 92, 115, 121, 123, 128, 131, 134, 139, 144, 148, 149, 154, 161, 162, 172, 176
regulatory loop, 63, 105
renal cell carcinoma, 30, 135, 139, 140, 141, 201
renal cell clear carcinoma, 133
replicative potential, 53, 60
reproducibility, 35
resistance, 60, 69, 76, 100, 101, 102, 105, 107, 117, 122, 128, 131, 137, 147, 157, 158, 159, 162, 174, 175, 189, 192, 194, 195, 200
retinoblastoma protein, 186, 201
retroviral transduction, 101
reverse transcriptase, 41, 60, 69, 199, 201
reverse transcription, 47, 48, 201
ribonucleoprotein assembly, 134
risk factor, 29, 73, 76, 107, 108, 167, 182
risk score, 109, 116
RNAHybrid, 37
ROS, 58, 60, 201

## S

screening, 61, 73, 78, 87, 112, 154, 158, 169, 176
self-assembling monolayer, 46, 201
self-renewal, 5, 12, 173, 196
self-sufficiency, 53, 55, 57
senescence, 59, 60, 61, 68, 69, 70

sensitivity, 35, 36, 39, 60, 77, 85, 89, 94, 95, 100, 108, 110, 111, 112, 117, 125, 128, 137, 138, 146, 150, 151, 155, 162, 168, 175, 194
sequence analysis, 34
sequence variants, 27, 134
serum, 15, 76, 77, 87, 94, 95, 102, 109, 115, 119, 120, 124, 125, 146, 158, 163, 164, 169, 170, 176, 177, 202
side effect, 85, 162
signal transducers, 9
signaling cascade, 9, 10
signaling pathways, 9, 10, 73, 74, 75, 76, 118, 137, 144, 189, 192, 193, 194
single nucleotide polymorphisms, 92, 202
siRNA, 4, 13, 18, 20, 22, 202
SMAD, 9, 21, 202
small cell lung cancer, 107, 116, 119, 121, 201
solid cancers, vii, 6, 55, 80, 126, 157, 190
specificity, 7, 11, 27, 36, 40, 46, 70, 77, 85, 110, 111, 112, 125, 146, 168, 175
S-phase, 58
splicing, 134
Sprouty2, 162, 163
sputum, 112, 120
squamous cell (epidermoid) carcinoma, 108
STarMIR, 38
stem-loop RT primer, 41
steroid receptor, 92
survival rate, 91, 134, 138, 157, 189
survivin, 62
susceptibility, 25, 27, 28, 30, 31, 32, 93, 102, 108, 109, 119, 144, 150, 176, 197
SYBR green, 41, 47

## T

tail sequence, 40
tamoxifen, 11, 99
TaqMan low density arrays, 47, 202
TaqMan PCR, 41
targeted therapy, 81, 186
TargetScan, 28, 37, 38, 76
taxol, 100, 105, 192, 195
telomere, 60, 61, 69, 70, 199
temozolomide, 192, 195, 201
terminator-based method, 35
the basal membrane, 57
therapeutical target, 73
therapy response, 25, 73, 74, 83, 84, 105, 161, 192
thrombospondin 1, 62, 75, 202
thyroid cancer, 182, 184, 186, 187, 188
thyroid gland, 181
tight junctions, 65

TIMP3, 64, 75, 150, 154, 193, 202
tissue sample, 33, 41, 43, 78, 89, 108, 110, 111, 128, 171
tissue-based diagnosis, 158
TNM, 79, 134, 159
Tomudex, 84
topotecan, 100
total RNA, 39, 41, 47, 48, 52, 94
total thyroidectomy, 182
transcription factor, 5, 6, 20, 57, 61, 64, 67, 70, 74, 198, 200, 201, 202
transcription profiling, 34
transcriptional unit, 59
transforming growth factor-β, 9
translational cancer research, 33, 43
transmembrane receptors, 55
transplantation, 144
trastuzumab, 99
TRBP, 2, 12, 14, 20, 22, 27, 76, 202
triple-negative, 92, 97, 99, 104
tropomyosin 1, 59, 64, 96, 104, 202
tubuligenesis, 62
tumor necrosis factor-related apoptosis inducing ligand, 58, 192, 202
tumor suppressor gene, 53, 54, 56, 59, 66, 69, 74, 104, 129, 139, 152, 153, 174
tumor suppressor p53, 9
tumor suppressor-like miRNAs, 10
tumor-derived miRNAs, 169
tumorigenesis, 18, 62, 66, 71, 86, 93, 96, 99, 122, 135, 144, 155, 158, 161, 168, 188
tumors-derived miRNAs, 111
tumorsphere formation, 173
TUNEL analysis, 60
TUT4, 11, 202

Twist, 6, 20, 64, 202
tyrosine kinase, 55, 62, 65, 70, 99, 183, 199

## U

universal primer, 40, 202
up-regulation, 55, 64, 98, 126, 129, 138, 150, 152, 175, 190, 194

## V

variant alleles, 29, 76, 93, 145
VEGF, 10, 62, 70, 98, 134, 144, 162, 202
VHL, 133, 137, 141, 202
vincristine, 175, 202
viral vector-encoded miRNAs, 100
Vogelstein model, 74

## W

Watson-Crick base pairing, 14, 46
well-differentiated thyroid carcinoma, 181, 184, 202
well-differentiated tumors, 78
Wnt/β-catenin, 74

## X

xenograft, 100, 150, 163

## Z

zinc-finger E-box binding homeobox, 75